ICSA Book Series in Statistics

Series Editors

Jiahua Chen, Department of Statistics, University of British Columbia, Vancouver, BC, Canada

Ding-Geng (Din) Chen, College of Health Solutions, Arizona State University, Tempe, AZ, USA

The ICSA Book Series in Statistics showcases research from the International Chinese Statistical Association that has an international reach. It publishes books in statistical theory, applications, and statistical education. All books are associated with the ICSA or are authored by invited contributors. Books may be monographs, edited volumes, textbooks and proceedings.

Wenqing He • Liqun Wang • Jiahua Chen •
Chunfang Devon Lin

Editors

Advances and Innovations in Statistics and Data Science

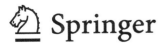 Springer

Editors
Wenqing He
Department of Statistical and Actuarial
Sciences
University of Western Ontario
London, ON, Canada

Liqun Wang
Department of Statistics
University of Manitoba
Winnipeg, MB, Canada

Jiahua Chen
Department of Statistics
University of British Columbia
Vancouver, BC, Canada

Chunfang Devon Lin
Department of Mathematics and Statistics
Queen's University
Kingston, ON, Canada

ISSN 2199-0980   ISSN 2199-0999   (electronic)
ICSA Book Series in Statistics
ISBN 978-3-031-08328-0   ISBN 978-3-031-08329-7   (eBook)
https://doi.org/10.1007/978-3-031-08329-7

This Springer imprint is published by the registered company Springer Nature Switzerland AG
The registered company address is: Gewerbestrasse 11, 6330 Cham, Switzerland

*To my wife Grace Y. Yi, my son Morgan He,
and my daughter Joy He, for their love and
support.*

Wenqing He, PhD

To my parents Lijun Huang and Xiuyong Lin.
Chunfang Devon Lin, PhD

Preface

This book is a compilation of the invited papers presented at or solicited papers from the invited speakers of the Fourth Symposium of the Canada Chapter of the International Chinese Statistical Association (ICSA-Canada) held at Queen's University, Kingston, Ontario, Canada, August 9–11, 2019 (https://icsa-canada-chapter.org/symposium2019/). The Symposium's theme was "Advances and Innovations in Statistics and Data Science," and the goal of the Symposium is to promote advances and innovations in statistics and data science and to offer the opportunity for researchers to exchange research ideas and disseminate their results. The Symposium has diverse topics and sessions in both statistics and data sciences, including statistical challenges in high-dimensional data, survival data, missing data and data with measurement error, longitudinal data and functional data analysis, and statistical inference for biomarkers.

This book aims to provide a platform for the research ideas presented at the Symposium to promote further advanced and innovative research in statistics and data science. In this book, we collected 15 articles which are divided into two parts. Part I includes six articles that discuss the advanced methodology in data science, while Part II contains nine papers that investigate a variety of development in statistical science.

Part I: Methodology Development in Data Science (Chapters 1–6)

In Chapter 1, Henry Linder and Yuping Zhang present an integrated, graphical regression model to endogenize the directed miRNA-gene target interactions and control their effects on signalling pathway disturbance. They identify prominent miRNA-gene interactions and propose a graphical representation of the targeting. The network is merged with signalling pathway networks to obtain a cross-functional graph representation of regulatory relationships between genes and miRNAs. Gene expression and miRNA expression are integrated, in tandem with graphical integration of epigenetic and transcriptomic data types, to estimate a statistical model.

Chapter 2 deals with feature screening commonly used to handle ultrahigh-dimensional data before being formally analyzed. Li-Pang Chen and Grace Y. Yi consider error-prone ultrahigh-dimensional survival data and propose a robust feature screening method. In addition, they develop an iterative algorithm to improve the performance of retaining all informative covariates. Theoretical results are established for the proposed method.

Controlling the false discovery rate (FDR) and maintaining the high sensitivity are key desiderata in post-selection inference in high-dimensional data analysis. In Chapter 3, Bangxin Zhao and Wenqing He propose a method to control the FDR and sensitivity simultaneously for high-dimensional post-selection inference using Least Angle Regression (LARS), termed Cosine PoSI. Cosine PoSI focuses on the geometric aspect of Least Angle Regression: in each step of the LARS algorithm, the proposed Cosine PoSI method makes use of the angle between the entering variable and current residual and treats this angle as a random variable that follows a cosine distribution. Given the collection of the possible angles, the variable selection path is stopped using a hypothesis testing based on the limiting distribution of the maximum angle that can be obtained through the order statistics of the cosine distribution. It is shown that both the sensitivity and the FDR can be controlled by using the stopping criteria.

When a population exhibits heterogeneity, a finite mixture model is often invoked to decompose the population into several different but homogeneous subpopulations. Contemporary practice favors learning the mixtures by maximizing the likelihood for statistical efficiency and the convenient EM-algorithm for numerical computation. Yet the maximum likelihood estimate (MLE) is not well defined for finite location-scale mixture in general. In Chapter 4, Qiong Zhang and Jiahua Chen investigate feasible alternatives to MLE, such as minimum distance estimators. Specifically, they use the Wasserstein distance that has intuitive geometric interpretation and is successfully employed in many new applications. They find that the minimum Wasserstein distance estimator (MWDE) is consistent, and derive a numerical solution under finite location-scale mixtures. The robustness of MWDE against outliers and mild model mis-specifications is studied. They found that the MWDE suffers some efficiency loss against a penalized version of MLE in general without a noticeable gain in robustness and reaffirmed the general superiority of the likelihood-based learning strategies, even for the non-regular finite location-scale mixtures.

Automatically ranking comments by relevance plays an important role in text mining. In Chapter 5, Yuyang Zhang and Hao Yu present a new text digitization method, the bag of word clusters model, by grouping semantic-related words as clusters using pre-trained word2vec word embeddings and representing each comment as a distribution of word clusters. This method extracts both semantic and statistical information from texts. They then propose an unsupervised ranking algorithm that identifies relevant comments by their distance to the "ideal" comment. This "ideal" comment is the maximum general entropy comment with respect to the global word cluster distribution. The "ideal" comment highlights aspects of a product that many other comments frequently mention and thus is regarded as a standard to judge a comment's relevance to this product.

Chapter 6 deals with statistical quality control for high-dimensional non-normal data. M. Rauf Ahmad and S. Ejaz Ahmed propose a modification to the limit of the Hotelling's T^2-statistic for statistical control under high-dimensional settings and evaluate its robustness to the normality assumption. The limit, evaluated for high-dimensional asymptotics, is shown to be robust under a few mild assumptions and a general multivariate model covering normality as a special case. Further, the limit holds without any dimension reduction or preprocessing.

Part II: Challenges in Statistical Analysis (Chapters 7–15)

In the functional linear regression models, many methods have been proposed and studied to estimate the slope function, while the functional predictors were observed in the entire domain. However, works on functional linear regression models with partially observed trajectories have received less attention. In Chapter 7, Yafei Wang, Tingyu Lai, Bei Jian, Linglong Kong, and Zhongzhan Zhang consider the scenario where individual functional predictors may be observed only on the part of the domain to fill the gap. Two methods are developed depending on whether the measurement error is presented in functional predictors. One is based on linear functionals of the observed part of the trajectory, and the other one uses conditional principal component scores.

In Chapter 8, Yanqing Sun and Fang Fang study several profile estimation methods for the generalized semiparametric varying-coefficient additive model for longitudinal data by utilizing the within-subject correlations. The model is flexible in allowing time-varying effects for some covariates and constant effects for others, and in having the option to choose different link functions which can be used to analyze both discrete and continuous longitudinal responses. They investigated the profile generalized estimating equation (GEE) approaches and the profile quadratic inference function (QIF) approach. The profile estimations are assisted with the local linear smoothing technique to estimate the time-varying effects. Several approaches that incorporate the within-subject correlations are investigated, including the quasi-likelihood (QL), the minimum generalized variance (MGV), the quadratic inference function, and the weighted least squares (WLS). The proposed estimation procedures can accommodate flexible sampling schemes. These methods provide a unified approach that works well for discrete longitudinal responses as well as for continuous longitudinal responses.

In Chapter 9, Riyadh Rustam Al-Mosawi and Xuewen Lu propose to estimate both the regression coefficients and the baseline survival function of the semiparametric linear transformation model with left-truncated and current status data using the Sieve maximum likelihood estimation method based on techniques of constrained Bernstein polynomials. They proved that the obtained estimators are semiparametrically efficient and asymptotically normally distributed based on the conditional likelihood given the truncation time, and the estimator for the nonparametric baseline survival function achieves the optimal rate of convergence.

Compositional data arise in many applications across various disciplines such as ecology, geology, demography, and economics. For some time, log-ratio methods have been a popular approach for analyzing compositional data and have motivated much of the recent research in the area. In Chapter 10, Michail Tsagris and Connie Stewart review two recently proposed transformations for data defined on the simplex. The first α transformation transforms the data from the simplex to a subset of Euclidean space, and the other one is a more complex transformation involving folding, resulting in data with Euclidean sample space. In both cases, the transformed data are assumed to follow a multivariate normal distribution, and the parameter α provides flexibility compared to the traditional log-ratio transformations.

The autoregressive conditional heteroscedasticity (ARCH) model and its various generalizations have been widely used to analyze economic and financial data. Although many variables like GDP, inflation, and commodity prices are imprecisely measured, research focusing on the mismeasured response processes in GARCH models is sparse. In Chapter 11, Mustafa Salamh and Liqun Wang study a dynamic model with ARCH error where the underlying process is latent and subject to additive measurement error. They show that, in contrast to the case of covariate measurement error, this model is identifiable by using the observations of the proxy process only, and no extra information is needed. They construct generalized method of moments (GMM) estimators for the unknown parameters, which are consistent and asymptotically normally distributed under general conditions. They also propose a procedure to test the presence of measurement error, which avoids the usual boundary problem of testing variance parameters.

Chapter 12 deals with skewed, truncated, or contaminated data with outliers. Sijia Xiang and Weixin Yao introduce a new regression tool, named modal regression, that aims to find the most probable conditional value (mode) of a dependent variable Y given covariates X rather than the mean that is used by the traditional mean regression. The modal regression can reveal new interesting data structure that is possibly missed by the conditional mean or quantiles. In addition, modal regression is resistant to outliers and heavy-tailed data, and can provide shorter prediction intervals when the data are skewed. Furthermore, unlike traditional mean regression, the modal regression can be directly applied to the truncated data. Modal regression could be a potentially very useful regression tool that can complement the traditional mean and quantile regressions.

The Galveston Bay Recovery Study conducted a longitudinal survey of residents of two counties in Texas in the aftermath of Hurricane Ike, which made landfall on September 13, 2008, and caused widespread damage. An important objective was to chart the extent of symptoms of post-traumatic stress disorder (PTSD) in the resident population over the following months. In Chapter 13, Mary E. Thompson, Gang Meng, Joseph Sedransk, Qixuan Chen, and Rebecca Anthopoulos model the course of the repeated PTSD measures as a function of individual characteristics and area segment, and to examine the analytical and visual evidence for spatial correlation of the area segment effect. The composite likelihood approach is used in the multilevel analysis to incorporate design information. The authors compare their proposed method with a Bayesian multilevel analysis and discuss the estimability of the model when the cluster level variation has spatial dependence.

Lasso regression has attracted significant attention in statistical learning and data science. However, there is sporadic work on constructing efficient data collection for regularized regression. In Chapter 14, Peter Chien, Xinwei Deng, and Chunfang Devon Lin propose an experimental design approach using nearly orthogonal Latin hypercube designs to enhance the variable selection accuracy of Lasso regression. Systematic methods for constructing such designs are presented.

In Chapter 15, Xinyi Ge, Yingwei Peng, and Dongsheng Tu present a selective overview of statistical methods for identifying the treatment-sensitive subsets of patients. Identifying a subset of patients who may benefit from or be sensitive to a specific type of treatment has become a critical research topic in clinical trials and other types of clinical research. Statistical methods are essential in helping clinical researchers to identify the subset. They consider first the cases where the outcome of the clinical studies is time-to-event or survival time, and the subset is defined by one continuous covariate, such as the expression level of a gene, or by multiple covariates which can be continuous or categorical, such as mutation statuses of multiple genes. The cases where the outcomes of the clinical studies are longitudinal or repeated measurements, such as patient-reported quality of life scores before, during, and after a treatment, are considered next. Gaps between the needs in clinical research and the methods available in statistical literature are identified, and future research topics to bridge these gaps are discussed based on this overview.

We have organized the book chapters to be self-contained, with their separate references, to provide readers with the complete materials for each topic.

We sincerely thank the organizations and individuals for their support of the Symposium. We owe a big thank you to the local organization team at Queen's University led by Drs. Devon Lin and Wenyu Jiang. We thank the program committee for organizing the eye-catching scientific sessions of the Symposium: Drs. Jiguo Cao at Simon Fraser University, Wenqing He at the University of Western Ontario, Linglong Kong at the University of Alberta, Longhai Li at the University of Saskatchewan, Xuewen Lu at the University of Calgary, Liqun Wang at the University of Manitoba, Lang Wu at the University of British Columbia, and Ying Zhang at Acadia University.

The editors would like to thank the authors of this book's chapters for their expertise, knowledge, and time contribution. Our sincere gratitude goes to the sponsors of the Fourth Symposium of the ICSA-Canada for their financial support: the Canadian Statistical Science Institute (CANSSI), the Department of Mathematics and Statistics, and the Faculty of Arts and Sciences at Queen's University. We are also grateful to the volunteers and staff of Queen's University for their assistance at the Symposium. Without their support, the Symposium, as well as this book, would not be possible.

We would also like to acknowledge the professional support from the publication team at Springer.

We welcome readers' comments and suggestions for the book. This book is a collective contribution from the authors. Please send your suggestions and comments to the chapter authors or any of the co-editors below. We will be delighted to pass your suggestions and comments to the chapter corresponding authors.

London, ON, Canada   Wenqing He
Winnipeg, MB, Canada   Liqun Wang
Vancouver, BC, Canada   Jiahua Chen
Kingston, ON, Canada   Chunfang Devon Lin
August 2022

Contents

Part I Methodology Development in Data Science

MiRNA–Gene Activity Interaction Networks (miGAIN): Integrated Joint Models of miRNA–Gene Targeting and Disturbance in Signaling Pathways 3
Henry Linder and Yuping Zhang

Robust Feature Screening for Ultrahigh-Dimensional Censored Data Subject to Measurement Error 23
Li-Pang Chen and Grace Y. Yi

Simultaneous Control of False Discovery Rate and Sensitivity Using Least Angle Regressions in High-Dimensional Data Analysis 55
Bangxin Zhao and Wenqing He

Minimum Wasserstein Distance Estimator Under Finite Location-Scale Mixtures 69
Qiong Zhang and Jiahua Chen

An Entropy-Based Comment Ranking Method with Word Embedding Clustering 99
Yuyang Zhang and Hao Yu

A Robust Approach to Statistical Quality Control for High-Dimensional Non-Normal Data 121
M. Rauf Ahmad and S. Ejaz Ahmed

Part II Challenges in Statistical Analysis

Functional Linear Regression for Partially Observed Functional Data ... 137
Yafei Wang, Tingyu Lai, Bei Jiang, Linglong Kong, and Zhongzhan Zhang

Profile Estimation of Generalized Semiparametric Varying-Coefficient Additive Models for Longitudinal Data with Within-Subject Correlations 159
Yanqing Sun and Fang Fang

Sieve Estimation of Semiparametric Linear Transformation Model with Left-Truncated and Current Status Data 181
Riyadh Rustam Al-Mosawi and Xuewen Lu

A Review of Flexible Transformations for Modeling Compositional Data 225
Michail Tsagris and Connie Stewart

Identifiability and Estimation of Autoregressive ARCH Models with Measurement Error 235
Mustafa Salamh and Liqun Wang

Modal Regression for Skewed, Truncated, or Contaminated Data with Outliers 257
Sijia Xiang and Weixin Yao

Spatial Multilevel Modelling in the Galveston Bay Recovery Study Survey 275
Mary E. Thompson, Gang Meng, Joseph Sedransk, Qixuan Chen, and Rebecca Anthopolos

Efficient Experimental Design for Lasso Regression 295
Peter Chien, Xinwei Deng, and Chunfang Devon Lin

A Selective Overview of Statistical Methods for Identification of the Treatment-Sensitive Subsets of Patients 311
Xinyi Ge, Yingwei Peng, and Dongsheng Tu

Index 331

Contributors

M. Rauf Ahmad Department of Statistics, Uppsala University, Uppsala, Sweden

S. Ejaz Ahmed Department of Mathematics and Statistics, Brock University, St. Catharines, ON, Canada

Riyadh Rustam Al-Mosawi Department of Mathematics, College of Computer Science and Mathematics, University of Thi-Qar, Thi-Qar, Iraq

Rebecca Anthopolos New York University, NY, USA

Jiahua Chen Department of Statistics, University of British Columbia, Vancouver, BC, Canada

Li-Pang Chen Department of Statistical and Actuarial Sciences, University of Western Ontario, London, ON, Canada
Department of Statistics, National Chengchi University, Taipei, Taiwan

Qixuan Chen Department of Biostatistics, Columbia University New York, NY, USA

Peter Chien Department of Statistics, University of Wisconsin-Madison, Madison, WI, SA

Xinwei Deng Department of Statistics, Virginia Tech, Blacksburg, VA, USA

Fang Fang Corporate Model Risk at Wells Fargo, Charlotte, NC, USA

Xinyi Ge Department of Mathematics and Statistics, Queen's University, Kingston, ON, Canada

Wenqing He Department of Statistical and Actuarial Sciences, University of Western Ontario, London, ON, Canada

Bei Jiang Department of Mathematical and Statistical Sciences, University of Alberta, Edmonton, AB, Canada

Linglong Kong Department of Mathematical and Statistical Sciences, Faculty of Science, University of Alberta, Edmonton, AB, Canada

Tingyu Lai Beijing University of Technology, Beijing, China

Chunfang Devon Lin Department of Mathematics and Statistics, Queen's University, Kingston, ON, Canada

Henry Linder Department of Statistics, University of Connecticut, Storrs, CT, USA

Xuewen Lu Department of Mathematics and Statistics, University of Calgary, Calgary, AB, Canada

Gang Meng Department of Statistics and Actuarial Sciences, University of Waterloo, Waterloo, ON, Canada

Yingwei Peng Departments of Public Health Sciences and Mathematics and Statistics, Queen's University, Kingston, ON, Canada

Mustafa Salamh Department of Statistics, Cairo University, Giza, Egypt

Joseph Sedransk University of Maryland, College Park, MD, USA

Connie Stewart Department of Mathematics and Statistics, University of New Brunswick, Saint John, NB, Canada

Yanqing Sun Department of Mathematics and Statistics, University of North Carolina at Charlotte, Charlotte, NC, USA

Michail Tsagris Department of Economics, University of Crete, Rethymnon, Greece

Mary E. Thompson Department of Statistics and Actuarial Sciences, University of Waterloo, Waterloo, ON, Canada

Dongsheng Tu Departments of Public Health Sciences and Mathematics and Statistics, Queen's University, Kingston, ON, Canada

Liqun Wang Department of Statistics, University of Manitoba, Winnipeg, MB, Canada

Yafei Wang Department of Statistics and Data Science, Faculty of Science, Beijing University of Technology, Beijing, China
Department of Mathematical and Statistical Sciences, Faculty of Science, University of Alberta, Edmonton, AB, Canada

Sijia Xiang School of Data Sciences, Zhejiang University of Finance and Economics, Hangzhou, China

Weixin Yao Department of Statistics, University of California at Riverside, Riverside, CA, USA

Grace Y. Yi Department of Statistical and Actuarial Sciences, University of Western Ontario, London, ON, Canada
Department of Computer Science, University of Western Ontario, London, ON, Canada

Hao Yu Department of Statistical and Actuarial Sciences, University of Western Ontario, London, ON, Canada

Qiong Zhang Department of Statistics, University of British Columbia, Vancouver, BC, Canada

Yuping Zhang Department of Statistics, University of Connecticut, Storrs, CT, USA

Yuyang Zhang Department of Statistical and Actuarial Sciences, University of Western Ontario, London, ON, Canada

Zhongzhan Zhang Beijing University of Technology, Beijing, China

Bangxin Zhao Department of Statistical and Actuarial Sciences, University of Western Ontario, London, ON, Canada

Part I
Methodology Development in Data Science

MiRNA–Gene Activity Interaction Networks (miGAIN): Integrated Joint Models of miRNA–Gene Targeting and Disturbance in Signaling Pathways

Henry Linder and Yuping Zhang

Abstract Omics data are now inexpensive to collect in vast quantities, across a wide variety of not only multiple data platform, but also distinct functional units. These bioinformatic datasets can enable scientific analysis of system-level cellular processes, including complex diseases such as cancers. Recent experimental research has found significant interactions between non-coding microRNAs (miRNAs) and genes. We propose an integrated, graphical regression model to endogenize the directed miRNA–gene target interactions and control for their effects in signaling pathway disturbance. We identify prominent miRNA–gene interactions and propose a graphical representation of the targeting. We merge this network with signaling pathway networks to obtain a cross-functional graph representation of regulatory relationships between genes and miRNAs. We integrate gene expression and miRNA expression, in tandem with graphical integration of epigenetic and transcriptomic data types, and estimate a statistical model. We find that our integration approach improves the statistical power, using a simulation study. We demonstrate our integrated model with an application to disturbance of the BRAF signaling pathway across 9 cancers. We find that integration of miRNA–gene targets clarifies the differential activity between healthy and tumor tissues, which in turn reflects different roles for the pathway across the different cancers.

Keywords Data integration · Network analysis · Statistical inference

1 Introduction

The widespread availability of genomic data has dramatically increased the scope of quantitative research into biology at the molecular, genomic, and systems levels. The diversity of data available for study improves the detail available to characterize the

H. Linder · Y. Zhang (✉)
Department of Statistics, University of Connecticut, Storrs, CT, USA
e-mail: matthew.linder@uconn.edu; yuping.zhang@uconn.edu

© The Author(s), under exclusive license to Springer Nature Switzerland AG 2022
W. He et al. (eds.), *Advances and Innovations in Statistics and Data Science*, ICSA
Book Series in Statistics, https://doi.org/10.1007/978-3-031-08329-7_1

functional processes of the genome. Significantly, these data may provide valuable new insight into the drivers of complex diseases. Multi-view datasets are now routinely collected in multiple modalities across separate biological structures, and large-scale research studies coordinate to improve the quality and quantity of data available to advance knowledge, treatment, and prevention.

To analyze these high-resolution omics data, robust methods are essential to ensure scientific rigor and validity. New experimental techniques should be complemented by statistical methods that reflect the biology in a sophisticated way. Increasingly, data is collected for genomic entities other than the gene, such as non-coding microRNAs (miRNAs).

Notably, miRNA research is fundamentally integrative in nature. Individual miRNAs are believed to target genes in a functional manner (Lewis et al. 2005), and it is often the case that single miRNAs target multiple genes. To model correlated gene activity due to a shared miRNA parent, miRNA–gene target interactions must be known and available to researchers. Early miRNA–gene target research validated individual targets experimentally, but the combinatoric problems introduced by large numbers of genes and miRNAs motivated meta-analytic and computational approaches. One such study of miRNA–gene targets was miRTarBase (Hsu et al. 2010), which identified gene targets for fewer than 700 miRNAs by manual aggregation of experimental evidence. Modern informatic methods permit large-scale analyses to identify miRNA targets. Frameworks such as miRTarBase and DIANA-miRPath (Vlachos et al. 2015) utilize web interfaces to access and explore association analyses between miRNAs and genes. DIANA-miRPath adapts methods originally applied to gene expression. In addition to Fisher's exact test, they also test for differential activity in miRNAs using the enrichment analysis method of Bleazard et al. (2015). Computational approaches have been used to identify targets, too. Hsu et al. (2011) proposed miRTar, a successor to miRTarBase that used gene set enrichment analysis for significance testing of differential activity. These are often applied to specific phenomena or systems. Other databases include DIANA-TarBase (Karagkouni et al. 2017) and TargetScan (Agarwal et al. 2015). Coll et al. (2015) used correlation analysis to identify miRNA–gene targets related to cirrhosis of liver tissue.

Integrative analysis unifies multiple data types into a single whole. However, real-world analysis is often highly restrictive in its assumptions and the sophistication of its representation of biological systems. In many cases, "integrated" analysis refers to qualitative aggregation of separate marginal analyses on different data types, as well as correlation analysis between data types. Early statistical analyses of miRNAs were characterized by straightforward statistical methods. The CORNA method of Wu and Watson (2009) applied hypergeometric and Fisher's exact tests to assess differential activity in miRNA–gene interactions and networks. Du and Zhang (2015) integrated methylation in a small-sample analysis of lung cancer that also included expression in genes and miRNAs. They used miRNA–gene target databases, but the interactions were excluded from gene enrichment analysis. Godard and van Eyll (2015) performed pathway analysis of miRNA in the context of Alzheimer's disease, also using a hypergeometric enrichment test. Their procedure also treated pathways as simple gene sets, thereby ignoring known structural information about the signaling pathways. Miao et al. (2017) analyzed the relationship between miRNAs and DNA methylation in sheep. They identified gene–miRNA networks on the basis of a correlation analysis but only applied a basic t-test for differential activity across gene sets, ignoring network topology. Moreover, their integration was largely restricted to correlation analysis to cluster genes targeted by the same miRNAs. Volinia and Croce (2013) analyzed gene expression and miRNA expression for a breast cancer dataset. Their analysis focused on survival outcomes, and the extent of their data integration was to include both genes and miRNAs as covariates, rather than a structural or model-based integration. Cava et al. (2014) considered copy number as well as gene and miRNA expression. But, genes and miRNAs were only heuristically integrated, by performing separate marginal analyses, as well as comparing up- and downregulation across the different data types.

This lack of a single coherent integration scheme is also found in miRNA analyses applied to cancer datasets. Enerly et al. (2011) studied miRNA suppression in a novel miRNA and gene expression breast tumor dataset. But, their integration was limited to correlation analysis and separate studies on each data type. Likewise, Yu et al. (2019) identified specific biomarkers with differential survival outcomes in lung cancer, and Li et al. (2018) used differential correlation analysis between miRNAs and genes in cancer, both using correlation analysis.

We address this lack of technical statistical methods for joint integrative analysis of data observed on genes and miRNAs. We identify prominent miRNA–gene interactions and construct a graphical model to represent the targets. We merge this network with signaling pathways to estimate pathway activity while controlling network effects and coexpression of genes due to the miRNAs. We extend the NetGSA regression model for analysis of signaling pathways, which was restricted to gene-level measurements, originally only gene expression (E) in Shojaie and Michailidis (2009) and Shojaie and Michailidis (2010). Zhang et al. (2017) extended the signaling pathway network to include gene methylation (M) and copy number (C), and we use their EMC-NetGSA model to integrate gene-level omics observations. In this chapter, we also incorporate miRNAs into the statistical model. Furthermore, we also introduce a semi-parametric bootstrap procedure to assess the robustness of the statistical inference.

This chapter proceeds as follows. In Sect. 2, we give an overview of the omics datasets we use for integrative analysis. In Sect. 3, we give details of the network integration and pathway model. In Sect. 4, we first perform simulation studies to examine the statistical level and power of the proposed method in Sect. 4.1 and then conduct a data analysis of pathway disturbance in the BRAF signaling pathway in 9 cancers in Sect. 4.2. Finally, we conclude our paper with discussion in Sect. 5.

2   Data

We consider a multi-platform omics dataset assembled from observations published by The Cancer Genome Atlas (TCGA). TCGA is an ongoing, international study funded by the National Cancer Institute (NCI) that collects tumorous tissue samples in patients with more than 30 distinct cancers (Tomczak et al. 2015). For each cancer, we obtained measurements of gene expression, copy number variation (CNV), and methylation, as well as miRNA expression. In order to analyze differential activity by cancer, we downloaded omics data for all tumor samples, as well as matched healthy control tissue samples. We describe in Sect. 4.2 our steps to aggregate methylation and copy number at the level of individual genes.

Unlike gene-level integration of methylation and copy number features, no standard, direct mapping exists between genes and miRNAs. Instead, we use resources on functional miRNA–gene targets to construct an integrated statistical model. Substantial work has been done to identify miRNA–gene targets. One resource that quantifies the degree of experimental evidence in support of a given miRNA–gene target interaction is mirDIP. Tokar et al. (2017) compiled the database as a meta-analysis to integrate predicted miRNA–gene targets from 30 separate sources of experimentally validated interactions. It includes information on the degree to which the source databases overlap in their conclusion.

3 Methods

We integrate the omics data described in the previous section through a statistical model across the four data types collected across miRNAs and genes. At a high level, we start with a known genetic signaling pathway, specified as a directed graph on vertices representing genes. We identify likely miRNA–gene targets and integrate these with directed edges. We use a similar approach to integrate gene methylation and copy number within each gene. Finally, the graph adjacency matrix of the fully integrated omics network is used to form a design matrix for a mixed linear model. This enables hypothesis testing for differential pathway activity between two populations.

We introduce our integrated graphical network constructively. We start with a genetic signaling pathway specifying known functional relationships between genes. We define a directed graph $\mathcal{G} = \{\mathcal{V}, \mathcal{E}\}$. Initially, $\mathcal{V}$ contains p graph vertices, and $\mathcal{E}$ contains the directed edges between elements of the genes $\mathcal{V}$ that comprise the signaling pathway. In general, the graph vertices in $\mathcal{V}$ represent biological features, while the edges in $\mathcal{E}$ represent the functional interactions.

Graph $\mathcal{G}$ can be represented by a $p \times p$ adjacency matrix, $\mathbf{A}_E^\star$. The subscript "E" emphasizes that the graph relations in $\mathbf{A}_E^\star$ specify relationships between vertices for gene expression. The element α_{jk} of $\mathbf{A}_E^\star$ is an indicator for the presence of a directed edge from vertex k to vertex j, for all $j, k = 1, \ldots, p$. α_{jk} is nonzero when gene j is conditionally dependent on gene k. For each gene, we observe gene expression as a vector $\mathbf{y}_{i1}$ of p elements, where $i = 1, \ldots, N$ indexes tissue samples.

Suppose the p pathway genes are targeted by g miRNAs, and for each sample, we observe a vector of g elements $\mathbf{y}_{i2}$, the values of which measure miRNA expression. We add g vertices to $\mathcal{V}$ integrated the miRNA–gene target interactions, and we construct the $p \times g$ graph adjacency matrix $\mathbf{A}^{\star}_{\text{mi}}$. The element $\tau_{j\ell} \in \mathbf{A}^{\star}_{\text{mi}}$ is an indicator value for miRNA ℓ targeting gene j, $j = 1, \ldots, p$, $\ell = 1, \ldots, g$. Each miRNA–gene target is represented by a directed edge which we add to $\mathcal{E}$.

We construct the $(p + g) \times (p + g)$ integrated adjacency matrix $\mathbf{A}^{\star}_{\text{miE}}$ that spans both the genetic pathway and the miRNA–gene targets and contains elements of 0 and 1:

$$\mathbf{A}^{\star}_{\text{miE}} = \begin{pmatrix} \mathbf{A}^{\star}_{\text{E}} & \mathbf{A}^{\star}_{\text{mi}} \\ \mathbf{O}_{g \times p} & \mathbf{O}_{g \times g} \end{pmatrix}, \tag{1}$$

where $\mathbf{O}_{m \times n}$ is a $m \times n$ matrix of zeros.

Moreover, for each gene in $\mathbf{y}_{i1}$, we also observe copy number and methylation, contained in the vectors $\mathbf{y}_{i3}$ and $\mathbf{y}_{i4}$, respectively. We adopt the EMC-NetGSA model (Zhang et al. 2017) to integrate $\{\mathbf{y}_{i1}, \mathbf{y}_{i3}, \mathbf{y}_{i4}\}$ by adding $2p$ vertices to $\mathcal{V}$, one for each gene for copy number and methylation, and $2p$ directed edges to $\mathcal{E}$, from the copy number and methylation vertices to their counterpart gene expression vertices. This produces a fully integrated adjacency matrix, $\mathbf{A}^{\star}_{\text{miEMC}}$:

$$\mathbf{A}^{\star}_{\text{miEMC}} = \begin{pmatrix} \mathbf{A}^{\star}_{\text{E}} & \mathbf{A}^{\star}_{\text{mi}} & \mathbf{I}_{p \times p} & \mathbf{I}_{p \times p} \\ \mathbf{O}_{(g+2p) \times p} & \mathbf{O}_{(g+2p) \times g} & \mathbf{O}_{(g+2p) \times p} & \mathbf{O}_{(g+2p) \times p} \end{pmatrix}. \tag{2}$$

In real-world datasets, individual elements of $\mathbf{y}_{i2}$, $\mathbf{y}_{i3}$, and $\mathbf{y}_{i4}$ may be missing across all N samples. An advantage of our unidirectional integration, which does not model directed interactions from genes to the other omics features, is that we may simply omit the columns and rows for the corresponding miRNA, copy number, and methylation features in $\mathbf{A}^{\star}_{\text{miEMC}}$ prior to the pathway analysis. Without loss of generality, we consider the full $(g + 3p) \times (g + 3p)$ adjacency matrix $\mathbf{A}^{\star}_{\text{miEMC}}$, with the knowledge that its true dimension q is such that $q \leq (g + 3p)$.

The network in Eq. 2 composes three distinct network layers: (1) the primary signaling network on elements of $\mathbf{y}_{i1}$; (2) the miRNA integration layer of directed relationships, possibly many-to-one, from miRNAs in $\mathbf{y}_{i2}$ to genes in $\mathbf{y}_{i1}$; and (3) a within-gene layer integrating copy number in $\mathbf{y}_{i3}$ and methylation in $\mathbf{y}_{i4}$. Therefore, the graph simultaneously provides for causal relationships between genes, allows correlation between genes, and reduces noise by controlling for epigenetic and transcriptional effects. Each of the three components is supported by scientific knowledge of the complex underlying biological processes.

For expositional clarity, define $m = (g + 3p)$, $\mathbf{y}_i = (\mathbf{y}'_{i1}, \mathbf{y}'_{i2}, \mathbf{y}'_{i3}, \mathbf{y}'_{i4})'$, $\mathbf{A}^{\star} \equiv \mathbf{A}^{\star}_{\text{miEMC}}$, and the elements of $\mathbf{A}^{\star}$ by δ_{jk}, $j, k = 1, \ldots, m$.

Gaussian graphical models formalize the conditional dependence of vertex j on vertex k as the partial correlation ρ_{jk} between gene-level random variables Y_j, Y_k, controlling for the effects of the remaining $(m - 2)$ vertices in $\mathcal{V}$. Writing the random variables for the remaining $(m - 2)$ vertices by $\mathcal{Z}$, $\rho_{jk} = \text{corr}(Y_{j \setminus \mathcal{Z}}, Y_{k \setminus \mathcal{Z}})$, where $Y_{j \setminus \mathcal{Z}} = Y_j - \mathcal{P}_{\mathcal{Z}} Y_j$ is the orthogonal complement of Y_j with respect to $\mathcal{Z}$, and $\mathcal{P}_{\mathcal{Z}}$ is a projection onto $\mathcal{Z}$ (Krämer et al. 2009).

We estimate ρ_{jk} with the sample partial correlation r_{jk}. We first estimate two separate regressions, one of Y_j on $\mathcal{Z}$ and the other of Y_k on $\mathcal{Z}$. Then, we estimate r_{jk} by the Pearson correlation coefficient between the residuals of the two regressions (Kim 2015). Finally, we form a weighted adjacency matrix $\mathbf{A}$ with elements $a_{jk} = r_{jk}\alpha_{jk}$, $j, k = 1, \ldots, m$. Elements of $\mathbf{A}$ thus take either the value 0, when no interaction exists, or a value in the interval $(-1, 1)$ corresponding to the strength of conditional association between two vertices with a functional interaction.

The effect of coexpression due to the graph topology $\mathcal{G}$ can be summarized by a transformation $\mathbf{\Lambda}$ of $\mathbf{A}$, called the influence matrix. As detailed in Shojaie and Michailidis (2009), in the special case of directed acyclic graphs (DAGs), it can be shown that $\mathbf{\Lambda} = (\mathbf{I}_m - \mathbf{A})^{-1}$. This definition extends to all graphs for which the adjacency matrix has eigenvalues all of which are smaller than 1 in magnitude. Shojaie and Michailidis (2010) extended the definition to non-DAG, non-substochastic graphs. They used a limit approximation to induce in arbitrary directed graphs the necessary eigenvalue properties of $\mathbf{A}$.

The NetGSA statistical model uses $\mathbf{\Lambda}$ to structure the mean of $\mathbf{y}_i$, by setting $\mathbb{E}\mathbf{y}_i = \mathbf{\Lambda}\boldsymbol{\beta}$ for an unknown vector of m regression coefficients $\boldsymbol{\beta}$. $\boldsymbol{\beta}$ is the network-adjusted activity parameter, giving the mean values for the m observed elements of $\mathbf{y}_i$, controlling for pass-through network effect due to $\mathcal{G}$. The influence matrix also structures the covariance of $\mathbf{y}_i$. The NetGSA model parameterizes variability in individuals' mean expression via a mixed effects linear regression model: $\mathbf{y}_i = \mathbf{\Lambda}\boldsymbol{\beta} + \mathbf{\Lambda}\boldsymbol{\gamma}_i + \boldsymbol{\epsilon}_i$, $\boldsymbol{\gamma}_i \sim N_m(\mathbf{0}_m, \sigma_\gamma^2 \mathbf{I}_m)$, $\boldsymbol{\epsilon}_i \sim N_m(\mathbf{0}_m, \sigma_\epsilon^2 \mathbf{I}_m)$, where $\boldsymbol{\gamma}_i$ is a sample-level random effect, and $i = 1, \ldots, N$.

In proposing the NetGSA model, Shojaie and Michailidis (2009) also proposed a hypothesis test for difference in mean vectors between two populations. Denote the population label for sample i by c_i, where $c_i \in \{C, T\}$, "C" corresponds to control, and "T" corresponds to treatment. In our pathway analysis of cancerous tumors, we assign healthy tissue samples the label of "control," and tumor tissues the label "treatment." We estimate separate weighted adjacency matrices $\mathbf{A}_C$, $\mathbf{A}_T$, yielding distinct influence matrices $\mathbf{\Lambda}_C$, $\mathbf{\Lambda}_T$, and population-specific mean parameters $\boldsymbol{\beta}_C$, $\boldsymbol{\beta}_T$.

We test for differential activity in subsets of the pathway features, corresponding to elements in $\boldsymbol{\beta}_C$, $\boldsymbol{\beta}_T$, using an indicator vector $\mathbf{b}$ for the omics features of interest. The NetGSA network contrast is $\boldsymbol{\ell} = (-\mathbf{b} \cdot \mathbf{b}\mathbf{\Lambda}_C, \mathbf{b} \cdot \mathbf{b}\mathbf{\Lambda}_T)$, and this yields a test statistic $T \propto \boldsymbol{\ell}\boldsymbol{\beta}$, $\boldsymbol{\beta} = (\boldsymbol{\beta}_{C'}, \boldsymbol{\beta}_{T'})'$. T follows a Student's t distribution with degrees of freedom estimated using Satterthwaite's approximation.

The above inference depends upon both the assumption of normality and the composition of the control population. In practice, the size of the healthy sample population is very small, and we may wish to assess the robustness of the inference to the specific control samples. Therefore, we propose a semi-parametric bootstrap test based on the principles discussed by MacKinnon (2009).

Specifically, we generate B pairwise bootstrap replicates under the null hypothesis of no difference in the network-adjusted mean parameters in the two populations. We randomly select pairs of population labels and omics observations, with replacement. If a sample contains fewer than 10 observations in the control (healthy) population, we re-generate the bootstrap sample. Because the distribution of the NetGSA test statistic is approximated using a function of the estimated variance, the distributions of the test statistic are not comparable between bootstrap replicates, as the degrees of freedom vary substantially. Instead, when the empirical p-value is nominally significant, we calculate a 95% bootstrap upper confidence bound. Inversely, for a p-value that is nominally not significant, we calculate a 5% bootstrap lower bound.

This bootstrap procedure offers a semi-parametric criterion for assessing the robustness of the outcome of a hypothesis test. The procedure still depends upon the underlying assumptions of the mixed linear model but instead addresses the robustness of the procedure to small sample sizes in the control population.

4 Results

First, we use a simulation study to demonstrate the improved power of our method due to the integration of miRNA–gene target information. We then apply our method to the TCGA dataset introduced in Sect. 2 for pathway analysis of the BRAF pathway.

4.1 Simulations

Our simulation study borrows the ideas on simulation designs in the EMC-NetGSA paper (Zhang et al. 2017). Broadly, we construct a pathway composed of a binary tree signaling pathway; we model miRNA–gene targets that drive correlated gene expression, and we integrate the methylation and copy number within genes. This supplies three separate layers of network information that may contribute to gene expression, and we examine the relationship between omics integration and statistical power.

We modeled a signaling pathway consisting of a five-level binary tree containing 31 genes. We integrated miRNA with directed edges from miRNA to corresponding genes. For every gene, we added three distinct miRNA vertices, i.e., each had out-degree 1. We then partitioned the genes in V into disjoint sets of two, proceeding from the root node. We assigned to each pair of genes one shared miRNA, i.e., with out-degree 2. Finally, we repeated this procedure for sets of three genes. We assigned each triplet one miRNA with out-degree 3. The network topology for the control population signaling pathway used the same integrated binary tree structure, with all edges in the tree's left branch removed. For EMC-NetGSA integration, we add G directed edges into each gene from two vertices representing methylation and copy number.

We set the correlation between expression vertices to 0.8 in the top third (two levels) of the tree; association is 0.5 in the middle third (third level); and association

0.2 in the final third (final level). We set the magnitude of the association strength between miRNA and their gene targets to 0.4. In the TCGA dataset, we found that the partial correlation coefficients between miRNA and expression were generally symmetric. Therefore, we assigned alternating edges from miRNAs to genes to have positive and negative association, respectively. This may be understood as simulating cases where miRNAs with multiple gene targets have the same sign for association, as well as different associations with different genes for a single miRNA. We set the association 0.5 between copy number and gene expression and -0.25 between methylation and expression.

We generated observation vectors $\mathbf{y}_i$, $i = 1, \ldots, N$, from the NetGSA linear mixed model, where $N = N_C + N_T$. The number of control samples was $N_C = 50$, and the number of treatment samples was $N_T = 150$. This reflects the imbalanced sample sizes in the real cancer datasets. We set the variance parameters as $\sigma_\gamma^2 = 5$ and $\sigma_\epsilon^2 = 0.5$.

Denoting the mean vectors for gene expression, miRNA expression, gene copy number, and gene methylation by $\boldsymbol{\beta}_{c1}, \boldsymbol{\beta}_{c2}, \boldsymbol{\beta}_{c3}, \boldsymbol{\beta}_{c4}$, we simulated two scenarios for the network-adjusted mean parameter $\boldsymbol{\beta}$. Here, $c \in \{C, T\}$ indexes the control and treatment populations. In the first scenario, we assigned $\boldsymbol{\beta}_{cj} = \mathbf{0}$, $c \in \{C, T\}$, $j = 1, 2, 3, 4$. In the second mean scenario, we held $\boldsymbol{\beta}_{Cj} = \mathbf{0}$ for all j. For the top two-thirds levels of the binary tree, we set $(\beta_{T1}, \beta_{T2}, \beta_{T3}, \beta_{T4}) = (0.25, 0.5, 1.0, 0.5)$. In the bottom third of the binary tree, we maintained $(\beta_{T1}, \beta_{T2}, \beta_{T3}, \beta_{T4}) = \mathbf{0}$, as in the first scenario.

For each simulated dataset, we tested four gene sets for differential activation: (1) the full binary tree; (2) the top third of the tree; (3) the top two-thirds of the tree; and (4) the bottom third of the tree. We estimated the miEMC-NetGSA model for the entire simulated dataset, as well as the NetGSA variants with the adjacency matrices $\mathbf{A}_{miE}$, $\mathbf{A}_{EMC}$, and $\mathbf{A}_E$, as well as the corresponding hypothesis test for each network. We ran 1000 replicates of the simulation. We calculated the power for each method by the proportion of hypothesis test p-values that were significant at the $\alpha = 0.05$ level, i.e., the proportion of replicates for which we reject the null hypothesis of no difference in pathway-adjusted mean parameters.

Figure 1 shows boxplots of the $-\log_{10} p$-values from the significance tests. The left-hand panel shows the results of the first mean scenario, in which no features are differentially expressed. The right-hand panel shows the second mean scenario, in which the top two-thirds of the binary tree signaling pathway are differentially expressed. We compare the performance of miEMC-NetGSA with the other integrated models described above.

The first mean scenario permits assessment of the false positive rate under different omics integration schemes. We observe that in all gene sets that we tested, all four NetGSA-based methods have low false positive rates. Most importantly, integration of miRNA with expression alone ("miE") does not cause an elevated false positive rate over the original NetGSA method. Likewise, although the false positive rate is somewhat elevated in miEMC-NetGSA, we observe that it is not elevated significantly over the existing EMC-NetGSA method. Therefore, we do not attribute to the miRNA integration a meaningful increase of the type I error rate.

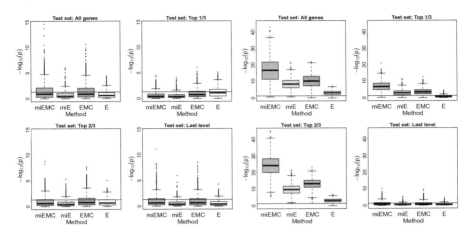

Fig. 1 Boxplots of $-\log_{10} p$-values from simulation study. The left-hand panel shows significance tests for four gene sets of interest, under the first mean scenario in which no omics features exhibit differential activation. The right-hand panel shows the second mean scenario, in which the top two-thirds of the simulated binary tree signaling pathway is differentially activated, but the final third is equal in the control and treatment populations. miEMC-NetGSA is shown in green, miE-NetGSA in yellow, EMC-NetGSA in blue, and NetGSA ("E") on expression only in white

Further, we note that the number of miRNAs is large relative to the number of genes. This causes the type I error rate to be *lower* for the methods that integrate miRNA–gene targets, shown in the test set of the top 1/3 genes. The reason is that the larger overall number of features provides increased accuracy to miEMC-NetGSA and miE integration, so more substantial information is available to the inference procedure than the methods with only gene-level network features.

The second mean scenario provides an assessment of the method's power. We observe that in the three test sets that contain differentially activated features, the power of models that integrate miRNA–gene targets dominates the gene-only analyses. In fact, an integrated model of miRNA and expression has power comparable to EMC-NetGSA integration of methylation and copy number, although miRNA–gene expression remains under-powered relative to EMC-NetGSA.

Also prominent is the increased power of the new method, which integrates both the miRNA–gene targets and gene copy number and methylation. Integration of miRNA reduces the type II error rate of the EMC-NetGSA model; equivalently, it increases the analytic power. Finally, the miRNA methods continue to exhibit low rates of type I errors for the gene set that is not differentially activated.

Taken in tandem, the results of the two simulation scenarios confirm the value of pathway analysis that integrates miRNA–gene targets. We find miRNA contributes to pathway analyses improved statistical power, relative to analyses conducted solely at the level of individual genes. At the same time, we find that miRNA integration does not artificially elevate the false positive rate. Finally, although the addition of miRNA to an expression-only analysis improves power, the increase is marginally less substantial than is provided by integrating copy number and methylation. But, our composition of these two integration schemes achieves the highest statistical power and does not noticeably increase the type I error rate.

4.2 Data Analysis

Prior to analysis, we formatted the dataset described in Sect. 2. We downloaded level 3 TCGA data for 33 cancers from the NCI Genomic Data Commons (Grossman et al. 2016), using the R package TCGA-Assembler, version 2.0.0 (Zhu et al. 2014; Wei et al. 2017).

Starting with gene expression data measured using RNASeqV2, we used a normalization of the read counts provided by TCGA, fragments per kilobase of transcript per million mapped reads upper quartile (FPKM-UQ) (Grossman et al. 2016). We further took a $\log_2$ transformation of the normalized read counts. We used CNV data with common germ-line copy number variants removed and averaged gene-level CNV across the corresponding DNA regions. We aggregated observed methylation beta values across CpG sites by gene and took the mean.

Similar to gene expression, miRNA expression data are available from TCGA in two formats: raw read counts and normalized reads per million (RPM). Raw read counts were collected on the miRNASeq platform, and the TCGA processing pipeline outlined by Chu et al. (2015) is consistent with procedures in comparable projects, such as ENCODE (ENCODE Project Consortium et al. 2012). After alignment and read trimming, a library of approximately 22 base pairs of mature strands was used with an insert length of approximately 22.

Typical miRNASeq analyses use methods traditionally developed for RNASeq. For example, Stokowy et al. (2014) employed RPM normalization and cited its original definition from Mortazavi et al. (2008), in the context of gene expression. They cited other work that applies RPM normalization to miRNASeq data, including Chen et al. (2013). Following RPM normalization but prior to the primary analysis, those authors applied a $\log_2$ transformation. Han et al. (2018) integrated gene and miRNA expression. They first applied FPKM-UQ normalization RNASeq gene expression values, then calculated RPM for miRNASeq values, and transformed logarithmically. TCGA provides RPM-normalized transformation of the data, so for our integrative analysis, we applied a $\log_2$ transformation to the RPM-normalized values. Empirically, we observed that this normalization was comparable to FPKM-UQ applied to the raw read counts.

To demonstrate our procedure, we performed data analysis of the BRAF pathway, a genetic signaling pathway previously studied by Zhang et al. (2017). The left-hand panel of Fig. 2 shows the network topology of the BRAF pathway. It consists of 10 genes—AKT1, BRAF, MAP2K1, MAP2K2, MAPK1, MTOR, NRAS, PIK3CA, PTEN, and RAF1—which are connected by 12 directed edges. The BRAF pathway is a DAG, and this property is preserved under integration with miRNA, copy number, and methylation.

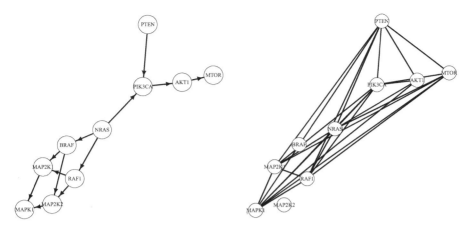

Fig. 2 Network diagrams for the BRAF signaling pathway. The left-hand network is the directed graph representing the BRAF genetic signaling pathway, consisting of 10 genes with 12 directed edges between. The right-hand network contains the same 10 gene vertices, but edges represent a shared miRNA parent. In other words, two genes that share an edge are both targets of a single miRNA and possibly several. The graph contains 25 such edges. miRNA–gene targets are chosen as those entries in the mirDIP database with an "very high" confidence score. Neither the NRAS nor PTEN genes are targeted by any other genes. MAP2K1, MAP2K2, MAPK1, and PIK3CA each have in-degree 2 from other genes. The remaining genes in the network each in-degree 1 from genes. The density of miRNA–gene targets is much higher: in-degree from miRNAs ranges from 10–50 (AKT1, MAP2K1, MTOR, PIK3CA, RAF1) to 143 (PTEN), and BRAF and MAP2K2 are not targeted by any miRNAs

The mirDIP database compiled by Tokar et al. (2017) aggregates predicted miRNA–gene target relationships from several experimentally validated sources. The database assigns each miRNA–gene pair found across any of the 30 sources a composite integrative score. The score, valued on the interval $[0, 1]$, quantifies the strength of experimental evidence that supports the existence of the interaction. The scores are stratified by the so-called confidence classes, expressed in the labels "very high," "high," "medium", and "low" confidence. These classes, respectively, represent the top 1% of scores (very high), the next 4% of scores (high), remainder of top 33% of scores (medium), and all other scores (low). The classes offer a discrete criterion for determining whether to include in $\mathbf{A}^{\star}_{miEMC}$ a specific miRNA–gene interaction. We downloaded their mirDIP unidirectional database, version 4.1, and we considered both 3' and 5' UTR miRNA entries for miRNAs that were also present in the TCGA dataset.

Figure 3 shows a scatter plot of the miRNA–gene target scores from mirDIP for all genes in the BRAF pathway. For a given gene, we identified all miRNAs in the database that target that gene. In the figure, the scores are grouped by gene and colored by confidence class: blue represents very high confidence, green is high confidence, yellow is medium confidence, and red is low confidence.

In our analysis, we used the subset of miRNA–gene targets for which the scores in Fig. 3 belong to the "very high" confidence class. We can construct the secondary

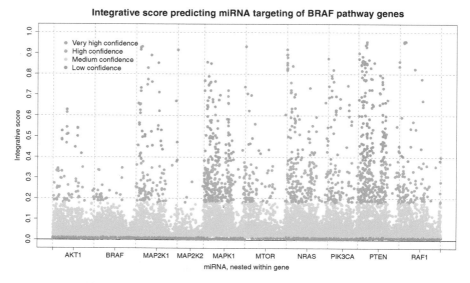

Fig. 3 miRNA–gene interaction scores for all miRNA in TCGA dataset that target any of the 10 genes that comprise the BRAF pathway. Scores are grouped by gene and colored by confidence class: very high, high, medium, and low confidence are colored blue, green, yellow, and red, respectively. For our data analysis, we included only miRNA–gene target interactions with "very high" confidence that the interaction exists, i.e., the blue scores

graph formed between genes that are both targeted by a mutual miRNA parent. Compared with the genetic signaling pathway, this secondary network has a far denser edge set: whereas the BRAF pathway contains 12 edges, the miRNA co-target graph contains 25 edges.

More generally, this larger edge set due to miRNA–gene targets indicates that miRNA integration substantially complexifies the network structure used as input for the pathway analysis. This contrasts with the underlying simplicity of the original graph: whereas the signaling pathway consists of 10 genes, miRNA integration introduces to the network 238 vertices for miRNA observations. Nearly, half of these miRNAs target multiple genes in the BRAF pathway.

The miRNA–gene target subnetwork, corresponding to the unweighted adjacency matrix $\mathbf{A}^{\star}_{mi}$ in Eq. 2, is shown in Fig. 4. This graph shows the subnetwork produced by the directed edges from miRNA vertices to genes, based on miRNA–gene targets. The number of miRNAs targeting a given gene varies substantially, from as many as 143 miRNAs targeting PTEN to as few as to 0. These in-degrees from miRNA vertices are given in the caption to Fig. 2.

Although most miRNAs in the TCGA dataset target a single gene in the BRAF pathway, 47% of the miRNAs target two or more genes. In the network diagram in Fig. 4, miRNAs and their edges are colored according to the degree of the miRNA node, that is, the number of genes in the BRAF pathway targeted by the miRNA. Although there are 128 miRNAs that target only a single gene, the remaining 110

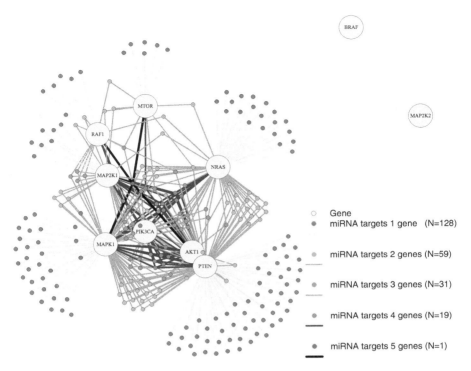

Fig. 4 Topology of subnetwork of the integrated BRAF signaling pathway corresponding to the unweighted adjacency matrix $\mathbf{A}^\star_{\mathrm{mi}}$ in Eq. 2, namely, the graph formed by miRNA–gene targets. All edges are directed from the miRNA vertex to the gene vertex. The miRNA node colors, edge widths, and edge colors correspond to the degree of the miRNA vertex, that is, the number of genes in the BRAF pathway targeted by a given miRNA. Gray graph nodes are genes, while colored graph nodes are miRNAs, targeting 1 gene (red), 2 genes (yellow), 3 genes (green), 4 genes (blue), and 5 genes (purple). The genes BRAF and MAP2K2 are not targeted by any genes. Darker edge colors correspond to higher out-degree of the associated miRNA

target multiple genes. This intricate structure is not balanced, in neither the in-degree of gene nodes nor the out-degree of miRNA nodes. The number of unique miRNAs that target each gene varies from 58 (PTEN) to 4 (PIK3CA); while one miRNA targets 5 genes, there are 19 that target 4, 31 that target 3, and 59 that target 2.

We obtained observations of gene expression, miRNA expression, methylation, and copy number from TCGA, as described in Sect. 2. Among the TCGA cancer studies, we restricted our analysis to the subset of cancers for which all 10 BRAF pathway genes were observed, and for which more than 10 samples were available in both the tumor and normal tissue sample populations. This yielded nine cancers for integrative pathway analysis of the BRAF pathway: bladder, breast, head and neck squamous cell, kidney renal clear cell and papillary cell, liver hepatocellular, thyroid, and uterine corpus endometrial carcinomas, and prostate adenocarcinoma. Sample sizes and proportional representation of the healthy samples were consistent across the nine cancers. For example, the bladder urothelial carcinoma dataset contained 341 samples of tumor tissue and 15 samples of healthy tissue. This corresponds to 356 total samples, 4% of which are healthy controls.

Within each cancer, we performed the same four NetGSA-based pathway analyses as in the simulation study: full integration of gene expression, miRNA expression, and gene-level methylation and copy number (miEMC-NetGSA); integration of gene and miRNA expression ("miE"); integration of gene expression, methylation, and copy number (EMC-NetGSA); and the original NetGSA for expression only ("E"). To correct for the multiple comparison problem, we adjusted p-values within each cancer using the method of Benjamini and Hochberg (1995) (BH).

The adjusted p-values are plotted in the top panel of Fig. 5. The pathway is significantly disturbed at the $\alpha = 0.05$ level across all cancers for both methods that integrate miRNA. However, the cancers diverge in their decision outcomes when only gene-level features are included. In head and neck squamous cell carcinoma (HNSC) and prostate adenocarcinoma (PRAD), both methods that integrate only gene-level features, namely, EMC-NetGSA and expression-only NetGSA, fail to reject the null hypothesis of no pathway disturbance, but miRNA integration confirms pathway disturbance. In bladder urothelial carcinoma (BLCA), thyroid carcinoma (THCA), and uterine corpus endometrial carcinoma (UCEC), the expression-only analysis does not reject the null hypothesis, while integration of any features beyond gene expression leads to the conclusion of pathway disturbance. In these cancers, integration of miRNA features leads to differential effects: in the bladder and thyroid cancers, miRNA integration causes a large increase in significance. Likewise, although the pathway is significantly disturbed in kidney renal clear cell carcinoma (KIRC) and liver hepatocellular carcinoma (LIHC), miRNA integration substantially increases the significance of the hypothesis test. The same is largely true of breast invasive carcinoma (BRCA). On the other hand, in the uterine cancer, the change in significance is less pronounced between gene-only and miRNA–gene integration. Similarly, kidney renal papillary cell carcinoma (KIRP) exhibits a lesser degree of differentiation between the significance of the three integrative methods.

Figure 5 also shows bar plots of the test statistics corresponding to the p-values. For most cancers with substantial increases in significance due to miRNA integration, bladder, breast, kidney renal clear cell, prostate, and thyroid correspond to test statistics with the same sign and distinctly greater magnitude than the gene-level analyses. The test statistics of kidney renal papillary cell carcinoma display a similar pattern in the relative magnitudes of the test statistics, despite the lesser differences in statistical significance between the EMC-NetGSA and the miRNA-NetGSA analyses. The liver and head and neck cancers have test statistics with the opposite sign from those six cancers, in conjunction with sign switches in the test statistics before and after miRNA integration. In contrast, the test statistics for the uterine cancer display test statistics with consistent signs, though the magnitude increases with miRNA integration.

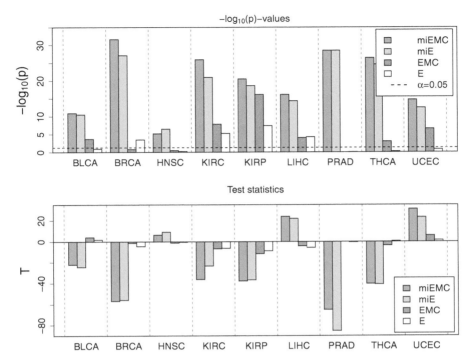

Fig. 5 *(Top)* Results of significance tests for pathway disturbance in the BRAF pathway, across 9 TCGA cancers. Barplots give values of $-\log_{10}$ p-values, after Benjamini–Hochberg adjustment for multiple comparisons. Full gene expression miRNA expression, and gene-level methylation and copy number are shown in green ("miEMC"); integration of gene and miRNA expression is in yellow ("miE"); integration of gene expression and gene-level methylation and copy number are in blue ("EMC"); and the original, expression-only NetGSA results are in white ("E"). The horizontal dotted line gives the significance threshold at the $\alpha = 0.05$ level. *(Bottom)* Test statistics for pathway disturbance in 9 TCGA cancers, for the BRAF pathway. Bar plot heights give the test statistic value. miEMC-NetGSA is in green, miE-NetGSA in yellow, EMC-NetGSA in blue, and NetGSA ("E") in white

Across the nine cancer types, we did not observe any apparent pattern in the relation between the test statistic signs and the relative significance of the tests. Relatively weaker significance in gene-level analyses sometimes corresponds to small test statistics with the same sign, as in breast and kidney renal clear cell cancers. But it also corresponds to sign changes in the test statistics, as in bladder, head and neck, and thyroid cancers. The head and neck, liver, and uterine cancers are notable for their inversion of the test statistic's sign in the miRNA analyses, relative to the other cancers. Despite the similarity between kidney renal papillary cell carcinoma and uterine corpus endometrial carcinoma in terms of p-values and relative significances of the four analyses, the kidney cancer test statistic sign is more comparable to the other kidney cancer, among others. The large magnitude of the prostate cancer test statistics under miRNA integration matches the sharp increase in significance.

Finally, we assessed the robustness of our inference to the assumptions, especially symmetric errors. Overdispersion can be a characteristic of RNASeq count data (Zhou et al. 2011), but this typically arises in the context of count data and the choice between Poisson and negative binomial distributions. Empirically, the transformations we apply to the raw counts induce symmetry, and the assumption of normality provides separate parameters for location and dispersion.

Furthermore, we applied the bootstrap method described in the previous section, with $B = 9999$, and found that the inference for the full miEMC-NetGSA integration and the partial miRNA–gene expression integration were both robust in all cancers, and the semi-parametric decision outcome matches that of the parametric test. On the other hand, the EMC-NetGSA tests were not robust in any cancers except the kidney cancers, and the expression-only tests for bladder and thyroid cancers were likewise inconclusive. Therefore, we conclude that the inferences we draw are robust to the model assumptions, and the evidence for pathway disturbance in the miRNA-integrated analyses is valid in the semi-parametric setting, as well.

These results indicate statistically meaningful contributions of the miRNA features to the pathway analysis. Moreover, they suggest the effect of miRNA integration does not lead deterministically to a specific decision outcome. In some cancers, miRNA integration reinforces the conclusions of pathway analysis using existing methods based solely on gene-level features. In others, the miRNAs identify a significant disturbance that is less apparent when the BRAF pathway is considered using only gene-level features. This may be due to the reduction in noise at the level of gene expression features using the augmented network, thereby accentuating the differential expression in the pathway. Finally, in all the cancers, the reduction of gene-level noise that is accomplished by the miRNA–gene target network effect clarifies the expression of pathway genes.

We have made publicly available the code to produce the results of our analysis at:

`https://github.com/Zhang-Data-Science-Research-Lab/miEMC-NetGSA-BRAF`

5 Discussion

In this chapter, we highlighted the importance of integrating miRNA measurements into network analysis of genetic signaling pathways. We proposed a statistical modeling approach that incorporates recent biological research on the functional relationships between protein-coding and non-coding RNAs. We identified significant miRNA–gene targets and constructed a graphical model of these interactions. We combined this graph with a signaling pathway graph to account for correlated coexpression in genes through a biological mechanism external to the signaling pathway of interest. We used a simulation study to show that an integrative model of miRNA–gene targets has higher statistical power than analysis that focuses only on gene-level features. At the same time, we demonstrated that our method does not increase the false discovery rate, relative to the existing methods. Our miEMC-NetGSA model offers a statistical framework for data integration and pathway analysis of multiple omics data types, obtains high power, and is grounded in current biological research.

Finally, we applied the miRNA–gene analysis to the BRAF signaling pathway on a large-scale cancer study. Although the genetic pathway itself consisted of only 12 edges on 10 vertices, we found that the fully integrated network of gene expression, miRNA expression, gene copy number, and gene methylation observations consisted of 268 vertices and 452 directed edges. The decision outcome in a hypothesis test for differential expression varied across the 9 cancers under consideration. In some cancers, integration of either miRNA or gene-level copy number and methylation led to higher significance, but the composition of all integrative features did not necessarily strengthen the significance. In other cancers, integration of miRNA–gene targets with expression confirmed the result of a gene expression-only analysis; while the integration of gene expression with methylation and copy number indicated strong significance, the further addition miRNA integration was in consensus with the expression-only and miRNA–gene analyses.

References

Agarwal, V., Bell, G.W., Nam, J.-W., & Bartel, D.P. (2015). Predicting effective microRNA target sites in mammalian mRNAs. elife, 4:e05005.

Benjamini, Y., & Hochberg, Y. (1995). Controlling the false discovery rate: a practical and powerful approach to multiple testing. *Journal of the Royal Statistical Society: Series B (Methodological), 57*(1), 289–300.

Bleazard, T., Lamb, J.A., & Griffiths-Jones, S. (2015). Bias in microRNA functional enrichment analysis. *Bioinformatics, 31*(10), 1592–1598.

Cava, C., Bertoli, G., Ripamonti, M., Mauri, G., Zoppis, I., Della Rosa, P. A., Gilardi, M. C., & Castiglioni, I. (2014). Integration of mRNA expression profile, copy number alterations, and microRNA expression levels in breast cancer to improve grade definition. *PLoS ONE, 9*(5), e97681.

Chen, M., Zhang, X., Liu, J., & Storey, K. B. (2013). High-throughput sequencing reveals differential expression of miRNAs in intestine from sea cucumber during aestivation. *PLoS One, 8*(10), e76120.

Chu, A., Robertson, G., Brooks, D., Mungall, A. J., Birol, I., Coope, R., Ma, Y., Jones, S., & Marra, M. A. (2015). Large-scale profiling of microRNAs for the cancer genome atlas. *Nucleic Acids Research, 44*(1), e3–e3.

Coll, M., El Taghdouini, A., Perea, L., Mannaerts, I., Vila-Casadesús, M., Blaya, D., Rodrigo-Torres, D., Affò, S., Morales-Ibanez, O., Graupera, I., et al. (2015). Integrative miRNA and gene expression profiling analysis of human quiescent hepatic stellate cells. *Scientific Reports, 5*, 11549.

Du, J., & Zhang, L. (2015). Integrated analysis of DNA methylation and microRNA regulation of the lung adenocarcinoma transcriptome. *Oncology Reports, 34*(2), 585–594.

ENCODE Project Consortium et al. (2012) An integrated encyclopedia of DNA elements in the human genome. *Nature, 489*(7414),57.

Enerly, E., Steinfeld, I., Kleivi, K., Leivonen, S.-K., Aure, M. R., Russnes, H. G., Rønneberg, J. A., Johnsen, H., Navon, R., Rødland, E., et al. (2011). miRNA-mRNA integrated analysis reveals roles for miRNAs in primary breast tumors. *PLoS One, 6*(2), e16915.

Godard, P., & van Eyll, J. (2015). Pathway analysis from lists of microRNAs: common pitfalls and alternative strategy. *Nucleic Acids Research, 43*(7), 3490–3497.

Grossman, R. L., Heath, A. P., Ferretti, V., Varmus, H. E., Lowy, D. R., Kibbe, W. A., & Staudt, L. M. (2016). Toward a shared vision for cancer genomic data. *New England Journal of Medicine, 375*(12), 1109–1112.

Han, S., Kim, D., Shivakumar, M., Lee, Y.-J., Garg, T., Miller, J. E., Kim, J. H., Kim, D., & Lee, Y. (2018). The effects of alternative splicing on miRNA binding sites in bladder cancer. *PLoS One, 13*(1):e0190708.

Hsu, S.-D., Lin, F.-M., Wu, W.-Y., Liang, C., Huang, W.-C., Chan, W.-L., Tsai, W.-T., Chen, G.-Z., Lee, C.-J., Chiu, C.-M., et al. (2010). miRTarBase: a database curates experimentally validated microRNA–target interactions. *Nucleic Acids Research, 39*(suppl_1), D163–D169.

Hsu, J. B. K., Chiu, C. M., Hsu, S. D., Huang, W. Y., Chien, C. H., Lee, T. Y., & Huang, H. D. (2011). miRTar: an integrated system for identifying miRNA-target interactions in human. *BMC Bioinformatics, 12*(1), 300.

Karagkouni, D., Paraskevopoulou, M. D., Chatzopoulos, S., Vlachos, I. S., Tastsoglou, S., Kanellos, I., Papadimitriou, D., Kavakiotis, I., Maniou, S., Skoufos, G., et al. (2017). DIANA-TarBase v8: a decade-long collection of experimentally supported miRNA–gene interactions. *Nucleic Acids Research, 46*(D1), D239–D245.

Kim, S. (2015). ppcor: an R package for a fast calculation to semi-partial correlation coefficients. *Communications for Statistical Applications and Methods, 22*(6), 665.

Krämer, N., Schäfer, J., & Boulesteix, A.-L. (2009). Regularized estimation of large-scale gene association networks using graphical Gaussian models. *BMC Bioinformatics, 10*(1), 384.

Lewis, B. P., Burge, C. B., & Bartel, D. P. (2005). Conserved seed pairing, often flanked by adenosines, indicates that thousands of human genes are microRNA targets. *Cell, 120*(1), 15–20.

Li, X., Yu, X., He, Y., Meng, Y., Liang, J., Huang, L., Du, H., Wang, X., & Liu, W. (2018). Integrated analysis of microRNA (miRNA) and mRNA profiles reveals reduced correlation between microRNA and target gene in cancer. *BioMed Research International, 2018*.

MacKinnon, J. G. (2009). Bootstrap hypothesis testing. *Handbook of Computational Econometrics, 183*, 213.

Miao, X., Luo, Q., Zhao, H., & Qin, X. (2017). An integrated analysis of miRNAs and methylated genes encoding mRNAs and lncRNAs in sheep breeds with different fecundity. *Frontiers in Physiology, 8*, 1049.

Mortazavi, A., Williams, B. A., McCue, K., Schaeffer, L., & Wold, B. (2008). Mapping and quantifying mammalian transcriptomes by RNA-seq. *Nature Methods, 5*(7), 621.

Shojaie, A., & Michailidis, G. (2009). Analysis of gene sets based on the underlying regulatory network. *Journal of Computational Biology, 16*(3), 407–426.

Shojaie, A., & Michailidis, G. (2010). Network enrichment analysis in complex experiments. *Statistical Applications in Genetics and Molecular Biology, 9*(1).

Stokowy, T., Eszlinger, M., Świerniak, M., Fujarewicz, K., Jarząb, B., Paschke, R., & Krohn, K. (2014). Analysis options for high-throughput sequencing in miRNA expression profiling. *BMC Research Notes, 7*(1), 144.

Tokar, T., Pastrello, C., Rossos, A. E. M., Abovsky, M., Hauschild, A.-C., Tsay, M., Lu, R., & Jurisica, I. (2017). mirDIP 4.1–integrative database of human microRNA target predictions. *Nucleic Acids Research, 46*(D1), D360–D370.

Tomczak, K., Czerwińska, P., & Wiznerowicz, M. (2015). The cancer genome atlas (TCGA): an immeasurable source of knowledge. *Contemporary Oncology, 19*(1A), A68.

Vlachos, I. S., Zagganas, K., Paraskevopoulou, M. D., Georgakilas, G., Karagkouni, D., Vergoulis, T., Dalamagas, T., & Hatzigeorgiou, A. G. (2015). DIANA-miRPath v3. 0: deciphering microRNA function with experimental support. *Nucleic Acids Research, 43*(W1), W460–W466.

Volinia, S., & Croce, C. M. (2013). Prognostic microRNA/mRNA signature from the integrated analysis of patients with invasive breast cancer. *Proceedings of the National Academy of Sciences, 110*(18), 7413–7417.

Wei, L., Jin, Z., Yang, S., Xu, Y., Zhu, Y., & Ji, Y. (2017). TCGA-assembler 2: software pipeline for retrieval and processing of TCGA/CPTAC data. *Bioinformatics, 34*(9), 1615–1617.

Wu, X., & Watson, M. (2009). CORNA: testing gene lists for regulation by microRNAs. *Bioinformatics, 25*(6), 832–833.

Yu, N., Yong, S., Kim, H. K., Choi, Y.-L., Jung, Y., Kim, D., Seo, J., Lee, Y. E., Baek, D., Lee, J., et al. (2019). Identification of tumor suppressor miRNAs by integrative miRNA and mRNA sequencing of matched tumor–normal samples in lung adenocarcinoma. *Molecular Oncology, 13*(6), 1356.

Zhang, Y., Linder, M. H., Shojaie, A., Ouyang, Z., Shen, R., Baggerly, K. A., Baladandayuthapani, V., & Zhao, H. (2017). Dissecting pathway disturbances using network topology and multi-platform genomics data. *Statistics in Biosciences*, 1–21.

Zhou, Y.-H., Xia, K., & Wright, F. A. (2011). A powerful and flexible approach to the analysis of RNA sequence count data. *Bioinformatics, 27*(19), 2672–2678.

Zhu, Y., Qiu, P., & Ji, Y. (2014). TCGA-assembler: open-source software for retrieving and processing TCGA data. *Nature Methods, 11*(6), 599.

Robust Feature Screening for Ultrahigh-Dimensional Censored Data Subject to Measurement Error

Li-Pang Chen and Grace Y. Yi

Abstract Feature screening is commonly used to handle ultrahigh-dimensional data prior to conducting a formal data analysis. While various feature screening methods have been developed in the literature, research gaps still exist. The existing methods usually make an implicit assumption that data are accurately measured. This requirement, however, is frequently violated in applications. In this chapter, we consider error-prone ultrahigh-dimensional survival data and propose a robust feature screening method. We develop an iteration algorithm to improve the performance of retaining all informative covariates. Theoretical results are established for the proposed method. Simulation studies are reported to assess the performance of the proposed method, together with an application of the proposed method to handle a mantle cell lymphoma microarray dataset.

Keywords Censored data · Distance correlation · Inverse Fourier transformation · Measurement error · Robustness · Screening · Ultrahigh-dimension

1 Introduction

With modern technologies, data with high dimensions and complex structures can be collected easily. One concern on high-dimensional data is the relevance and

L.-P. Chen
Department of Statistical and Actuarial Sciences, University of Western Ontario, London, ON, Canada

Department of Statistics, National Chengchi University, Taipei, Taiwan
e-mail: lchen723@nccu.edu.tw

G. Y. Yi (✉)
Department of Statistical and Actuarial Sciences, University of Western Ontario, London, ON, Canada

Department of Computer Science, University of Western Ontario, London, ON, Canada
e-mail: gyi5@uwo.ca

© The Author(s), under exclusive license to Springer Nature Switzerland AG 2022
W. He et al. (eds.), *Advances and Innovations in Statistics and Data Science*, ICSA Book Series in Statistics, https://doi.org/10.1007/978-3-031-08329-7_2

usefulness of the associated variables. It is important to preprocess data by excluding unimportant variables before performing a formal analysis of the data (e.g., Chen & Chen 2008).

Various methods of feature screening have been developed in the literature. For example, Fan & Lv (2008) proposed the sure independent screening (SIS) procedure for ultrahigh-dimensional linear models by utilizing the Pearson correlation. Hall & Miller (2009) developed the bootstrap procedure to rank the predictor importance based on the Pearson correlation between the response and the covariates. Fan et al. (2009) and Fan & Song (2010) ranked the importance of each predictor using the marginal likelihood method. To explore a flexible setting with model misspecification, Zhu et al. (2011) and Li et al. (2012) proposed model-free feature screening procedures to capture informative covariates for ultrahigh-dimensional data. Yi et al. (2021) developed a screening method for settings where both the sample size and the dimension of variables are large. To make robust feature screening, Xue & Liang (2017) implemented cumulative distribution functions of responses and covariates to the Henze–Zirkler test statistics, where the normal distribution assumption was imposed.

Concerning high-dimensional survival data, Fan et al. (2010) proposed the SIS method for the Cox model. Song et al. (2014) explored the censored rank independence screening procedure. Yan et al. (2017) developed the Spearman rank correlation screening method. Zhang et al. (2020) used the distance correlation to describe the correlation of covariates with survival or censoring times. To avoid the impact of outliers and make robust inference, Chen et al. (2018) modified the distance correlation by incorporating the cumulative distribution functions of survival times and covariates. Hao et al. (2019) proposed to rank the covariance for the cumulative distribution function of the covariates and the survivor function of the survival time.

Even though different feature screening methods have been developed for ultrahigh-dimensional data, research gaps still exist. One issue is the *accuracy* of feature screening. Conventional feature screening methods rank the importance of each predictor through marginal measures, which may fail to detect truly important covariates that are marginally independent of the response due to their correlations with other covariates. An example can be found in Sect. 4.2.2 of Fan & Lv (2008). To overcome this problem, Fan & Lv (2008) proposed the iterative SIS method. Zhong & Zhu (2015) developed the iterated distance correlation to improve the accuracy of variable screening. For survival data, Hao et al. (2019) proposed the robust projection to update the selection of variables that are falsely excluded by conventional feature screening methods. A second issue concerns measurement error, an issue receiving little attention in the context of feature screening, though Chen (2019) proposed a feature screening method for data with measurement error. However, Chen (2019) considered only the case with classical additive error where the normal distribution is assumed.

In this chapter, we develop a model-free feature screening method by utilizing the cumulative distribution functions of survival times and covariates. To eliminate measurement error effects, we employ the inverse Fourier transformation that allows us to consider a broad class of measurement error models. Theoretical results are established to justify the validity of the proposed method. Moreover, we propose an iterated procedure to improve the accuracy of feature screening.

The remainder is organized as follows. In Sect. 2, we introduce the basic framework, together with the distance correlation method under the error-free setting. In Sect. 3, we propose the inverse Fourier transformation approach to address the feature of mismeasured covariates and establish theoretical results. In Sect. 4, we describe the iterative feature screening procedure to accommodate the case where important covariates are falsely excluded using the method in Sect. 3. Empirical studies, including simulation results and real-data analysis, are provided in Sect. 5. We conclude the article with discussions in Sect. 6.

2 Notation and Framework

2.1 Survival Data

For any individual, let T denote the failure time, and let C represent the associated censoring time. Write $Y = \min\{T, C\}$ and let $\delta = \mathbb{I}(T \leq C)$ be the censoring indicator, where $\mathbb{I}(\cdot)$ is the indicator function. Let $X = \left(X_{(1)}, \cdots, X_{(p)}\right)^\top$ denote the p-dimensional random vector of possibly associated covariates. Let $\tau > 0$ be a finite value representing the length of the study period, where $P(T < \tau) > 0$. Conditional on the covariates X, T and C are assumed to be independent.

Let

$$I = \left\{j : T \text{ is associated with } X_{(j)} \text{ for } j = 1, \cdots, p\right\}$$

denote the *active set* containing all the relevant covariates for the response T, and let $q = |I|$. Let I^c be the complement of I that contains all the covariates in X that are irrelevant to the response T. Let $X_I = \left\{X_{(j)} : j \in I\right\}$ denote the vector containing all the active covariates, and let $X_{I^c} = \left\{X_{(j)} : j \in I^c\right\}$ be the vector containing all the irrelevant covariates. We consider settings where the dimension p of the covariates is ultrahigh relative to the sample size, denoted n, with $p = \exp\left\{O(n^r)\right\}$ for some $r > 0$ (e.g., Fan & Lv 2008) and where $q < n$. Our goal is to develop a feature screening procedure to exclude irrelevant covariates as much as possible, while retaining the covariates in I to output a reduced dataset for a further formal analysis. Suppose that we have a sample $\left\{(T_i, X_i, \delta_i, C_i) : i = 1, \cdots, n\right\}$, where the $(T_i, X_i, \delta_i, C_i)$ have the same distribution as (T, X, δ, C). Write $Y_i = \min\{T_i, C_i\}$ for $i = 1, \cdots, n$.

2.2 Distance Correlation of Two Random Variables

For the following development, we now briefly review the distance correlation method of Székely et al. (2007). For two random vectors U and V of dimension d_U and d_V, respectively, let $\phi_U(s) = E\left\{\exp\left(\mathbf{i}s^\top U\right)\right\}$ and $\phi_V(t) = E\left\{\exp\left(\mathbf{i}t^\top V\right)\right\}$, respectively, denote their characteristic functions, and let $\phi_{U,V}(s,t) = E\left[\exp\left\{\mathbf{i}\left(s^\top U + t^\top V\right)\right\}\right]$ be the joint characteristic function of U and V, where $\mathbf{i}$ is the imaginary unit with $\mathbf{i}^2 = -1$, and s and t are $d_U \times 1$ and $d_V \times 1$ vectors of real numbers, respectively. For any complex function $\phi(t)$ consisting of a real part and an imaginary part with $\mathbf{i}$, let $\bar{\phi}(\cdot)$ denote its conjugate with $\mathbf{i}$ replaced by $-\mathbf{i}$, and define $\|\phi(t)\|^2 = \phi(t)\bar{\phi}(t)$.

Define the *distance covariance* between U and V as

$$\mathrm{dcov}(U, V) = \int_{\mathbb{R}^{d_U}} \int_{\mathbb{R}^{d_V}} \left\|\phi_{U,V}(s,t) - \phi_U(s)\phi_V(t)\right\|^2 w(s,t)\,ds\,dt,$$

where

$$w(s,t) = \left\{c_{d_U} c_{d_V} \|s\|_{d_U}^{1+d_U} \|t\|_{d_V}^{1+d_V}\right\}^{-1};$$

for a given d, $c_d = \pi^{(1+d)/2}/\Gamma\{(1+d)/2\}$ with $\Gamma(t)$ being the gamma function; and $\|a\|_d = \left(a_1^2 + \cdots + a_d^2\right)^{1/2}$ represents the Euclidean norm for a d-dimensional vector $a = (a_1, \cdots, a_d)^\top \in \mathbb{R}^d$.

Székely et al. (2007) showed that $\mathrm{dcov}(U, V)$ can be alternatively written as

$$\mathrm{dcov}(U, V) = J_1 + J_2 - 2J_3, \tag{1}$$

where

$$J_1 = E\left(\left\|U - \widetilde{U}\right\|_{d_U} \left\|V - \widetilde{V}\right\|_{d_V}\right),$$

$$J_2 = E\left(\left\|U - \widetilde{U}\right\|_{d_U}\right) E\left(\left\|V - \widetilde{V}\right\|_{d_V}\right),$$

$$J_3 = E\left\{E\left(\left\|U - \widetilde{U}\right\|_{d_U}\Big| U\right) E\left(\left\|V - \widetilde{V}\right\|_{d_V}\Big| V\right)\right\},$$

and $(\widetilde{U}, \widetilde{V})$ is an independent copy of (U, V).

The distance correlation (DC) between U and V is defined as

$$\mathrm{dcorr}(U, V) = \frac{\mathrm{dcov}(U, V)}{\sqrt{\mathrm{dcov}(U, U)\mathrm{dcov}(V, V)}}. \tag{2}$$

Székely et al. (2007) proved that two random vectors U and V are independent if and only if $\mathrm{dcorr}(U, V) = 0$. This property shows that the distance correlation is useful to characterize the association between random variables, which is the basis for our following development.

2.3   Feature Screening for Censored Data with Precise Measurements

In the absence of censoring, it is straightforward to employ the distance correlation between the covariates and the survival times to determine the active set $\mathcal{I}$. However, right censoring makes the direct implementation of this method impossible. Further, as indicated by Chen et al. (2018), covariates may exhibit heavy-tailed distributions and contain outliers. To alleviate the issues, we consider the transformed random variables using cumulative distribution functions which are known to be bounded and monotone.

To be specific, modifying (2), we propose the *functional distance correlation* for $X_{(j)}$ and Y, given by

$$
\begin{aligned}
\omega_j &\triangleq \mathrm{dcorr}\{F_{X_{(j)}}(X_{(j)}), F(Y)\} \\
&= \frac{\mathrm{dcov}\{F_{X_{(j)}}(X_{(j)}), F(Y)\}}{\sqrt{\mathrm{dcov}\{F_{X_{(j)}}(X_{(j)}), F_{X_{(j)}}(X_{(j)})\}\mathrm{dcov}\{F(Y), F(Y)\}}}
\end{aligned}
\tag{3}
$$

for $j = 1, \ldots, p$, where $F(t) = P(T \leq t)$ is the cumulative distribution function of the failure time T and $F_{X_{(j)}}(x) = P(X_{(j)} \leq x)$ is the cumulative distribution function of the jth covariate. While the formulation (3) applies to both continuous and discrete covariates, in this chapter, we focus on continuous covariates only. Therefore, $F_{X_{(j)}}(x)$ can be written as $F_{X_{(j)}}(x) = \int_{-\infty}^{x} f_{X_{(j)}}(u)du$, where $f_{X_{(j)}}(x)$ is the probability density function of $X_{(j)}$.

Similar to the idea of using the distance correlation to do feature screening (e.g., Li et al. 2012; Chen et al. 2018; Zhang et al. 2020), we use the functional distance correlation ω_j for $j = 1, \cdots, p$ to screen the covariates. A smaller value of ω_j indicates a weaker correlation between the jth covariate and the survival time, and thus, ranking all the ω_j for $j = 1, \cdots, p$ allows us to screen out the covariates of little relevance to the survival time.

To implement this idea, we estimate (3) using the sample data. First, we may express the three terms $\mathrm{dcov}(\cdot, \cdot)$ in (3) using their equivalent forms, as suggested by (1) with relevant quantities modified. Since estimation of $\mathrm{dcov}\{F_{X_{(j)}}(X_{(j)}), F_{X_{(j)}}(X_{(j)})\}$ and $\mathrm{dcov}\{F(Y), F(Y)\}$ can be obtained analogously to that of $\mathrm{dcov}\{F_{X_{(j)}}(X_{(j)}), F(Y)\}$, we describe the latter case only. Similar to (1), $\mathrm{dcov}\{F_{X_{(j)}}(X_{(j)}), F(Y)\}$ can be estimated by its empirical counterpart from the sample data:

$$
\widehat{\mathrm{dcov}}\{\widehat{F}_{X_{(j)}}(X_{(j)}), \widehat{F}(Y)\} = \widehat{M}_{j,1} + \widehat{M}_{j,2} - 2\widehat{M}_{j,3}
\tag{4}
$$

with

$$\widehat{M}_{j,1} = \frac{1}{n^2} \sum_{i=1}^{n} \sum_{k=1}^{n} \left\{ \left| \widehat{F}_{X_{(j)}}(X_{i(j)}) - \widehat{F}_{X_{(j)}}(X_{k(j)}) \right| \left| \widehat{F}(Y_i) - \widehat{F}(Y_k) \right| \right\},$$

$$\widehat{M}_{j,2} = \left\{ \frac{1}{n^2} \sum_{i=1}^{n} \sum_{k=1}^{n} \left| \widehat{F}_{X_{(j)}}(X_{i(j)}) - \widehat{F}_{X_{(j)}}(X_{k(j)}) \right| \right\} \left\{ \frac{1}{n^2} \sum_{i=1}^{n} \sum_{k=1}^{n} \left| \widehat{F}(Y_i) - \widehat{F}(Y_k) \right| \right\},$$

$$\widehat{M}_{j,3} = \frac{1}{n} \sum_{i=1}^{n} \left[\left\{ \frac{1}{n} \sum_{k=1}^{n} |\widehat{F}_{X_{(j)}}(X_{i(j)}) - \widehat{F}_{X_{(j)}}(X_{k(j)})| \right\} \left\{ \frac{1}{n} \sum_{l=1}^{n} |\widehat{F}(Y_i) - \widehat{F}(Y_l)| \right\} \right],$$

where $X_{i(j)}$ represents the jth element of X_i,

$$\widehat{F}(t) = 1 - \prod_{i=1}^{n} \left\{ 1 - \frac{1}{\sum_{k=1}^{n} \mathbb{I}(Y_k \geq Y_i)} \right\}^{\delta_i \mathbb{I}(Y_i \leq t)}$$

is the Kaplan–Meier estimator of $F(t)$, and

$$\widehat{F}_{X_{(j)}}(x) = \int_{-\infty}^{x} \widehat{f}_{X_{(j)}}(u) du \tag{5}$$

is the estimator of $F_{X_{(j)}}(x)$ with $\widehat{f}_{X_{(j)}}(u)$ being the nonparametric estimate of $f_{X_{(j)}}(u)$.

Consequently, using (4) gives the final estimator of (3)

$$\widetilde{\text{dcorr}}\{\widehat{F}_{X_{(j)}}(X_{(j)}), \widehat{F}(Y)\} = \frac{\widehat{\text{dcov}}\{\widehat{F}_{X_{(j)}}(X_{(j)}), \widehat{F}(Y)\}}{\sqrt{\widehat{\text{dcov}}\{\widehat{F}_{X_{(j)}}(X_{(j)}), \widehat{F}_{X_{(j)}}(X_{(j)})\}\widehat{\text{dcov}}\{\widehat{F}(Y), \widehat{F}(Y)\}}}.$$

In this chapter, we take $\widehat{f}_{X_{(j)}}(u)$ as the kernel estimator, given by

$$\widehat{f}_{X_{(j)}}(u) = \frac{1}{nh} \sum_{i=1}^{n} K\left(\frac{u - X_{i(j)}}{h} \right), \tag{6}$$

with h being a bandwidth and $K(\cdot)$ being a kernel function satisfying the following conditions (e.g., Wand & Jones 1995):

(C1) $\int_{-\infty}^{\infty} K(u)du = 1$; $K(u) \geq 0$; $K(u)$ is symmetric; $\int_{-\infty}^{\infty} u^r K(u)du$ is finite for all $r \in \mathbb{N}$.

(C2) $h = o(n^{-\frac{1}{5}})$.

Condition (C1) is standard for implementing the kernel estimation, in which the requirement of $\int_{-\infty}^{\infty} u^r K(u)du$ to be finite for $r \in \mathbb{N}$ is satisfied by commonly used kernel functions listed in Wand & Jones (1995). Condition (C2) is regarded as the optimal bandwidth in the sense of Wand and Jones (1995, Sect. 2.5), and thus, we take h as of the rate of $n^{-1/5}$ in the following development.

3 Feature Screening for Censored Data with Error-Prone Covariates

3.1 Measurement Error Model

We consider the setting where for $i = 1, \cdots, n$, X_i is not precisely observed, but instead, a surrogate, denoted X_i^*, is observed for X_i. Let Σ_{X^*} and Σ_X denote the covariance matrices of X_i^* and X_i, respectively. Here we focus on the classical measurement error model (e.g., Carroll et al. 2006; Yi 2017)

$$X_i^* = X_i + \epsilon_i \tag{7}$$

for $i = 1, \cdots, n$, where ϵ_i is the noise term with mean zero and covariance matrix Σ_ϵ, and ϵ_i is independent of $\{X_i, T_i, C_i\}$.

Let $f_\epsilon(\cdot)$ denote the probability density function of ϵ_i that may or may not have unknown parameters. In the following development, we consider three scenarios:

Scenario I: The distribution $f_\epsilon(\cdot)$ of ϵ_i in (7) is completely known, and hence, no unknown parameters are involved.
This is the simplest case to develop a screening procedure with measurement error effects incorporated. In this instance, the covariance matrix Σ_ϵ is uniquely determined by the distribution $f_\epsilon(\cdot)$.

Scenario II: The functional form of the density function $f_\epsilon(\cdot)$ is known, but its associated parameters are unknown yet repeated surrogate measurements are available to estimate Σ_ϵ.
That is, we have replicates of X_i^*, denoted X_{ir}^*, which follow

$$X_{ir}^* = X_i + \epsilon_{ir}$$

for $i = 1, \cdots, n$ and $r = 1, \cdots, n_i$ with $n_i \geq 2$, where ϵ_{ir} is independent of $\{X_i, T_i, C_i\}$ and $\epsilon_{ir} \sim (0, \Sigma_\epsilon)$. Using the method of moments, we estimate Σ_ϵ by

$$\widehat{\Sigma}_\epsilon = \frac{\sum_{i=1}^{n} \sum_{r=1}^{n_i} \left(X_{ir}^* - \bar{X}_{i\cdot}^*\right)\left(X_{ir}^* - \bar{X}_{i\cdot}^*\right)^\top}{\sum_{i=1}^{n} (n_i - 1)}, \tag{8}$$

where $\bar{X}^*_{i\cdot} = \frac{1}{n_i} \sum_{r=1}^{n_i} X^*_{ir}$.

Scenario III: Both functional form of $f_\epsilon(\cdot)$ and its associated parameters are unknown, but external validation data are available.

Suppose that $\mathcal{M}$ is the subject set for the main study containing measurements $\{(T_i, C_i, \delta_i, X^*_i) : i \in \mathcal{M}\}$ for n subjects and that $\mathcal{V}$ is the subject set for the external validation study containing measurements $\{(X_i, X^*_i) : i \in \mathcal{V}\}$ for m subjects, where $\mathcal{M}$ and $\mathcal{V}$ do not overlap. Assume that the main study and the validation study share the same measurement error model (7); this is the so-called *transportability* assumption (e.g., Yi et al. 2015).

With the availability of external validation data, $f_{\epsilon_{(j)}}(\cdot)$ for $j = 1, \cdots, p$ and Σ_ϵ can be estimated. For $i \in \mathcal{V}$ and $j = 1, \cdots, p$, the jth component of ϵ_i is given by $\epsilon_{i(j)} = X^*_{i(j)} - X_{i(j)}$, which is known. Then adopting the estimator (6) with $X_{i(j)}$ replaced by $\epsilon_{i(j)}$ and n replaced by m gives an estimate of the probability density function $f_{\epsilon_{i(j)}}(\cdot)$ of $\epsilon_{i(j)}$:

$$\widehat{f}_{\epsilon_{(j)}}(u) = \frac{1}{mh} \sum_{i \in \mathcal{V}} K\left(\frac{u - \epsilon_{i(j)}}{h}\right).$$

Thus, the corresponding characteristic function $\phi_{\epsilon_{(j)}}(u)$ is estimated by $\widehat{\phi}_{\epsilon_{(j)}}(u) = \int_{-\infty}^{\infty} \exp(iux) \widehat{f}_{\epsilon_{(j)}}(x) dx$. In addition, applying the least squares regression method gives the estimator of Σ_ϵ:

$$\widehat{\Sigma}_\epsilon = \frac{1}{m-1} \sum_{i \in \mathcal{V}} (X^*_i - X_i)(X^*_i - X_i)^\top. \tag{9}$$

3.2 Feature Screening with Measurement Error Effects Accommodated

In the presence of measurement error in covariates, the method in Sect. 2.3 cannot apply because the estimator (5) cannot be directly calculated due to the unavailability of the X_i. In this subsection, we derive an estimator (5) using the observed surrogate X^*_i. First, we re-express the probability density function $f_{X_{(j)}}(x)$ by the *inverse Fourier* transformation, given by

$$f_{X_{(j)}}(x) = \frac{1}{2\pi} \int_{-\infty}^{\infty} \exp(-iux) \phi_{X_{(j)}}(u) du, \tag{10}$$

where $\phi_{X_{(j)}}(u)$ is the characteristic function of $X_{(j)}$.

For $j = 1, \cdots, p$, let $\phi_{X^*_{(j)}}(u)$ and $\phi_{\epsilon_{(j)}}(u)$ denote the characteristic functions of $X^*_{(j)}$ and $\epsilon_{(j)}$, respectively, where $X^*_{(j)}$ and $\epsilon_{(j)}$ are the jth component of X^* and ϵ, respectively; and X^* and ϵ follow the same distribution as X^*_i and ϵ_i, respectively. Then model (7) yields that

$$\phi_{X^*_{(j)}}(u) = \phi_{X_{(j)}}(u)\phi_{\epsilon_{(j)}}(u),$$

and thus, $\phi_{X_{(j)}}(u) = \dfrac{\phi_{X^*_{(j)}}(u)}{\phi_{\epsilon_{(j)}}(u)}$, assuming $\phi_{\epsilon_{(j)}}(u) \neq 0$. Then (10) becomes

$$f_{X_{(j)}}(x) = \frac{1}{2\pi} \int_{-\infty}^{\infty} \exp(-\mathbf{i}ux) \frac{\phi_{X^*_{(j)}}(u)}{\phi_{\epsilon_{(j)}}(u)} du. \tag{11}$$

To emphasize that (11) is expressed in terms of the surrogate $X^*_{(j)}$, we let $f_{adj,j}(x)$ to replace $f_{X_{(j)}}(x)$ in the left-hand side of (11).

Next, to implement (11), we need to calculate $\phi_{X^*_{(j)}}(u)$ and $\phi_{\epsilon_{(j)}}(u)$, where $\phi_{\epsilon_{(j)}}(u)$ is derived from the distribution $f_{\epsilon_{(j)}}(\cdot)$ of $\epsilon_{(j)}$, the jth marginal distribution derived from $f_\epsilon(\cdot)$.

It now remains to calculate $\phi_{X^*_{(j)}}(u)$, which is given by

$$\phi_{X^*_{(j)}}(u) = \int_{-\infty}^{\infty} \exp(\mathbf{i}ux)\, f_{X^*_{(j)}}(x)dx, \tag{12}$$

where $f_{X^*_{(j)}}(x)$ denotes the probability density function of $X^*_{(j)}$. Since $X^*_{(j)}$ is observable, then the probability density function of $X^*_{(j)}$ can be estimated by the kernel estimation, given by

$$\widehat{f}_{X^*_{(j)}}(x) = \frac{1}{nh} \sum_{i=1}^{n} K\left(\frac{x - X^*_{i(j)}}{h}\right), \tag{13}$$

where h and $K(\cdot)$ are described for (6). In our numerical examination, we specify $K(u)$ to be the normal kernel and h can be estimated by the cross-validation method (e.g., Wand & Jones 1995).

Consequently, with $f_{X^*_{(j)}}(x)$ in (12) replaced by $\widehat{f}_{X^*_{(j)}}(x)$, $\phi_{X^*}(u)$ can be estimated by

$$\widehat{\phi}_{X^*_{(j)}}(u) = \int_{-\infty}^{\infty} \exp(\mathbf{i}ux)\, \widehat{f}_{X^*_{(j)}}(x)dx$$

$$= \int_{-\infty}^{\infty} \exp(\mathbf{i}ux) \frac{1}{nh} \sum_{i=1}^{n} K\left(\frac{x - X^*_{i(j)}}{h}\right) dx.$$

Let $z = \frac{x - X^*_{i(j)}}{h}$; then applying the change of variables yields

$$\widehat{\phi}_{X^*_{(j)}}(u) = \int_{-\infty}^{\infty} \frac{1}{n} \sum_{i=1}^{n} \exp\left(iu X^*_{(j)} + iuhz\right) K(z) \, dz$$

$$= \left\{\int_{-\infty}^{\infty} \exp(iuhz) K(z) dz\right\} \times \left\{\frac{1}{n} \sum_{i=1}^{n} \exp\left(iu X^*_{i(j)}\right)\right\}. \qquad (14)$$

Combining (11) and (14) gives an estimator of (11):

$$\widehat{f}_{adj,j}(x) = \frac{1}{2\pi} \int_{-\infty}^{\infty} \exp(-iux) \frac{\widehat{\phi}_{X^*_{(j)}}(u)}{\phi_{\epsilon_{(j)}}(u)} du, \qquad (15)$$

and thus, an adjusted estimator of the cumulative distribution function $F_{X_{(j)}}(x)$ in terms of $X^*_{(j)}$ is

$$\widehat{F}_{adj,j}(x) = \int_{-\infty}^{x} \widehat{f}_{adj,j}(u) du. \qquad (16)$$

Therefore, the functional distance correlation (3) can be estimated using the observed surrogate $X^*_{(j)}$ together with the outcome Y, given by

$$\widehat{\omega}_j \triangleq \widehat{dcorr}\{\widehat{F}_{adj,j}(X^*_{(j)}), \widehat{F}(Y)\}$$

$$= \frac{\widehat{dcov}\{\widehat{F}_{adj,j}(X^*_{(j)}), \widehat{F}(Y)\}}{\sqrt{\widehat{dcov}\{\widehat{F}_{adj,j}(X^*_{(j)}), \widehat{F}_{adj,j}(X^*_{(j)})\}\widehat{dcov}^*\{\widehat{F}(Y), \widehat{F}(Y)\}}}, \qquad (17)$$

where $\widehat{dcov}\{\widehat{F}_{adj,j}(X^*_{(j)}), \widehat{F}(Y)\}$ is determined by (4) with $\widehat{F}_{X_{(j)}}(x)$ replaced by (16).

Remark The development here extends the discussion of Chen (2019) who assumed that $f_\epsilon(\cdot)$ is the probability density function of a normal distribution under Scenarios I, II, and III. With the jth noise term $\epsilon_{(j)}$ assuming a normal distribution with mean zero and variance $\sigma^2_{\epsilon_{(j)}}$, we have that the characteristic function is given by $\phi_{\epsilon_{(j)}}(u) = \exp\left(-\frac{1}{2}u^2 \sigma^2_{\epsilon_{(j)}}\right)$, and thus, (15) becomes

$$\widehat{f}_{adj,j}(x) = \frac{1}{2\pi} \int_{-\infty}^{\infty} \exp\left(-iux + \frac{1}{2}u\sigma^2_{\epsilon_{(j)}}\right) \widehat{\phi}_{X^*_{(j)}}(u) du.$$

In contrast, if $\epsilon_{(j)}$ follows a t distribution with degrees of freedom $v > 1$, then the corresponding characteristic function is given by Dreiera & Kotzb (2002):

$$\phi_{\epsilon_{(j)}}(u) = \frac{2^v v^{v/2}}{\Gamma(v)} \int_0^\infty \exp\left\{-v^{1/2}(2x + |u|)\right\} \times \{x(x + |u|)\}^{(v-1)/2} \, dx, \quad (18)$$

and substituting (18) into (15) yields $\widehat{f}_{adj,j}(x)$.

3.3 Asymptotic Results

To establish theoretical results of the proposed method, we impose the following additional conditions:

(C3) There exists a positive constant w_0 such that for all $0 < w \leq 2w_0$,

$$\sup_p \max_{1 \leq j \leq p} E\left\{\exp\left(w\|X_{(j)}\|_1^2\right)\right\} < \infty \quad \text{and} \quad E\left\{\exp\left(w\|Y\|_q^2\right)\right\} < \infty.$$

(C4) The minimum of the functional distance correlations for the active covariates satisfies

$$\min_{j \in I} |\omega_j| \geq 2cn^{-\zeta}$$

for some constants $c > 0$ and $0 \leq \zeta < 1/2$.

(C5) There exists a positive constant v_0 such that $\lim_{p \to \infty} \left(\min_{j \in I} |\omega_j| - \max_{j \in I^c} |\omega_j|\right) > v_0$, assuming the limits exists.

(C6) The covariates X_i^* for $i = 1, \cdots, n$ are bounded.

Condition (C3) is used to examine the boundedness of the difference $|\widehat{\omega}_j - \omega_j|$ between (3) and its estimator (17). Condition (C4) says that the marginal DC of active covariates cannot be too small, which is similar to Condition 3 of Fan & Lv (2008). Condition (C5) basically requires the signal carried by the active covariates to be stronger than that displayed by inactive covariates for at least a fixed amount if the dimension p goes to infinty. This condition was also imposed by other authors (e.g., Cui et al. 2015). Condition (C6) indicates the finite boundedness of surrogate measurements of the covariates.

Theorem 1 *Under regularity conditions (C3) and (C5) and the assumptions of Lemmas 1 and 2 in Appendix A, we have that for c and ζ described in Condition (C4), there exists a constant $D > 0$ such that*

$$P\left(\max_{j=1,\cdots,p} |\widehat{\omega}_j - \omega_j| \geq cn^{-\zeta}\right) = O\left\{p\exp\left(-Dn^{1-2\zeta}\right)\right\}. \quad (19)$$

Moreover,

$$P\left(\max_{j\in\mathcal{I}^c}|\widehat{\omega}_j| \geq \min_{j\in\mathcal{I}}|\widehat{\omega}_j|\right) = O\left\{\exp\left(-\frac{1}{4}Dnv_0^2\right)\right\}, \tag{20}$$

where v_0 is the constant described in Condition (C5).

Equation (19) in Theorem 1 indicates ω_j is close to its estimate with a large probability. Similar to the discussion in Li et al. (2012) and Chen et al. (2018), (19) shows that the proposed method is able to handle the non-polynomial (NP) dimensionality of order $\log p = o(n^{1-2\zeta})$ for some constant $0 \leq \zeta < 1/2$. Equation (20) in Theorem 1 ensures that the proposed estimator (17) has the ranking consistency property, similar to that discussed by Cui et al. (2015) and Hao et al. (2019).

Theorem 2 *Suppose that Conditions (C3)–(C4) and the assumptions of Lemmas 1 and 2 in Appendix A hold. Let*

$$\widehat{\mathcal{I}} = \left\{j : |\widehat{\omega}_j| \geq cn^{-\zeta} \text{ for } j = 1, \cdots, p\right\} \tag{21}$$

for c and ζ described in Condition (C4). Then for a sufficiently large n, $\widehat{\mathcal{I}}$ has the sure screening property:

$$P\left(\mathcal{I} \subseteq \widehat{\mathcal{I}}\right) \geq 1 - O\left\{q\exp\left(-Dn^{1-2\zeta}\right)\right\},$$

where D and ζ are the constants described in Theorem 1.

The sure screening property in Theorem 2 shows that with a large probability, the true active set is included in the estimated active set. This property is important which is commonly required for any sensible screening procedure (e.g., Fan & Lv 2008; Li et al. 2012; Chen et al. 2018).

While (21) allows us to establish the sure screening property of the procedure, it does not tell us exactly about the choice of a suitable threshold value because c and ζ are unknown. In the actual implementation, we often rank the covariates by the values of the $\widehat{\omega}_j$ for $j = 1, \cdots, p$ and then retain, say, $\widetilde{q}$ covariates with the first $\widetilde{q}$ largest $\widehat{\omega}_j$. A common choice of $\widetilde{q}$ is $\widetilde{q} = \left\lfloor \frac{n}{\log n} \right\rfloor$, where $\lfloor \cdot \rfloor$ stands for the floor function (e.g., Li et al. 2012; Cui et al. 2015; Yan et al. 2017; Chen et al. 2018; Chen 2019).

4 Iteration Algorithm

While Theorem 2 shows that using (21) to do screening has a large probability for retaining active covariates when n is sufficiently large and regularity conditions are satisfied, it does not ensure a good performance in some settings. Typically, when some covariates possess strong correlations, unimportant covariates may be likely to be retained due to their correlations with the important covariates. On the other hand, some covariates may only have a weak marginal association with the response variable, but they have a strong joint effect on the change of the response. This phenomenon was discussed in Sect. 4.2.2 of Fan & Lv (2008). As a remedy, we now add extra steps to modify the procedure that uses (17) to do screening.

The key idea is to construct the residuals in terms of the retained variables in $\widehat{\mathcal{I}}$ and then use those residuals to identify highly dependent variables in the inactive set $\widehat{\mathcal{I}}^c$. Similar to Chen (2019), we take the "residual" as the projection of the distribution for variables in the inactive set $\widehat{\mathcal{I}}$ onto the orthogonal space of the distribution of variables selected in the active set $\widehat{\mathcal{I}}$. To present the idea explicitly, we perform the following iteration algorithm:

Step 1:   *Initial determination of the active set.*
First, we use (17) to select q_1 variables, where q_1 is a positive integer specified to be smaller than $\widetilde{q}$. Let $\widehat{\mathcal{I}}_1$ denote the estimated active set containing the selected q_1 variables. Now decompose the measurement error model (7) as

$$X^*_{i,\widehat{\mathcal{I}}_1} = X_{i,\widehat{\mathcal{I}}_1} + \epsilon_{i,\widehat{\mathcal{I}}_1} \tag{22a}$$

$$X^*_{i,\widehat{\mathcal{I}}_1^c} = X_{i,\widehat{\mathcal{I}}_1^c} + \epsilon_{i,\widehat{\mathcal{I}}_1^c}, \tag{22b}$$

where $X^*_i = \left(X^{*\top}_{i,\widehat{\mathcal{I}}_1}, X^{*\top}_{i,\widehat{\mathcal{I}}_1^c} \right)^\top$, $X_i = \left(X^\top_{i,\widehat{\mathcal{I}}_1}, X^\top_{i,\widehat{\mathcal{I}}_1^c} \right)^\top$, and $\epsilon_i = \left(\epsilon^\top_{i,\widehat{\mathcal{I}}_1}, \epsilon^\top_{i,\widehat{\mathcal{I}}_1^c} \right)^\top$. The covariance matrix Σ_ϵ is also decomposed accordingly:

$$\Sigma_\epsilon = \begin{pmatrix} \Sigma_{\epsilon_{\widehat{\mathcal{I}}_1}} & \Sigma_{\epsilon_{\widehat{\mathcal{I}}_1 \widehat{\mathcal{I}}_1^c}} \\ \Sigma^\top_{\epsilon_{\widehat{\mathcal{I}}_1 \widehat{\mathcal{I}}_1^c}} & \Sigma_{\epsilon_{\widehat{\mathcal{I}}_1^c}} \end{pmatrix},$$

where $\Sigma_{\epsilon_{\widehat{\mathcal{I}}_1}}$ is the $q_1 \times q_1$ covariance matrix based on (22a), $\Sigma_{\epsilon_{\widehat{\mathcal{I}}_1^c}}$ is the $(p - q_1) \times (p - q_1)$ covariance matrix based on (22b), and $\Sigma_{\epsilon_{\widehat{\mathcal{I}}_1 \widehat{\mathcal{I}}_1^c}}$ is the $q_1 \times (p - q_1)$ covariance matrix based on the interaction of (22a) and (22b).

Step 2:   *Improvement.*
Corresponding to (22a) and (22b), we define $\mathcal{F}_{\widehat{\mathcal{I}}_1}$ as the $n \times q_1$ matrix with the entry (i, j) being $\widehat{F}_{adj,j}(X^*_{i(j)})$ for $j \in \widehat{\mathcal{I}}_1$ and $i = 1, \cdots, n$, where $\widehat{F}_{adj,j}(x)$ is the proposed estimated function in (16) and $X^*_{i(j)}$ the jth component of X^*_i. Similarly, let $\mathcal{F}_{\widehat{\mathcal{I}}_1^c}$ be the $n \times (p - q_1)$ matrix with the entry (i, j) being $\widehat{F}_{adj,j}(X^*_{i(j)})$ for $j \in \widehat{\mathcal{I}}_1^c$ and $i = 1, \cdots, n$. $\mathcal{F}_{\widehat{\mathcal{I}}_1}$ and $\mathcal{F}_{\widehat{\mathcal{I}}_1^c}$ essentially reflect informative and noninformative variables in $\widehat{\mathcal{I}}_1$ and $\widehat{\mathcal{I}}_1^c$, respectively.

Next, define the predictor residual matrix

$$\mathcal{F}_{\text{new}} = \left\{ I_n - \mathcal{F}_{\widehat{\mathcal{I}}_1} \left(\mathcal{F}_{\widehat{\mathcal{I}}_1}^\top \mathcal{F}_{\widehat{\mathcal{I}}_1} \right)^{-1} \mathcal{F}_{\widehat{\mathcal{I}}_1}^\top \right\} \mathcal{F}_{\widehat{\mathcal{I}}_1^c}, \qquad (23)$$

where I_n represents the $n \times n$ identity matrix, and the inverse matrix $\left(\mathcal{F}_{\widehat{\mathcal{I}}_1}^\top \mathcal{F}_{\widehat{\mathcal{I}}_1} \right)$ is assumed to exist. Noting that $\mathcal{F}_{\text{new}}$ can be regarded as the residual of linearly regressing $\mathcal{F}_{\widehat{\mathcal{I}}_1^c}$ on $\mathcal{F}_{\widehat{\mathcal{I}}_1}$, suggesting that $\mathcal{F}_{\text{new}}$ contains the covariate information in $\widehat{\mathcal{I}}_1^c$ and is uncorrelated with $\mathcal{F}_{\widehat{\mathcal{I}}_1}$. Therefore, implementing (17) with $\widehat{F}_{adj,j}(X_{(j)})$ replaced by $\mathcal{F}_{\text{new}}$ enables us to further select variables from $\widehat{\mathcal{I}}_1^c$. Suppose that we select q_2 such variables, and let $\widehat{\mathcal{I}}_2$ denote the resulting active set containing q_2 variables.

Step 3:   *Update of the active set.*
    Repeat Step 2 for $(N-1)$ times such that $\widetilde{q} = q_1 + q_2 + \cdots + q_N$. Then the resulting estimated active set is given by $\widehat{\mathcal{I}} = \bigcup_{k=1}^{N} \widehat{\mathcal{I}}_k$, where N is a positive integer.

Here we make several comments. In the absence of measurement error, Zhong & Zhu (2015) considered to regress variables in the inactive set onto the variables in the active set to eliminate the potential correlation among the variables and then detect variables that are falsely excluded by the initial feature screening method. When measurement error occurs in covariates, Chen (2019) took the similar strategies of Zhong & Zhu (2015) and employed the conditional expectation method to eliminate measurement error effects. Unlike Zhong & Zhu (2015) and Chen (2019) who directly used the variables to produce "residuals," our strategy (23) implements the estimated cumulative distribution functions, and we expect that this treatment is more likely to yield more robust results than the procedures considered by Zhong & Zhu (2015) and Chen (2019). In addition, different from Chen (2019) that needs an additional step to correct for measurement error effects, (23) directly builds in the error effects correction in the implementation procedure.

In applications, the choices N and $\{q_1, \cdots, q_N\}$ are not unique but user-specified (e.g., Zhong & Zhu 2015; Hao et al. 2019). In our numerical studies, we take $N = 2$ and set $q_1 = \left\lfloor \frac{3}{4}\widetilde{q} \right\rfloor$.

5   Numerical Studies

5.1   *Simulation Setup*

Let $X = \left(X_{(1)}, \cdots, X_{(p)} \right)^\top$ be generated from the normal distribution with mean zero and the covariance matrix Σ_X with the diagonal elements one, where $p = 2000$.

We examine two parts in this section. In Part 1, the entry (k, l) in Σ_X is set to be $\rho^{1+|k-l|}$ with $\rho = 0.5$ or 0.8 for $k, l = 1, \cdots, p$ and $k \neq l$, and the failure time T is generated from one of the following two models:

M1: $\lambda(t|X) = (\log t) \exp\left(X^\top \beta\right)$ with $\beta = (1_4^\top, 0_{p-4}^\top)^\top$.

M2: $T = \exp\left(X^\top \beta - 1\right) \sin^2\left(X^\top \beta\right) + \varpi$ with $\beta = (1_4^\top, 0_{p-4}^\top)^\top$, and the noise term ϖ follows a lognormal distribution with mean zero and variance one, where 1_d is the d-dimensional unit vector, and 0_d represents the d-dimensional zero vector.

Model M1 is the Cox proportional hazards model with the baseline hazards function $\log t$, and Model M2 is the nonlinear transformation model considered by Hao et al. (2019).

In Part 2, we consider the case similar to that considered in an example in Sect. 4.2.2 of Fan & Lv (2008): for $k \neq l$, the (k, l) element of Σ_X is set as ρ if $k \neq 4, l \neq 4$, and $\sqrt{\rho}$ otherwise, where we consider $\rho = 0.5$ or 0.8. Given the covariates, the failure time is generated from one of the following models:

M3:

$$T = \exp\left(X_{(1)} + X_{(2)} + X_{(3)} - 3\sqrt{\rho}X_{(4)} + \varpi\right), \tag{24}$$

where ϖ follows the standard extreme value distribution.

M4: T is given by (24), where ϖ follows the standard logistic distribution.

Models M3 and M4 are modified from linear models in Sect. 4.2.2 of Fan & Lv (2008), which were also considered by Chen et al. (2018), Hao et al. (2019), and Zhang et al. (2020).

For Parts 1 and 2, the censoring time C is generated from the uniform distribution $U(0, \tau_C)$, where τ_C is a constant such that the censoring rate is approximately 50%. As a result, we have $Y = \min\{T, C\}$ and $\delta = \mathbb{I}(T \leq C)$. We repeat data generation for $i = 1, \cdots, n$ independently and obtain the data $\left\{(Y_i, \delta_i, X_i) : i = 1, \cdots, n\right\}$, where we consider the sample size $n = 400$.

Finally, to generate the observed surrogate X_i^* for $i = 1, \cdots, n$, we take the measurement error model (7) for two scenarios of ϵ_i, where the components of ϵ_i are independent. In the first scenario, ϵ_i follows the normal distribution with mean zero and the diagonal matrix Σ_ϵ with all diagonal elements being σ_ϵ, where $\sigma_\epsilon = 1.5$, 2, or 3. In the second scenario, $\epsilon_{i(j)}$ follows the t distribution with the degrees of freedom v, where $j = 1, \cdots, p$, and v is specified as 6, 4, or 3, yielding the variance $\frac{v}{v-2} = 1.5, 2$, or 3, respectively. Finally, we repeat simulation 1000 times in each setting.

5.2   Simulation Results

From Models M1–M4, the $X_{(j)}$ with $j = 1, 2, 3, 4$ are informative variables, so the main goal is to retain them in implementing the screening procedure. For the data generated in Part 1, we use the robust feature screening method in Sect. 3.2; and for the data in Part 2, we implement the iteration procedure in Sect. 4. To assess the impact of the measurement error effects on feature screening, we examine the naive method using (17) with $\widehat{F}_{adj,j}(X^{*}_{(j)})$ replaced by the empirical cumulative distribution function of $X^{*}_{(j)}$. In addition, we compare the methods to the corrected DC method proposed by Chen (2019).

To evaluate the finite-sample performance of the proposed method, we report the proportion, denoted $\mathcal{P}_s$, for *each active covariate to be retained* in 1000 simulations and the proportion, denoted $\mathcal{P}_a$, for *all active covariates to be retained* in 1000 simulations. Here we present the results only for the case with known Σ_ϵ and omit the study for the cases with unknown Σ_ϵ as discussed in Sect. 3.1 due to the similarity in results. Numerical results for Part 1 are summarized in Table 1, and results for Part 2 are given in Table 2, where "Naive" represents the naive method, "DC" is the corrected DC method (Chen 2019), and "Proposed" is the proposed method.

We see that without suitable correction of measurement error effects, the naive method fails to retain all important variables, while the DC and proposed methods are able to keep those four variables with a high possibility. Comparing two error effect-corrected methods, we observe that when the noise term ϵ_i follows the normal distribution, both the DC and proposed methods keep truly important variables with a proportion near one. However, when the distribution of ϵ_i is non-normal, the proportion of retaining truly informative variables based on the DC method becomes less satisfactory. On the contrary, the proposed method still keeps all important variables with a proportion close to one. Moreover, regarding the trajectory of the model, the proposed method outperforms the DC method in Model M2 whose relationship between the response and the covariates is relatively oscillatory.

In summary, the simulation results confirm that the proposed method is successful in accounting for measurement error effects regardless of the distribution of the noise term and is robust in retaining important variables.

5.3   Analysis of Mantle Cell Lymphoma Microarray Data

In this subsection, we apply the proposed method to study the mantle cell lymphoma microarray dataset analyzed by Rosenwald et al. (2003). The dataset contains survival times of 92 patients together with gene expression measurements of 8810 genes for each patient. As 6330 gene expressions contain missing values, we remove them and consider the subset of the remaining 2480 gene expressions. During the study period, 64 patients died of mantle cell lymphoma, and the remaining 28

Table 1 Simulation results of feature screening for Part 1

Model	ρ	σ_ϵ	Method	$\epsilon_i \sim$ Normal $\mathcal{P}_s$ $X_{(1)}$	$X_{(2)}$	$X_{(3)}$	$X_{(4)}$	$\mathcal{P}_a$	$\epsilon_i \sim t(v)$ $\mathcal{P}_s$ $X_{(1)}$	$X_{(2)}$	$X_{(3)}$	$X_{(4)}$	$\mathcal{P}_a$
M1	0.5	1.5	Naive	0.001	0.002	0.002	0.001	0.001	0.000	0.000	0.000	0.000	0.000
			DC	1.000	0.998	1.000	1.000	0.998	0.833	0.876	0.855	0.853	0.840
			Proposed	1.000	0.999	1.000	1.000	0.999	0.998	0.996	0.997	0.997	0.996
		2	Naive	0.000	0.002	0.000	0.001	0.000	0.000	0.000	0.000	0.000	0.000
			DC	1.000	0.997	0.998	1.000	0.997	0.830	0.869	0.853	0.852	0.837
			Proposed	1.000	0.999	1.000	1.000	0.999	0.998	0.996	0.997	0.997	0.996
		3	Naive	0.000	0.000	0.000	0.001	0.000	0.000	0.000	0.000	0.000	0.000
			DC	1.000	0.997	0.997	0.998	0.997	0.827	0.858	0.844	0.846	0.830
			Proposed	1.000	0.998	1.000	1.000	0.998	0.997	0.996	0.996	0.996	0.996
	0.8	1.5	Naive	0.000	0.000	0.000	0.001	0.001	0.000	0.000	0.000	0.000	0.000
			DC	1.000	0.998	0.998	1.000	0.998	0.845	0.867	0.860	0.855	0.846
			Proposed	1.000	0.999	1.000	1.000	0.999	1.000	0.998	0.998	0.997	0.997
		2	Naive	0.000	0.000	0.000	0.000	0.000	0.000	0.000	0.000	0.000	0.000
			DC	0.998	0.997	0.997	1.000	0.997	0.838	0.864	0.856	0.847	0.839
			Proposed	1.000	0.999	1.000	1.000	0.999	0.998	0.996	0.997	0.997	0.996
		3	Naive	0.000	0.000	0.000	0.001	0.000	0.000	0.000	0.000	0.000	0.000
			DC	0.998	0.997	0.997	0.996	0.996	0.833	0.845	0.836	0.841	0.835
			Proposed	1.000	0.998	0.998	1.000	0.998	0.998	0.997	0.996	0.997	0.996
M2	0.5	1.5	Naive	0.001	0.000	0.000	0.000	0.000	0.000	0.000	0.000	0.000	0.000
			DC	0.951	0.958	0.963	0.969	0.951	0.836	0.846	0.847	0.847	0.836
			Proposed	1.000	0.998	0.998	1.000	0.998	0.998	0.997	0.998	0.997	0.997
		2	Naive	0.000	0.000	0.000	0.000	0.000	0.000	0.000	0.000	0.000	0.000
			DC	0.950	0.955	0.962	0.963	0.950	0.834	0.844	0.845	0.844	0.834
			Proposed	1.000	0.997	0.997	0.998	0.997	0.996	0.996	0.995	0.996	0.995
		3	Naive	0.000	0.000	0.000	0.000	0.000	0.000	0.000	0.000	0.000	0.000
			DC	0.946	0.951	0.957	0.957	0.944	0.830	0.839	0.841	0.838	0.830
			Proposed	1.000	0.997	0.997	0.998	0.998	0.996	0.995	0.995	0.995	0.995
	0.8	1.5	Naive	0.000	0.000	0.000	0.000	0.000	0.000	0.000	0.000	0.000	0.000
			DC	0.953	0.956	0.960	0.966	0.953	0.831	0.844	0.844	0.843	0.831
			Proposed	1.000	0.999	0.998	0.999	0.998	0.998	0.998	0.998	0.997	0.997
		2	Naive	0.000	0.000	0.000	0.000	0.000	0.000	0.000	0.000	0.000	0.000
			DC	0.949	0.951	0.954	0.957	0.951	0.830	0.840	0.841	0.841	0.831
			Proposed	1.000	0.997	0.998	0.998	0.997	0.996	0.997	0.997	0.996	0.996
		3	Naive	0.000	0.000	0.000	0.000	0.000	0.000	0.000	0.000	0.000	0.000
			DC	0.945	0.947	0.950	0.953	0.943	0.826	0.831	0.833	0.833	0.831
			Proposed	1.000	0.996	0.997	0.997	0.996	0.996	0.996	0.997	0.996	0.996

$t(v)$: The t distribution with the degrees of freedom v

Table 2 Simulation results of feature screening for Part 2

Model	ρ	σ_ϵ	Method	$\epsilon_i \sim$ Normal					$\epsilon_i \sim t(v)$				
				$\mathcal{P}_s$					$\mathcal{P}_s$				
				$X_{(1)}$	$X_{(2)}$	$X_{(3)}$	$X_{(4)}$	$\mathcal{P}_a$	$X_{(1)}$	$X_{(2)}$	$X_{(3)}$	$X_{(4)}$	$\mathcal{P}_a$
M3	0.5	1.5	Naive	0.000	0.000	0.000	0.000	0.000	0.000	0.000	0.000	0.000	0.000
			DC	1.000	1.000	1.000	1.000	1.000	0.874	0.878	0.870	0.872	0.870
			Proposed	1.000	1.000	1.000	1.000	1.000	1.000	0.998	0.998	1.000	0.997
		2	Naive	0.000	0.000	0.000	0.000	0.000	0.000	0.000	0.000	0.000	0.000
			DC	1.000	1.000	1.000	1.000	1.000	0.869	0.874	0.866	0.867	0.865
			Proposed	1.000	1.000	1.000	1.000	1.000	0.997	0.997	0.998	1.000	0.997
		3	Naive	0.000	0.000	0.000	0.000	0.000	0.000	0.000	0.000	0.000	0.000
			DC	1.000	1.000	1.000	1.000	1.000	0.866	0.870	0.863	0.863	0.863
			Proposed	1.000	1.000	1.000	1.000	1.000	0.996	0.997	0.997	1.000	0.996
	0.8	1.5	Naive	0.000	0.000	0.000	0.000	0.000	0.000	0.000	0.000	0.000	0.000
			DC	1.000	1.000	1.000	1.000	1.000	0.870	0.875	0.870	0.870	0.870
			Proposed	1.000	1.000	1.000	1.000	1.000	1.000	0.998	0.998	0.998	0.997
		2	Naive	0.000	0.000	0.000	0.000	0.000	0.000	0.000	0.000	0.000	0.000
			DC	1.000	1.000	1.000	1.000	1.000	0.866	0.870	0.865	0.865	0.865
			Proposed	1.000	1.000	1.000	1.000	1.000	0.997	0.997	0.998	0.998	0.996
		3	Naive	0.000	0.000	0.000	0.000	0.000	0.000	0.000	0.000	0.000	0.000
			DC	1.000	1.000	1.000	1.000	1.000	0.860	0.861	0.860	0.860	0.860
			Proposed	1.000	1.000	1.000	1.000	1.000	0.996	0.997	0.996	0.997	0.996
M4	0.5	1.5	Naive	0.000	0.000	0.000	0.000	0.000	0.000	0.000	0.000	0.000	0.000
			DC	1.000	1.000	1.000	1.000	1.000	0.879	0.881	0.878	0.878	0.878
			Proposed	1.000	1.000	1.000	1.000	1.000	1.000	0.999	0.998	1.000	0.998
		2	Naive	0.000	0.000	0.000	0.000	0.000	0.000	0.000	0.000	0.000	0.000
			DC	1.000	1.000	1.000	1.000	1.000	0.879	0.877	0.876	0.878	0.876
			Proposed	1.000	1.000	1.000	1.000	1.000	0.999	0.998	0.998	1.000	0.998
		3	Naive	0.000	0.000	0.000	0.000	0.000	0.000	0.000	0.000	0.000	0.000
			DC	1.000	1.000	1.000	1.000	1.000	0.876	0.877	0.876	0.875	0.875
			Proposed	1.000	1.000	1.000	1.000	1.000	0.997	0.997	0.998	0.999	0.997
	0.8	1.5	Naive	0.000	0.000	0.000	0.000	0.000	0.000	0.000	0.000	0.000	0.000
			DC	1.000	1.000	1.000	1.000	1.000	0.875	0.876	0.875	0.875	0.875
			Proposed	1.000	1.000	1.000	1.000	1.000	1.000	0.999	0.998	0.998	0.998
		2	Naive	0.000	0.000	0.000	0.000	0.000	0.000	0.000	0.000	0.000	0.000
			DC	1.000	1.000	1.000	1.000	1.000	0.870	0.872	0.871	0.871	0.870
			Proposed	1.000	1.000	1.000	1.000	1.000	0.998	0.997	0.997	0.996	0.996
		3	Naive	0.000	0.000	0.000	0.000	0.000	0.000	0.000	0.000	0.000	0.000
			DC	1.000	1.000	1.000	1.000	1.000	0.868	0.867	0.867	0.869	0.866
			Proposed	1.000	1.000	1.000	1.000	1.000	0.996	0.995	0.997	0.995	0.995

$t(v)$: The t distribution with the degrees of freedom v

patients were censored, yielding the censoring rate 30%. As commented by Chen & Yi (2021a), gene expressions are usually measured with error, and it is imperative to account for this feature in data analysis.

Since the dataset has no additional information to characterize the degree of measurement error, to implement the proposed method, we conduct sensitivity analyses to address the measurement error effects, a commonly used strategy for exploring the impacts of different magnitudes of measurement error (e.g., Chen & Yi 2020, 2021a,b). Let Σ_X and Σ_{X^*} denote the covariance matrices of X_i and X_i^*, respectively, and let σ_{Xlk}, σ_{X^*lk}, and $\sigma_{\epsilon lk}$ denote the entry (l, k) of Σ_X, Σ_{X^*}, and Σ_ϵ, respectively. Measurement error model (7) suggests that σ_{Xlk} is smaller than σ_{X^*lk} for all l and k. To consider possible representative scenarios, we use the sample covariance $\widehat{\Sigma}_{X^*}$ to estimate Σ_{X^*} and take σ_{Xlk} as $\sigma_{Xlk} = 0.9\widehat{\sigma}_{X^*lk}$, where $\widehat{\sigma}_{X^*lk}$ is the entry (l, k) of $\widehat{\Sigma}_{X^*}$. To specify $\sigma_{\epsilon lk}$, we use the reliability ratio $R_{lk} = \frac{\sigma_{Xlk}}{\sigma_{X^*lk}} = \frac{\sigma_{Xlk}}{\sigma_{Xlk}+\sigma_{\epsilon lk}}$ to guide us:

$$\sigma_{\epsilon lk} = (R_{lk}^{-1} - 1)\widehat{\sigma}_{X^*lk}. \tag{25}$$

For ease of exposition, we take R_{lk} as a common constant for all l and k and let R denote it. Then (25) gives $\Sigma_\epsilon = (R^{-1} - 1)\widehat{\Sigma}_{X^*}$. When Σ_ϵ is given, the distribution of the noise term $\epsilon_{(j)}$ for $j = 1, \cdots, 2480$ is specified as a normal or a t distribution with degrees of freedom specified as $\left\lfloor \frac{2\sigma_{\epsilon jj}}{\sigma_{\epsilon jj}-1} \right\rfloor$.

Set $\widetilde{q} = \left\lfloor \frac{92}{\log 92} \right\rfloor = 20$, indicating that we aim to retain 20 variables with the first 20 largest $\widehat{\omega}_j$. For the feature screening method in Sect. 3.2, we directly choose $\widetilde{q}$ gene expressions; for the iteration method in Sect. 4, we take $N = 2$, where we retain the first $q_1 = 15$ gene expressions in Step 1, and then select the remaining $\widetilde{q} - q_1 = 5$ gene expressions in Step 2.

Noting that the feature screening results are similar for different values of R, to ease presentation, we summarize 20 selected genes' ID numbers for the case with $R = 0.85$ in Table 3, where "FS" represents the feature screening method in Sect. 3.2 and "IFS" stands for the iteration method in Sect. 4. In comparison, we use the naive method by directly implementing (13) rather than (15) as in the proposed method to do feature screening, and let "nFS" and "nIFS" be the naive feature screening method and the naive iteration method in Sects. 3.2 and 4, respectively. It is interesting that genes "29854," "27116," "24721," and "22155" are retained regardless of the specification of the distribution for the noise term, while other genes may be retained or excluded, depending on the distribution form of the noise term. For example, "26050" is retained if a normal distribution is assumed for the noise term, but it is excluded if a noise term assumes a t distribution; on the contrary, "25230" is retained if the noise term assumes a t distribution, but it is excluded if a normal distribution is assumed for the noise term. Regarding the iteration method, we observe that genes "23970," "16835," and "31992" are retained regardless of the specification of the distribution for the noise term. On the other hand, genes "26692"

Table 3 Sensitivity analyses of mantle cell lymphoma microarray data: the results of feature screening

	Normal		t distribution		Naive	
	FS	IFS	FS	IFS	nFS	nIFS
1	29854	29854	29854	29854	29598	29598
2	27116	27116	27116	27116	33027	33027
3	22155	22155	24721	24721	16787	16787
4	24721	24721	22155	22155	32583	32583
5	17230	17230	17545	17545	16121	16121
6	16528	16528	15936	15936	32049	32049
7	17545	17545	24819	24819	17548	17548
8	24819	24819	26050	26050	27361	27361
9	15936	15936	34524	34524	24610	24610
10	34524	34524	15936	15936	30282	30282
11	26050	26050	28726	28726	23970	23970
12	25230	25234	25230	25230	16835	16835
13	31935	31935	17176	17176	31992	31992
14	30575	30575	17927	17927	32259	32259
15	26692	26692	27019	27019	31895	31895
16	25234	31895	24850	31895	28726	29930
17	25055	23970	25055	23970	17176	24319
18	30157	16835	30157	16835	17927	31098
19	33570	31992	24545	31992	27019	27998
20	24734	32259	27998	31098	24850	24545

FS: The proposed feature screening method in Sect. 3.2
IFS: The proposed iteration method in Sect. 4
nFS: The naive feature screening method by implementing (13) to Sect. 3.2
nIFS: The naive iteration method by implementing (13) to Sect. 4

and "32259" are retained when the noise term is specified as a normal distribution but are excluded when the noise term assumes a t distribution, and genes "27019" and "31098" are retained when the noise term is assumed to follow a t distribution but are excluded if a normal distribution is assumed. Finally, we observe that without the error correction step, the genes retained by the naive methods have little in common with those obtained from the proposed methods.

To further explore the relationship between the response and the selected genes, we fit the Cox model to those data with the selected genes obtained, respectively, from the FS and IFS methods under the normal or t distribution specified previously for the measurement error, model, with $R = 0.85$:

$$\lambda(t|X_{\widehat{\mathcal{I}}}) = \lambda_0(t) \exp\left(X_{\widehat{\mathcal{I}}}^\top \beta\right), \tag{26}$$

where $\lambda_0(t)$ is the unspecified baseline hazard function, $X_{\widehat{\mathcal{I}}}$ is the vector of selected genes with $\widehat{\mathcal{I}}$ representing the estimated active set of genes listed in Table 3, and β is the vector of associated parameters.

To correct for the measurement error effects, we apply the insertion method proposed by Chen & Yi (2021b) to estimate β. The analysis results, including estimates (EST), standard errors (S.E.), and p-values, are summarized in Table 4. For those genes that are commonly selected under different distributions for the measurement error term, their estimates are stable and significant at the significant level 0.05. On the contrary, genes "25055" and "33570," which are retained by FS but excluded by IFS, are insignificant. The last five genes, retained by IFS, are all significant with small p-values.

6 Discussion

Ultrahigh-dimensional data analysis has received growing attention, where one of the prime concerns is to screen variables by retaining informative ones and excluding unimportant ones before conducting a formal analysis. While many methods have been developed to do feature screening, little attention is directed to deal with noisy data with measurement error.

In this chapter, we propose a robust feature screening method to handle ultrahigh-dimensional censored data subject to covariate measurement error, which generalizes to the procedure proposed by Chen (2019). The proposed method utilizes cumulative distribution functions to construct the distance correlation for the robustness. To improve the performance and retain truly important variables that may be falsely excluded by an initial feature screening procedure, we further develop the robust iteration procedure. Theoretical results and numerical examinations confirm the satisfactory performance of the proposed method.

There are some possible extensions and applications. For example, the development here is directed to continuous covariates subject to measurement error; it is interesting to develop robust approaches to handle binary and count variables with measurement error. The formula of the inverse Fourier transformation is developed for the classical measurement error model (7). It is also useful to explore screening procedures under other more complex measurement error models as outlined in Yi (2017, Sect. 2.6). In addition to considering right censoring for survival data, other characteristics of data, such as left truncation (e.g., Chen & Yi 2020, 2021b) and network structures in covariates (e.g., Chen & Yi 2021a), are of interest to be incorporated in feature screenings.

Acknowledgments The authors thank the co-editors and a referee for their helpful comments on the initial version. This research was supported by the Natural Sciences and Engineering Research Council of Canada (NSERC). Yi is Canada Research Chair in Data Science (Tier 1). Her research was undertaken, in part, thanks to funding from the Canada Research Chairs program.

Table 4 Sensitivity analyses for the mantle cell lymphoma microarray data: estimation results under the Cox model

| | Normal | | | | | | t distribution | | | | | |
| | FS | | | IFS | | | FS | | | IFS | | |
	EST	S.E.	p-value	EST	S.E.	p-value	EST	S.E.	p-value	EST	S.E.	p-value
1	1.377	0.493	0.005	1.414	0.413	0.001	1.398	0.475	0.003	1.423	0.424	0.001
2	1.104	0.337	0.001	1.003	0.287	0.000	1.097	0.320	0.001	1.036	0.293	0.000
3	0.812	0.398	0.041	0.760	0.385	0.048	−0.967	0.306	0.002	−0.938	0.294	0.001
4	−0.953	0.321	0.003	−0.944	0.287	0.001	0.847	0.378	0.041	0.813	0.369	0.048
5	−1.082	0.245	0.000	−1.108	0.276	0.000	−1.091	0.123	0.000	−1.114	0.120	0.000
6	1.395	0.258	0.000	1.234	0.260	0.000	0.988	0.366	0.007	0.980	0.405	0.016
7	−1.101	0.110	0.000	−1.106	0.134	0.000	−1.588	0.496	0.001	−1.571	0.491	0.001
8	−1.468	0.567	0.010	−1.372	0.487	0.005	−0.456	0.087	0.000	−0.435	0.091	0.000
9	0.969	0.381	0.011	0.979	0.446	0.028	−1.096	0.377	0.004	−1.079	0.263	0.000
10	−1.103	0.382	0.004	−1.070	0.156	0.000	0.957	0.338	0.005	0.966	0.343	0.005
11	−0.335	0.093	0.000	−0.305	0.121	0.012	0.898	0.101	0.000	0.923	0.125	0.000
12	1.285	0.437	0.003	1.200	0.222	0.000	1.117	0.405	0.006	1.208	0.366	0.001
13	−1.148	0.124	0.000	−1.070	0.083	0.000	1.037	0.118	0.000	1.095	0.123	0.000
14	−0.653	0.188	0.001	−0.769	0.178	0.000	−0.789	0.153	0.000	−0.774	0.148	0.000
15	−0.865	0.395	0.029	−0.969	0.464	0.037	0.858	0.236	0.000	0.811	0.210	0.000
16	0.726	0.307	0.018	1.582	0.170	0.000	0.664	0.231	0.004	1.453	0.186	0.000
17	0.254	0.434	0.558	1.195	0.396	0.003	0.281	0.402	0.485	1.142	0.378	0.003
18	0.728	0.257	0.005	0.560	0.209	0.007	0.711	0.233	0.002	0.537	0.186	0.004
19	−0.295	0.208	0.156	−0.982	0.216	0.000	0.133	0.304	0.662	−0.978	0.207	0.000
20	0.519	0.315	0.099	1.283	0.379	0.001	0.413	0.346	0.233	0.878	0.295	0.003

FS: The proposed feature screening method in Sect. 3.2
IFS: The proposed iterated feature screening method in Sect. 4

Appendix

A. Technical Lemmas

In this appendix, we provide some lemmas that are useful to derive the main theorems. The first lemma is the probabilistic bound of the estimated survivor function.

Lemma 1 *Let $H(t) = P(Y_i > t)$ denote the cumulative distribution function of Y_i, where $Y_i = \min\{T_i, C_i\}$. Suppose that there is a finite time point τ, such that $H(\tau) > \eta$ for a positive constant η. Then for $\xi > 2^7 n^{-1} \eta^{-2}$, there exist positive constants κ_1 and κ_2 such that*

$$P\left(\sup_{t \in [0,\tau]} |\widehat{F}(t) - F(t)| > \xi\right) \leq \kappa_1 \exp\left(-n\xi^2 \eta^4 \kappa_2\right). \tag{A.1}$$

This lemma is Theorem 2 of Földes & Rejtö (1981). The second lemma is about the probabilistic bound of the estimator (16).

Lemma 2 *Under regularity conditions (C1) and (C2), for any $\xi^* > 0$, we have*

$$P\left(\sup_x |\widehat{F}_{adj,j}(x) - F_{X_{(j)}}(x)| > \xi^*\right) \leq \kappa_3 \exp\left\{-\frac{2n^2 \xi^{*2}}{G^2} + o(n^{-\frac{1}{5}})\right\} \tag{A.2}$$

for some positive constants G and κ_3.

Proof We first write

$$\widehat{f}_{adj,j}(x) - f_{X_{(j)}}(x) = \left\{\widehat{f}_{adj,j}(x) - f_{adj,j}(x)\right\} + \left\{f_{adj,j}(x) - f_{X_{(j)}}(x)\right\}$$

$$= \widehat{f}_{adj,j}(x) - f_{adj,j}(x), \tag{A.3}$$

because $f_{adj,j}(x)$ is just a different symbol of the inverse Fourier transformation of $f_{X_{(j)}}(x)$, i.e., $f_{adj,j}(x) - f_{X_{(j)}}(x) = 0$. Therefore, the remaining task is to examine $\widehat{f}_{adj,j}(x) - f_{adj,j}(x)$. By (11) and (15), we have

$$\widehat{f}_{adj,j}(x) - f_{adj,j}(x) = \frac{1}{2\pi} \int_{-\infty}^{\infty} \frac{\exp(-\mathbf{i}ux)}{\phi_{\epsilon_{(j)}}(u)} \left\{\widehat{\phi}_{X_{(j)}^*}(u) - \phi_{X_{(j)}^*}(u)\right\} du. \tag{A.4}$$

Note that $\phi_{X_{(j)}^*}(u) = E\left\{\exp\left(\mathbf{i}u X_{i(j)}^*\right)\right\}$ and $\widehat{\phi}_{X_{(j)}^*}(u)$ is given by (14); then

$$\widehat{\phi}_{X_{(j)}^*}(u) - \phi_{X_{(j)}^*}(u)$$

$$= \left\{ \frac{1}{n} \sum_{i=1}^{n} \exp\left(\mathrm{i} u X_{i(j)}^*\right) \right\} \int_{-\infty}^{\infty} \exp\left(\mathrm{i} u h z\right) K(z) dz - E\left\{ \exp\left(\mathrm{i} u X_{i(j)}^*\right) \right\}. \quad (A.5)$$

By Conditions (C1) and (C2) and the finiteness of $\int_{-\infty}^{\infty} u^r K(u) du$ for all $r \in \mathbb{N}$, applying the Taylor series expansion of the exponential function gives that $\int_{-\infty}^{\infty} \exp\left(\mathrm{i} u h z\right) K(u) du = 1 + o(n^{-\frac{1}{5}})$. Combining with (A.5) gives

$$\widehat{\phi}_{X_{(j)}^*}(u) - \phi_{X_{(j)}^*}(u) = \frac{1}{n} \sum_{i=1}^{n} \exp\left(\mathrm{i} u X_{i(j)}^*\right) - E\left\{ \exp\left(\mathrm{i} u X_{i(j)}^*\right) \right\} + o(n^{-\frac{6}{5}}). \quad (A.6)$$

Let $Z_i = \exp\left(\mathrm{i} u X_{i(j)}^*\right)$, which is a complex random variable. By Theorem 1.2 of Isaev and McKay (2016), we have

$$\left| E\left[\exp\{Z_i - E(Z_i)\} \right] - 1 \right| \le \exp\left(\frac{G^2}{8} \right) - 1, \quad (A.7)$$

where G is some constant with $G > \mathrm{diam} Z \triangleq \inf\{c \in \mathbb{R}^+ : P\left(|Z_1 - Z_2| > c\right) = 0\}$. Note that $\widehat{\phi}_{X_{(j)}^*}(u) = \frac{1}{n} \sum_{i=1}^{n} Z_i$; then by (A.6), for any $\xi_2 > 0$ and $\nu > 0$,

$$P\left(\left| \widehat{\phi}_{X_{(j)}^*}(u) - \phi_{X_{(j)}^*}(u) \right| \ge \xi_2 \right)$$

$$\le P\left(\frac{1}{n} \sum_{i=1}^{n} \left| Z_i - E(Z_i) \right| \ge \xi_2 + o(n^{-\frac{6}{5}}) \right)$$

$$= P\left[\exp\left(\nu \sum_{i=1}^{n} \left| Z_i - E(Z_i) \right| \right) \ge \exp\left\{ \nu n \xi_2 + o(n^{-\frac{1}{5}}) \right\} \right]$$

$$\le \exp\left\{ -\nu n \xi_2 + o(n^{-\frac{1}{5}}) \right\} E\left\{ \exp\left(\nu \sum_{i=1}^{n} \left| Z_i - E(Z_i) \right| \right) \right\}$$

$$= \left[\exp\left\{ -\nu n \xi_2 + o(n^{-\frac{1}{5}}) \right\} \right] \times \left[\prod_{i=1}^{n} E\left\{ \exp\left(\nu \left| Z_i - E(Z_i) \right| \right) \right\} \right]$$

$$= \exp\left\{ \frac{n \nu^2 G^2}{8} - \nu n \xi_2 + o(n^{-\frac{1}{5}}) \right\}, \quad (A.8)$$

where the third step is due to Markov's inequality, the fourth step is by the independence of the X_i^*, and the last step comes from (A.7) with Z_i replaced by νZ_i, so that with constant νG satisfying $\nu G > \inf\{\nu c : P\left(\nu |Z_1 - Z_2| > \nu c\right) = 0\}$, we have $E\{\exp\left(\nu |Z_i - E(Z_i)|\right)\} \le \exp\left(\frac{\nu^2 G^2}{8} \right)$.

To get the best upper bound, we take the right-hand side of (A.8) as the function of ν and then minimize it. Specifically, let $\varphi(\nu) = \frac{n\nu^2 G^2}{8} - \nu n\xi_2 + o(n^{-\frac{1}{5}})$. Since $\varphi(\nu)$ is a quadratic function, it is easy to check that $\nu^* \triangleq \underset{\nu}{\arg\min}\, \varphi(\nu) = \frac{4\xi_2}{G^2}$. Then replacing ν by ν^* in (A.8) yields

$$P\left(\left|\widehat{\phi}_{X_{(j)}^*}(u) - \phi_{X_{(j)}^*}(u)\right| \geq \xi_2\right) \leq \exp\left\{-\frac{2n\xi_2^2}{G^2} + o(n^{-\frac{1}{5}})\right\}. \tag{A.9}$$

Moreover, by (A.4) and (A.9), we observe that with a probability greater than $1 - \exp\left\{-\frac{2n\xi_2^2}{G^2} + o(n^{-\frac{1}{5}})\right\}$,

$$\sup_x \left|\widehat{f}_{adj,j}(x) - f_{X_{(j)}}(x)\right| = \sup_x \left|\widehat{f}_{adj,j}(x) - f_{adj,j}(x)\right|$$

$$\leq \sup_x\left\{\frac{1}{2\pi}\int_{-\infty}^{\infty}\frac{\exp(-\mathbf{i}ux)}{\phi_{\epsilon_{(j)}}(u)}\left|\widehat{\phi}_{X_{(j)}^*}(u) - \phi_{X_{(j)}^*}(u)\right|du\right\}$$

$$\leq \left(\sup_x\frac{1}{2\pi}\int_{-\infty}^{\infty}\frac{\exp(-\mathbf{i}ux)}{\phi_{\epsilon_{(j)}}(u)}du\right)\xi_2,$$

where the first equality is due to (A.3), the last step comes from (A.9), and the improper integral $\int_{-\infty}^{\infty}\frac{\exp(-\mathbf{i}ux)}{\phi_{\epsilon_{(j)}}(u)}du$ is shown to converge to a finite value (e.g., Marsden & Hoffman 1999, Proposition 4.3.9).

In other words,

$$P\left\{\sup_x\left|\widehat{f}_{adj,j}(x) - f_{X_{(j)}}(x)\right| \geq \left(\sup_x\frac{1}{2\pi}\int_{-\infty}^{\infty}\frac{\exp(-\mathbf{i}ux)}{\phi_{\epsilon_{(j)}}(u)}du\right)\xi_2\right\}$$

$$\leq \exp\left\{-\frac{2n\xi_2^2}{G^2} + o(n^{-\frac{1}{5}})\right\}.$$

Specifying $\xi^* = \left(\sup_x\frac{1}{2\pi}\int_{-\infty}^{\infty}\frac{\exp(-\mathbf{i}ux)}{\phi_{\epsilon_{(j)}}(u)}du\right)\xi_2$ gives that

$$P\left(\sup_x\left|\widehat{f}_{adj,j}(x) - f_{X_{(j)}}(x)\right| \geq \xi^*\right) \leq \kappa_3\exp\left\{-\frac{2n\xi^{*2}}{G^2} + o(n^{-\frac{1}{5}})\right\},$$

where $\kappa_3 \triangleq \exp\left\{\frac{2n\xi^{*2}}{G^2} - \frac{2n\xi_2^2}{G^2}\right\}$, which is positive. Thus, by the definition of the cumulative distribution function and (16), we conclude the desired result (A.2). $\square$

B. Proofs of Main Theorems

B.1 Proof of Theorem 1

Part 1 *We prove* (19).

Since ω_j and $\widehat{\omega}_j$ are formulated in terms of $\mathrm{dov}(\cdot, \cdot)$ and the associated estimates, to show the desired result, it suffices to examine $\mathrm{dov}(\cdot, \cdot)$ and its estimates.

Let $\omega_j^* \triangleq \widehat{\mathrm{dcov}}(F_{X_{(j)}}(X_{(j)}), F(Y)) = \widetilde{M}_{j,1} + \widetilde{M}_{j,2} - 2\widetilde{M}_{j,3}$, where $\widetilde{M}_{j,k}$ with $k = 1, 2, 3$ has the same form as $\widehat{M}_{j,k}$ in (4) with $\widehat{F}_{X_{(j)}}(X_{(j)})$ and $\widehat{F}(Y)$ replaced by $F_{X_{(j)}}(X_{(j)})$ and $F(Y)$, respectively. Therefore, the difference between $\widehat{\omega}_j$ and ω_j can be expressed as

$$\widehat{\omega}_j^* - \omega_j = \left(\widehat{\omega}_j^* - \omega_j^*\right) + \left(\omega_j^* - \omega_j\right). \tag{B.1}$$

Similar to the derivation of Li et al. (2012), we can show that

$$P\left(\max_{j=1,\cdots,p} \left|\omega_j^* - \omega_j\right| > \xi\right) = O\left\{p \exp\left(-\widetilde{c}_1 n \xi^2\right)\right\} \tag{B.2}$$

for some positive constants $\widetilde{c}_1$ and ξ.

On the other hand, we examine $\widehat{\omega}_j - \omega_j^*$ by writing

$$\widehat{\omega}_j - \omega_j^* = \left(\widehat{M}_{j,1} - \widetilde{M}_{j,1}\right) + \left(\widehat{M}_{j,2} - \widetilde{M}_{j,2}\right) - 2\left(\widehat{M}_{j,3} - \widetilde{M}_{j,3}\right). \tag{B.3}$$

Since the derivations of $\widehat{M}_{j,2} - \widetilde{M}_{j,2}$ and $\widehat{M}_{j,3} - \widetilde{M}_{j,3}$ are similar to those of $\widehat{M}_{j,1} - \widetilde{M}_{j,1}$, we only present the argument for the latter case.

By adding and subtracting $\frac{1}{n^2} \sum_{i=1}^{n} \sum_{k=1}^{n} \left\{ \left|\widehat{F}_{adj,j}(X_{i(j)}) - \widehat{F}_{adj,j}(X_{k(j)})\right| |F(Y_i) - F(Y_k)| \right\}$, we obtain that

$$\widehat{M}_{j,1} - \widetilde{M}_{j,1}$$

$$= \left[\widehat{M}_{j,1} - \frac{1}{n^2} \sum_{i=1}^{n} \sum_{k=1}^{n} \left\{ \left|\widehat{F}_{adj,j}(X_{i(j)}) - \widehat{F}_{adj,j}(X_{k(j)})\right| |F(Y_i) - F(Y_k)| \right\}\right]$$

$$+ \left[\frac{1}{n^2} \sum_{i=1}^{n} \sum_{k=1}^{n} \left\{ \left|\widehat{F}_{adj,j}(X_{i(j)}) - \widehat{F}_{adj,j}(X_{k(j)})\right| |F(Y_i) - F(Y_k)| \right\} - \widetilde{M}_{j,1}\right]$$

$$= \frac{1}{n^2} \sum_{i=1}^{n} \sum_{k=1}^{n} \left\{ \left|\widehat{F}_{adj,j}(X_{i(j)}) - \widehat{F}_{adj,j}(X_{k(j)})\right| \left(\left|\widehat{F}(Y_i) - \widehat{F}(Y_k)\right| - |F(Y_i) - F(Y_k)|\right) \right\}$$

$$+ \frac{1}{n^2} \sum_{i=1}^{n} \sum_{k=1}^{n} \left\{ |F(Y_i) - F(Y_k)| \left(\left|\widehat{F}_{adj,j}(X_{i(j)}) - \widehat{F}_{X_{(j)}}(X_{k(j)})\right|\right. \right.$$

$$- \left| F_{adj,j}(X_{i(j)}) - F_{X_{(j)}}(X_{k(j)}) \right| \Big) \Big\}$$

$$\triangleq S_1 + S_2. \tag{B.4}$$

First, we examine S_1. Since $\widehat{F}_{adj,j}(x)$ is the estimated cumulative distribution function with $0 \leq \widehat{F}_{adj,j}(x) \leq 1$, then for any i and k, we have that

$$\left| \widehat{F}_{adj,j}(X_{i(j)}) - \widehat{F}_{adj,j}(X_{k(j)}) \right| \leq 1. \tag{B.5}$$

By the triangle inequality, we have that

$$\left| \widehat{F}(Y_i) - \widehat{F}(Y_k) \right| - |F(Y_i) - F(Y_k)| \leq \left| \widehat{F}(Y_i) - F(Y_i) \right| + \left| \widehat{F}(Y_k) - F(Y_k) \right|. \tag{B.6}$$

Then by (B.6), we have that

$$P \left\{ \left| \left| \widehat{F}(Y_i) - \widehat{F}(Y_k) \right| - |F(Y_i) - F(Y_k)| \right| > \xi \right\}$$

$$\leq P \left\{ \left(\left| \widehat{F}(Y_i) - F(Y_i) \right| + \left| \widehat{F}(Y_k) - F(Y_k) \right| \right) > \xi \right\}$$

$$\leq P \left\{ \sup_{t \in [0,\tau]} \left| \widehat{F}(t) - F(t) \right| + \sup_{t \in [0,\tau]} \left| \widehat{F}(t) - F(t) \right| > \xi \right\}$$

$$= P \left\{ 2 \sup_{t \in [0,\tau]} \left| \widehat{F}(t) - F(t) \right| > \xi \right\}$$

$$= P \left\{ \sup_{t \in [0,\tau]} \left| \widehat{F}(t) - F(t) \right| > \frac{\xi}{2} \right\}$$

$$\leq \kappa_1 \exp \left(-\frac{1}{4} n \xi^2 \eta^4 \kappa_2 \right), \tag{B.7}$$

where the last step is due to Lemma 1 with ξ in the right-hand side of (A.1) replaced by $\frac{\xi}{2}$. Therefore, combining (B.5) and (B.7) gives

$$P \left(|S_1| > \xi \right) \leq \kappa_1 \exp \left(-\frac{1}{4} n \xi^2 \eta^4 \kappa_2 \right). \tag{B.8}$$

Next, we examine S_2 in a similar manner. Similar to (B.5), we have that

$$|F(Y_i) - F(Y_k)| \leq 1. \tag{B.9}$$

Similar to the arguments for (B.7), we obtain that

$$P\left\{\left|\left|\widehat{F}_{adj,j}(X_{i(j)}) - \widehat{F}_{X_{(j)}}(X_{k(j)})\right| - \left|F_{adj,j}(X_{i(j)}) - F_{X_{(j)}}(X_{k(j)})\right|\right| > \xi\right\}$$

$$\leq \kappa_3 \exp\left\{-\frac{n\xi^2}{2G^2} + o(n^{-\frac{1}{5}})\right\}. \tag{B.10}$$

Therefore, combining (B.9) and (B.10) yields

$$P\left(|S_2| > \xi\right) \leq \kappa_3 \exp\left\{-\frac{n\xi^2}{2G^2} + o(n^{-\frac{1}{5}})\right\}. \tag{B.11}$$

Finally, combining (B.4), (B.8), and (B.11), the probabilistic bound of $\widehat{M}_{j,1} - \widetilde{M}_{j,1}$ is given by

$$P\left(\left|\widehat{M}_{j,1} - \widetilde{M}_{j,1}\right| > \xi\right) = P\left(|S_1 + S_2| > \xi\right) \tag{B.12}$$

$$\leq P\left(|S_1| + |S_2| > \xi\right)$$

$$\leq P\left(|S_1| > \frac{\xi}{2}\right) + P\left(|S_2| > \frac{\xi}{2}\right)$$

$$\leq \kappa_1 \exp\left(-\frac{1}{16}n\xi^2\eta^4\kappa_2\right) + \kappa_3 \exp\left\{-\frac{n\xi^2}{8G^2} + o(n^{-\frac{1}{5}})\right\}.$$

Furthermore, similar derivations show that

$$P\left(\left|\widehat{M}_{j,2} - \widetilde{M}_{j,2}\right| > \xi\right) \leq \kappa_1 \exp\left(-\frac{1}{16}n\xi^2\eta^4\kappa_2\right)$$

$$+ \kappa_3 \exp\left\{-\frac{n\xi^2}{8G^2} + o(n^{-\frac{1}{5}})\right\} \tag{B.13}$$

and

$$P\left(\left|\widehat{M}_{j,3} - \widetilde{M}_{j,3}\right| > \xi\right) \leq \kappa_1 \exp\left(-\frac{1}{16}n\xi^2\eta^4\kappa_2\right)$$

$$+ \kappa_3 \exp\left\{-\frac{n\xi^2}{8G^2} + o(n^{-\frac{1}{5}})\right\}. \tag{B.14}$$

Noting that the upper bounds in (B.12)–(B.14) are dominated by $\exp\left(-c^*n\xi^2\right)$ for certain constant c^*, we apply (B.12)–(B.14) to (B.3) and obtain that

$$P\left(\left|\widehat{\omega}_j - \omega_j^*\right| > \xi\right) = O\left\{\exp\left(-\widetilde{c}_2 n\xi^2\right)\right\} \tag{B.15}$$

for some $\tilde{c}_2 > 0$. Thus, combining (B.2) and (B.15) with (B.1) and specifying $\xi = cn^{-\zeta}$ for the constants c and ζ described in Condition (C4) yield the desired result.

Part 2 *We prove* (20).
Let $J = \min_{j \in I} |\omega_j| - \max_{j \in I^c} |\omega_j|$. The left-hand side of (20) can be expressed as

$$P\left(\max_{j \in I^c} |\widehat{\omega}_j| \geq \min_{j \in I} |\widehat{\omega}_j|\right) = P\left(\max_{j \in I^c} |\widehat{\omega}_j| - \max_{j \in I^c} |\omega_j| \geq \min_{j \in I} |\widehat{\omega}_j| - \max_{j \in I^c} |\omega_j|\right)$$

$$= P\left(\max_{j \in I^c} |\widehat{\omega}_j| - \max_{j \in I^c} |\omega_j| \geq \min_{j \in I} |\widehat{\omega}_j| - \min_{j \in I} |\omega_j| + J\right)$$

$$\leq P\left(\max_{j \in I^c} |\widehat{\omega}_j - \omega_j| + \max_{j \in I} |\widehat{\omega}_j - \omega_j| \geq J\right)$$

$$\leq P\left(2 \max_{j=1,\cdots,p} |\widehat{\omega}_j - \omega_j| \geq J\right)$$

$$= O\left\{\exp\left(-\frac{1}{4}Dnv_0^2\right)\right\},$$

where the last step comes from the result in Part 1 and Condition (C5). □

B.2 Proof of Theorem 2

Similar to the derivations of Li et al. (2012), one can obtain that

$$\left\{\max_{j \in I} |\widehat{\omega}_j - \omega_j| \leq cn^{-\zeta}\right\} \subseteq \{I \subseteq \widehat{I}\}.$$

It gives

$$P\left(I \subseteq \widehat{I}\right) \geq 1 - P\left(\max_{j \in I} |\widehat{\omega}_j - \omega_j| \leq cn^{-\zeta}\right)$$

$$\geq 1 - qP\left(|\widehat{\omega}_j - \omega_j| \leq cn^{-\zeta}\right)$$

$$\geq 1 - O\left\{q\exp\left(-Dn^{1-2\zeta}\right)\right\},$$

where the last step comes from Theorem 1. □

References

Carroll, R. J., Ruppert, D., Stefanski, L. A., & Crainiceanu, C. M. (2006). *Measurement Error in Nonlinear Model*. New York: CRC Press.

Chen, L.-P. (2019). Iterated feature screening based on distance correlation for ultrahigh-dimensional censored data with covariates measurement error. arXiv:1901.01610.

Chen, J., & Chen, Z. (2008). Extended Bayesian information criteria for model selection with large model spaces. *Biometrika, 95*, 759–771.

Chen, L.-P., & Yi, G. Y. (2020). Model selection and model averaging for analysis of truncated and censored data with measurement error. *Electronic Journal of Statistics, 14*, 4054–4109.

Chen, L.-P., & Yi, G. Y. (2021a). Analysis of noisy survival data with graphical proportional hazards measurement error models. *Biometrics*. https://doi.org/10.1111/biom.13331

Chen, L.-P., & Yi, G. Y. (2021b). Semiparametric methods for left-truncated and right-censored survival data with covariate measurement error. *Annals of the Institute of Statistical Mathematics, 73*, 481–517. https://doi.org/10.1007/s10463-020-00755-2

Chen, X., Chen, X., & Wang, H. (2018). Robust feature screening for ultra-high dimensional right censored data via distance correlation. *Computational Statistics and Data Analysis, 119*, 118–138.

Cui, H., Li, R., & Zhong, W. (2015). Model-free feature screening for ultrahigh dimensional discriminant analysis. *Journal of the American Statistical Association, 110*, 630–641.

Dreiera, I., & Kotzb, S. (2002). A note on the characteristic function of the t-distribution. *Statistics and Probability Letters, 57*, 221–224.

Fan, J., & Lv, J. (2008). Sure independence screening for ultrahigh dimensional feature space (with discussion). *Journal of the Royal Statistical Society, Series B, 70*, 849–911.

Fan, J., & Song, R. (2010). Sure independence screening in generalized linear models with NP-dimensionality. *The Annals of Statistics, 38*, 3567–3604.

Fan, J., Samworth, R., & Wu, Y. (2009). Ultrahigh dimensional feature selection: beyond the linear model. *Journal of Machine Learning Research, 10*, 1829–1853.

Fan, J., Feng, Y., & Wu, Y. (2010). Ultrahigh dimensional variable selection for Cox's proportional hazards model. *IMS Collect, 6*, 70–86.

Földes, A., & Rejtö, L. (1981). A LIL type result for the product limit estimator. *Z. Wahrscheinlichkeitstheorie verw. Gebiete, 56*, 75–86.

Hall, P., & Miller, H. (2009). Using generalized correlation to effect variable selection in very high dimensional problems. *Journal of Computational and Graphical Statistics, 18*, 533–550.

Hao, M., Lin, Y., Liu, X., & Tang, W. (2019). Robust feature screening for high-dimensional survival data. *Journal of Applied Statistics, 46*, 979–994.

Isaev, M., & McKay, B. D. (2016). On a bound of Hoeffding in the complex case. *Electronic Communications in Probability, 21*, 1–7.

Li, R., Zhong, W., & Zhu, L. (2012). Feature screening via distance correlation learning. *Journal of the American Statistical Association, 107*, 1129–1139.

Marsden, J. E., & Hoffman, M. J. (1999). *Basic complex analysis*. New York: W. H. Freeman.

Rosenwald, A., Wright, G., Chan, W. C., Connors, J. M., Campo, E., Fisher, R. I., Gascoyne, R. D., Muller-Hermelink, H. K., Smeland, E. B., & Staudt, L. M. (2003). The proliferation gene expression signature is a quantitative integrator of oncogenic events that predicts survival in mantle cell lymphoma. *Cancer Cell, 3*, 185–197.

Song, R., Lu, W., Ma, S., & Jeng, X. (2014). Censored rank independence screening for high-dimensional survival data. *Biometrika, 101*, 799–814.

Székely, G. J., Rizzo, M. L., & Bakirov, N. K. (2007). Measuring and testing dependence by correlation of distances. *The Annals of Statistics, 35*, 2769–2794.

Wand, M.P. & Jones, M.C. (1995). *Kernel Smoothing*. Chapman & Hall, London.

Xue, J., & Liang, F. (2017). A robust model free feature screening method for ultrahigh dimensional data. *Journal of Computational and Graphical Statistics, 26*, 803–813.

Yan, X., Tang, N., & Zhao, X. (2017). The Spearman rank correlation screening for ultrahigh dimensional censored data. arXiv:1702.02708v1.

Yi, G. Y. (2017). *Statistical Analysis with Measurement Error and Misclassication: Strategy, Method and Application*. Springer.

Yi, G.Y., He, W., & Caroll, R.J. (2021). Feature screening with large-scale and high-dimensional survival data. *Biometrics*. http://doi.org/10.1111/biom.13479

Yi, G. Y., Ma, Y., Spiegelman, D., & Carroll, R. J. (2015). Functional and structural methods with mixed measurement error and misclassification in covariates. *Journal of the American Statistical Association, 110*, 681–696.

Zhang, J., Liu, Y., & Cui, H. (2020). Model-free feature screening via distance correlation for ultrahigh dimensional survival data. *Statistical Papers*. https://doi.org/10.1007/s00362-020-01210-3

Zhong, W., & Zhu, L. (2015). An iterative approach to distance correlation-based sure independence screening. *Journal of Statistical Computation and Simulation, 85*, 2331–2345.

Zhu, L., Li, L., Li, R., & Zhu, L. (2011). Model-free feature screening for ultrahigh-dimensional data. *Journal of the American Statistical Association, 106*, 1464–1475.

Simultaneous Control of False Discovery Rate and Sensitivity Using Least Angle Regressions in High-Dimensional Data Analysis

Bangxin Zhao and Wenqing He

Abstract Controlling the false discovery rate (FDR) and maintaining the high sensitivity are key desiderata in post-selection inference in high-dimensional data analysis. *Least Angle Regression* (LARS) is an efficient variable selection method, and it provides a solution path along which the entered predictors always have the same absolute correlation with the current residual. In this chapter, we propose a new method to control the FDR and sensitivity simultaneously for high-dimensional post-selection inference using least angle regression, termed *Cosine PoSI*. *Cosine PoSI* focuses on the geometric aspect of *least angle regression*: in each step of the LARS algorithm, the proposed *Cosine PoSI* method makes use of the angle between the entering variable and the current residual and treats this angle as a random variable that follows a cosine distribution. Given the collection of the possible angles, the variable selection path is stopped using hypothesis testing based on the limiting distribution of the maximum angle that can be obtained through the order statistics of the cosine distribution. We show that both the sensitivity and the FDR can be controlled by using the stopping criteria. Simulation studies and a real-data analysis are conducted to assess the effectiveness of the proposed method.

Keywords False discovery rate · High-dimensional data · Least angle regression · Sensitivity

1 Introduction

In high-dimensional data analysis, the assumption of sparsity is often taken, and therefore, the variable selection is usually conducted to obtain the possible important variables that may have real effects on the response. The inference of the final model is conducted based on the selected variables and is therefore affected by

B. Zhao · W. He (✉)
Department of Statistical and Actuarial Sciences, University of Western Ontario, London, ON, Canada
e-mail: bzhao49@uwo.ca; whe@stats.uwo.ca

© The Author(s), under exclusive license to Springer Nature Switzerland AG 2022
W. He et al. (eds.), *Advances and Innovations in Statistics and Data Science*, ICSA Book Series in Statistics, https://doi.org/10.1007/978-3-031-08329-7_3

the selection procedure for the important variables. In this aspect, methods from classical statistical inference theory may be invalid due to the stochastic components in the high-dimensional structure. Some recent developments on making inference while doing variable selection using LASSO and forward-type regression can be found in the literature. Relatively recent approaches on *post-selection inference* were discussed in Berk et al. (2013), Lockhart et al. (2014), and Lee et al. (2016). Berk et al. (2013) tackled a valid *post-selection inference* (PoSI) problem by forming statistical tests and obtaining confidence intervals in linear models after selecting a subset of variables in a data-driven fashion. Lockhart et al. (2014) and Lee et al. (2016) illustrated the post-selection inference of LASSO by forming exact hypothesis tests and constructing confidence intervals, respectively.

Assuming the relationship between the response and the predictor variables can be postulated through a linear model:

$$\mathbf{Y} = \mathbf{X}\boldsymbol{\beta} + \boldsymbol{\epsilon}, \tag{1}$$

where $\mathbf{X} \in \mathbb{R}^{n \times p}$, $\mathbf{X}_i \in \mathbb{R}^{p \times 1}$ is the ith column vector of $\mathbf{X}$, $cov(\mathbf{X}_i) = \Sigma$, $i = 1, \ldots, n$, $\boldsymbol{\beta} \in \mathbb{R}^p$ is the vector of the coefficient of the respective covariates, and $\boldsymbol{\epsilon} \sim N(0, \sigma^2 I)$ is the noise in the model.

For high-dimensional data analysis with $p > n$, variables selection is often applied to obtain variables that have real relationship with the response through regularization:

$$\hat{\boldsymbol{\beta}} = \arg \min_{\boldsymbol{\beta}} \left\{ \|Y - \mathbf{X}\boldsymbol{\beta}\|_2^2 + p_\lambda(\boldsymbol{\beta}) \right\},$$

where $p_\lambda(\boldsymbol{\beta})$ is the penalty function of the coefficients $\boldsymbol{\beta}$ and $\lambda \geq 0$ is a tuning parameter. Many regularization methods with different penalty functions have been proposed in the literature. For example, LASSO regularization (Tibshirani 1996), or an L_1 penalty, takes the absolute value of the coefficients as the penalty

$$\hat{\boldsymbol{\beta}} = \arg \min_{\boldsymbol{\beta}} \left\{ \|Y - \mathbf{X}\boldsymbol{\beta}\|_2^2 + \lambda\|\boldsymbol{\beta}\|_1 \right\}. \tag{2}$$

The LASSO solution path $\hat{\boldsymbol{\beta}}(\lambda)$ can be viewed as a continuous piecewise linear function of the tuning parameter λ with a sequence of decreasing knots, i.e., $\lambda_1 \geq \lambda_2 \geq \cdots \geq \lambda_n \geq 0$. To choose a predictor that enters the LASSO solution path at a given knot, Lockhart et al. (2014) proposed a covariance test statistic. Let $\mathcal{M}_k = \{j_1, \ldots, j_k\}$ be the LASSO solution path with increasing complexity controlled by the tuning parameter λ. The corresponding tuning parameter at each step is λ_i, $i = 1, \ldots, k$. Note that $\lambda_0 = \infty$ corresponds to $\mathcal{M}_0 = \emptyset$. The j_kth ($j_k \geq 2$) predictor is added into the model after obtaining the solution path $\mathcal{M}_{k-1}$. Let the estimates of the coefficient $\boldsymbol{\beta}$ at the end of the $k - 1$th step be $\hat{\boldsymbol{\beta}}(\lambda_k)$. If we refit the LASSO by using just the variables in $\mathcal{M}_{k-1}$ with the tuning parameter λ_k, the estimates at the end of this step are $\hat{\boldsymbol{\beta}}_{\mathcal{M}_{k-1}}(\lambda_k)$. The *covariance test statistic* of the j_kth predictor proposed in Lockhart et al. (2014) is then defined as

$$\mathbf{T}_{j_k} = \frac{1}{\sigma^2} \cdot \left(\langle \mathbf{Y}, \mathbf{X}\hat{\boldsymbol{\beta}}(\lambda_k) \rangle - \langle \mathbf{Y}, \mathbf{X}_{\mathcal{M}_{k-1}} \hat{\boldsymbol{\beta}}_{\mathcal{M}_{k-1}}(\lambda_k) \rangle \right). \tag{3}$$

The statistic $\mathbf{T}_{j_k}$ measures how much contribution $\mathbf{X}_{j_k}$ made to improve the fitted model over the interval $(\lambda_{k-1}, \lambda_k)$. At a high probability, a larger value of $\mathbf{T}_{j_k}$ determines bigger contribution of the variable $\mathbf{X}_{j_k}$ in the model $\mathcal{M}_{k-1} \bigcup \{j_k\}$. Under the null hypothesis that all truly important variables are contained in the model $\mathcal{M}_{k-1} \bigcup \{j_k\}$, $\mathbf{T}_{j_k} \xrightarrow{d} \exp(1)$, as $n, p \to \infty$.

Lee et al. (2016) discussed a general scheme for post-selection inference that yields exact p-values and confidence intervals in the Gaussian case. Recall the linear model (1) with $\boldsymbol{\mu} = \mathbf{X}\boldsymbol{\beta}$ and $\boldsymbol{\epsilon} \sim N(\mathbf{0}, \sigma^2 I)$. Under the deterministic design matrix setting, $\mathbf{y} \sim N(\boldsymbol{\mu}, \sigma^2 I)$. For a given matrix M and vector b, a set of linear inequalities in $\mathbf{y}$, i.e., $\{M\mathbf{y} \leq b\}$, can be used for variable selection. Let $\mathcal{M}$ be the current solution set and $\eta = \mathbf{X}_{\mathcal{M}}(\mathbf{X}_{\mathcal{M}}^T \mathbf{X}_{\mathcal{M}})^{-1} e_j$, $j = 1, 2, \ldots, |\mathcal{M}|$, where e_j is a vector having 1 for the jth element and 0's elsewhere. Inferences about $\eta^T \boldsymbol{\mu}$ conditional on $\{M\mathbf{y} \leq b\}$ can be made using a truncated normal distribution.

This property provides the possibility of constructing a $1 - \alpha$ level selection interval for $\eta^T \boldsymbol{\mu}$, which can be obtained by solving the inequalities $\eta^T \boldsymbol{\mu}$ such that $P(\eta^T \boldsymbol{\mu}) \geq 1 - \alpha/2$ and $P(\eta^T \boldsymbol{\mu}) \leq \alpha/2$, respectively.

The path-based regression algorithms are widely used in high-dimensional statistics Fan & Lv (2010), such as forward-type regression, LASSO (Tibshirani 1996), LARS (Efron et al. 2004), SIS (Fan & Lv 2008), and DTCCS (Zhao et al. 2021). To obtain a final model using these methodologies, variables are added either one by one as in LARS and LASSO, or one group after another as in DTCCS. For the LASSO method, the number of non-zero variables in the "best" final model only depends on a single tuning parameter, which means that a sequence of "knots" of tuning parameters determine different final models. For the DTCCS, the candidate model size is predetermined, and a group of monotone values of tuning parameters is used to form a final model.

Since the final model is determined by either the tuning parameter as in LASSO or the predetermined number of variables in the final model as in DTCCS, there might be unimportant variables being selected in the final model. The false discovery rate (FDR) can be used to assess the final model (G'Sell et al. 2016; Li & Barber 2017). Let $\mathcal{M}_k = \{j_1, \ldots, j_k\}$ be the important variable solution set with increasing complexity. G'Sell et al. (2016) proposed the "ForwardStop" testing procedures and a stopping point $\hat{k}$ to control the FDR. Li and Barber (2017) develop a family of "accumulation tests" to choose a cutoff $\hat{k}$ to evaluate the model adequacy and control the FDR. On one side, we would like the model to be simple (parsimony principle), but on the other side, the model should fit the date well (adequacy principle). There is often a trade-off between these two aspects, and the FDR can be used to control the trade-off. A conservative FDR control may induce an oversimplified model. We follow the family of "accumulation tests" and propose a method to control the FDR and maintain a high sensitivity simultaneously for high-dimensional post-selection inference using least angle regression.

The rest of this chapter is organized as follows. Section 2 introduces the inference background and the new method that can control the FDR and sensitivity simultaneously. Numerical studies are reported in Sect. 3 to show the superb of the proposed method in high-dimensional settings even when strong multicollinearity exists in the predictors. The conclusion and discussion are described in Sect. 4.

2 Methodology

2.1 Cosin Distribution

Recall linear model (1) with $\mu = \mathbf{X}\beta$ and $\epsilon \sim N(\mathbf{0}, \sigma^2\mathbf{I})$. Under the deterministic design matrix setting, $\mathbf{Y} \sim N(\mu, \Sigma)$. Assuming that σ^2 is known. For a fixed matrix $\mathbf{X}_{n \times p}$ of the predictor variables, we assume that all the predictors have been standardized to have mean 0 and unit length, and the response is also centered. We consider the forward procedure to obtain the solution path in the LARS context. Note that we only consider the procedure of adding variables and ignore the possibility of deleting variables.

Let $\mathcal{M}_k$ be the active set that contains the entered predictors along the LARS solution path, X_{j_k} be the j_kth predictor entering into the path, and s_{j_k} be the sign of the correlation between the X_{j_k} and the residual from the previous step. Following Efron et al. (2004), define the matrix

$$X_{\mathcal{M}_k} = (\ldots s_{j_k} X_{j_k} \ldots)_{j_k \in \mathcal{M}_k}. \tag{4}$$

Let $S_{\mathcal{M}_k}$ be the vector containing the signs in the active set with the entering order and $X_S = X_{\mathcal{M}_k} S_{\mathcal{M}_k}$ be the corresponding submatrix formed by extracting the columns of $\mathbf{X}$ in the same order.

Let

$$G_{\mathcal{M}_k} = X_{\mathcal{M}_k}^T X_{\mathcal{M}_k} \quad \text{and} \quad A_{\mathcal{M}_k} = (1_{\mathcal{M}_k}^T G_{\mathcal{M}_k}^{-1} 1_{\mathcal{M}_k})^{-1/2}, \tag{5}$$

where $1_{\mathcal{M}_k}$ being a vector of 1s with length being equal to the cardinality of $\mathcal{M}_k$, denoted as $|\mathcal{M}_k|$.

The direction of LARS solution path is

$$v_{\mathcal{M}_k} = X_{\mathcal{M}_k}(X_{\mathcal{M}_k}^T X_{\mathcal{M}_k})^{-1} 1_{\mathcal{M}_k}, \tag{6}$$

and then the unit equiangular vector can be defined as

$$u_{\mathcal{M}_k} = \frac{v_{\mathcal{M}_k}}{\|v_{\mathcal{M}_k}\|}, \tag{7}$$

where $\|v_{\mathcal{M}_k}\| = 1/A_{\mathcal{M}_k}$. Hence, $X^T_{\mathcal{M}_k} u_{\mathcal{M}_k} = A_{\mathcal{M}_k} 1_{\mathcal{M}_k}$. The correlation vector between the equiangular direction and all predictors can be calculated by

$$a = X^T u_{\mathcal{M}_k}. \tag{8}$$

Let $S^T_{\mathcal{M}_k} X^T_{\mathcal{M}_k} u_{\mathcal{M}_k}$ be a subvector of a for $|\mathcal{M}_k| < n$. At the kth stage of selecting the entering predictor, let $\hat{C}_k$ be the largest absolute value of the correlation between the entering variables and the current residual Z_k. LARS finds the predictor that has the smallest angle with the current residual, and proceeds in the direction of $u_{\mathcal{M}_k}$, which has the same angle with all X_{j_k}'s, $j_k \in \mathcal{M}_k$, in a step size of $\hat{\gamma}$ until the next predictor earns its "most correlated" position. By the end of each stage, LARS updates the mean function, i.e.,

$$\hat{\mu}_{\mathcal{M}_{k+1}} = \hat{\mu}_{\mathcal{M}_k} + \hat{\gamma} u_{\mathcal{M}_k}, \tag{9}$$

where

$$\hat{\gamma} = \min_{l \notin \mathcal{M}_k}{}^+ \left\{ \frac{\hat{C}_k - \hat{c}_l}{A_{\mathcal{M}_k} - a_l}, \frac{\hat{C}_k + \hat{c}_l}{A_{\mathcal{M}_k} + a_l} \right\}, \tag{10}$$

where $\hat{c}_l$ is the current correlation of the lth remaining predictor variable and $\min^+$ indicates the smallest positive value. The mean function $\hat{\mu}$ can be written as

$$\hat{\mu}_{\mathcal{M}_k} = U_{\mathcal{M}_k} \Gamma_{\mathcal{M}_k}, \tag{11}$$

where $U_{\mathcal{M}_k} = (\mathbf{u}_1, \mathbf{u}_2, \cdots, \mathbf{u}_k)$ and $\Gamma_{\mathcal{M}} = (\hat{\gamma}_1, \hat{\gamma}_2, \ldots, \hat{\gamma}_k)^T$. Denote $\hat{\beta}(\hat{C}_k)$ as the regression coefficients of the active predictors at stage k, $\hat{\beta}(\hat{C}_k) = (X^T_S X_S)^{-1} X^T_S U_{\mathcal{M}_k} \Gamma_{\mathcal{M}_k}$. The current correlation can also be expressed as the score vector of the least squares criterion with entering predictor:

$$\hat{C}_k = -\frac{s_{j_k}}{2} \frac{\partial}{\partial \beta_{j_k}} \sum_{i=1}^{n} (y_i - x_i^T \beta)^2 \Big|_{\beta = \hat{\beta}(\hat{C}_k)}. \tag{12}$$

Define $\theta(X_{j_k}, Z_k)$ as the angle between the vector X_{j_k} and Z_k. Since X_{j_k} is standardized, we have

$$\cos\{\theta(X_{j_k}, Z_k)\} = \frac{\|X^T Z_k\|_\infty}{\|Z_k\|_2} = \frac{\hat{C}_k}{\|Z_k\|_2}. \tag{13}$$

In general, $|\cos\{\theta(X_{j_k}, Z_k)\}|$, $k = 1, 2, 3, \ldots$, diminish stochastically. LARS solution path ends at a predetermined step or when the angle $\theta(X_{j_k}, Z_k)$ is very close to $\frac{\pi}{2}$, i.e., the remaining variable is almost orthogonal to the current residual.

Lemma 1 *For $A_{M_k} \geq 1$, the sequence $|\cos\{\theta(X_{j_k}, Z_k)\}|$, $k = 1, 2, \ldots, n - 1$, is non-increasing along the LARS solution path.*

Proof For simplicity, we use θ_k to denote $\theta(X_{j_k}, Z_k)$.

Note that $\hat{C}_k$ declines with k increases (Efron et al. 2004). Showing $1 \geq \frac{\hat{C}_1}{\|Z_1\|_2} \geq \frac{\hat{C}_2}{\|Z_2\|_2} \geq \cdots$ is equivalent to show $\frac{\hat{C}_k}{\hat{C}_{k+1}} \geq \frac{\|Z_k\|_2}{\|Z_{k+1}\|_2} \geq 1$, for $k = 1, 2, \ldots$.

By Eq. (9), $Z_k - Z_{k+1} = \hat{\gamma}_k u_{M_k}$. Hence, $\hat{\gamma}_k^2 = (Z_k - Z_{k+1})^T (Z_k - Z_{k+1})$, for $k = 1, 2, \ldots$.

From Eq. (5), (8), (9), and (12), we obtain

$$\hat{C}_k - \hat{C}_{k+1} = \hat{\gamma}_k A_k \geq \hat{\gamma}_k = \|Z_k - Z_{k+1}\|_2 \geq \|Z_k\|_2 - \|Z_{k+1}\|_2.$$

The last inequality is based on the triangle inequalities. We can obtain $\frac{\hat{C}_k}{\hat{C}_{k+1}} \geq \frac{\|Z_k\|_2}{\|Z_{k+1}\|_2}$, that is, $|\cos(\theta_k)| \geq |\cos(\theta_{k+1})|$, for $k = 1, 2, \ldots, n - 1$.

Note that in the traditional linear regression model with intercept, $(1/A_{M_k})^2$ is the first element of the diagonal of hat matrix, which is always bounded by $\frac{1}{n}$ and 1. $\square$

Lemma 2 *For $Z(\neq 0) \in \mathbb{R}^n$, the following events are equivalent:*

$$\{\|Z_{k+1}\|_2 \cos\theta_{k+1} \leq \|Z_k\|_2 \cos\theta_k \leq \|Z_{k-1}\|_2 \cos\theta_{k-1}\} = \{\theta_{k-1} \leq \theta_k \leq \theta_{k+1}\}.$$

Proof The event in the left hand is equivalent to $\{\hat{C}_{k+1} \leq \hat{C}_k \leq \hat{C}_{k-1}\}$, for $k = 2, 3, \ldots$, which has the monotone property as shown in Efron et al. (2004). The monotonicity of θ's and the one-to-one correspondence of $\hat{C}_k$ and θ_k, $k = 2, 3, \ldots$ have been verified in Lemma 1. Hence, the above events are equivalent.

Recall in the linear regression model (1), negligible or zero value of residual $e_i = y_i - \mathbf{x}_i^T \hat{\boldsymbol{\beta}}$ shows a good prediction. In the LARS context, the absolute value of the corresponding angle at each knot is bounded by $\frac{\pi}{2}$, and no more predictor will enter the model once the angle is "big" enough. We consider the angle close to $\frac{\pi}{2}$ to be "big" enough.

We can make inference using the angle by assuming the angles follow a (truncated) cosine distribution. We connect the angle θ_k of each LARS solution path to the incremental null hypothesis that measures whether M_k statistically surpasses M_{k-1} or not. The limiting distribution of the maximum angle can be used to do an efficient and robust significance test for each predictor variable.

We propose a truncated cosine distribution in a data-driven fashion. Let $\theta_{(1)}$ and $\theta_{(n)}$ be the minimum and maximum order statistics of θ's, respectively. Under the domain of $[\theta_{(1)}, \theta_{(n)}]$, we defined the following (truncated) cosine distribution with the density function:

$$f(\theta) = \begin{cases} \dfrac{1}{2b} \cos\left(\dfrac{\theta - a}{b}\right) & \text{if } \theta_{(1)} \leq \theta \leq \theta_{(n)}, \\[4mm] 0 & \text{otherwise,} \end{cases} \tag{14}$$

where the location parameter $a = (\theta_{(1)} + \theta_{(n)})/2$ and the scale parameter $b = (\theta_{(n)} - \theta_{(1)})/\pi$.

Its cumulative density function (CDF) is given by

$$F(\theta) = \begin{cases} 0 & \text{if } \theta < \theta_{(1)}, \\[3mm] \sin^2\left(\dfrac{\theta - a}{2b} + \dfrac{\pi}{4}\right) & \text{if } \theta_{(1)} \leq \theta \leq \theta_{(n)}, \\[3mm] 1 & \text{if } \theta > \theta_{(n)}. \end{cases} \tag{15}$$

This CDF, $F(\theta)$, of cosine distribution can be used to do hypotheses testing of whether "$\mathcal{M}_k$ improves over $\mathcal{M}_{k-1}$" by the following theorem.

Theorem 1 *Assume that the covariate vectors $\mathbf{X}_j$'s, $j = 1, \ldots, p$, are linearly independent in the LARS solution path. Let $\theta_{(j)}$, $j = 1, \ldots, n$, be the corresponding angle at each knot $\hat{C}_j$ in the first n steps. a and b are defined in Eq. (14). If Lemma 1 and 2 hold:*

$$\frac{n}{2b^2}\left(\frac{\pi}{2} - \theta_{(n)}\right)^2 \xrightarrow{d} \chi_2^2 \text{ as } n \to \infty, \tag{16}$$

where χ_2^2 denotes a chi-square random variable with $df = 2$.

Proof We know that $\theta_{(j)}$'s, $j = 1, \ldots, n$, are monotone increasing. Hence, $\theta_{(1)}$ and $\theta_{(n)}$ can be considered as the minimum and maximum order statistics of θ's. As the dimension increases, $\frac{\pi}{2} - \theta_{(n)}$ will diminish stochastically.

Let $\tilde{\theta}_n = \frac{n}{2b^2}(\frac{\pi}{2} - \theta_{(n)})^2$. From the CDF of the cosine distribution Eq. (15) and the basic trigonometric formula, the distribution of $\tilde{\theta}_n$ can be derived as follows:

$$\begin{aligned} P(\tilde{\theta}_n \leq g) &= P\left\{\frac{n}{2b^2}\left(\frac{\pi}{2} - \theta_{(n)}\right)^2 \leq g\right\} \\[3mm] &= P\left\{\theta_{(n)} \geq \frac{\pi}{2} - b \cdot \left(\frac{2g}{n}\right)^{1/2}\right\} \\[3mm] &= 1 - \sin^{2n}\left[\frac{\frac{\pi}{2} - b \cdot \left(\frac{2g}{n}\right)^{1/2} - a}{2b} + \frac{\pi}{4}\right] \end{aligned}$$

$$= 1 - \cos^{2n} \left[\frac{1}{2} \left(\frac{2g}{n} \right)^{1/2} + \frac{\pi}{4} - \frac{\pi}{4b} + \frac{a}{2b} \right], \text{ over } 0 \le g \le \frac{n\pi^2}{8b^2}.$$

Therefore, the limiting distribution of $\tilde{\theta}_n$ is obtained as

$$\lim_{n \to \infty} P(\tilde{\theta}_n \le g) = 1 - \lim_{n \to \infty} \cos^{2n} \left[\frac{1}{2} \left(\frac{2g}{n} \right)^{1/2} + \frac{\pi}{4} - \frac{\pi}{4b} + \frac{a}{2b} \right]$$

$$\approx 1 - e^{-g/2}, \ g \ge 0,$$

since $\cos^{2n} \left[\frac{1}{2b} (\frac{2g}{n})^{1/2} + \frac{\pi}{4} - \frac{\pi}{4b} + \frac{a}{2b} \right] \approx (1 - \frac{g}{4n})^{2n} = e^{-g/2}$ as $n \to \infty$.

Hence, $\tilde{\theta}_n \overset{d}{\to} \chi_2^2$.

The limiting distribution of $\tilde{\theta}_n$ determines if the corresponding angle at knot $\hat{C}_k$ is "big" enough. A sequence of p-values can be obtained by using the above property $P(\chi_2^2 > \tilde{\theta}_j)$, $j = 1, \ldots, n$.

2.2 Selection Criteria

Definition 1 (Family of "Accumulation Tests," Li & Barber, 2017) Let $\mathcal{M}_m$ be the model that includes the first m entries. For an integer $k \in \{1, \ldots, m\}$, a sequence of null hypotheses, H_j, $j = 1, 2, \ldots, k$, measures whether model $\mathcal{M}_j$ statistically surpasses $\mathcal{M}_{j-1}$ or not. Suppose there is a sequence of uniformly distributed p-values, $p_1, p_2, \ldots, p_k \in [0, 1]$ corresponding to the hypotheses H_j. For a given function $\phi : [0, 1] \mapsto [0, \infty)$ satisfying $\int_{t=0}^{1} \phi(t) dt = 1$, where ϕ is termed "accumulation function," the "accumulation tests" determine the stopping point $\hat{k}$ to control FDR at level α

$$\hat{k}_\phi = \max \left\{ k \in \{1, \ldots, m\} : \frac{1}{k} \sum_{j=1}^{k} \phi(p_j) \le \alpha \right\}. \tag{17}$$

We suggest using $\phi(x) = \frac{x}{\sqrt{1-x^2}}$ to choose the stopping point $\hat{k}_\phi$. Testing the hypothesis H_0 : the jth angle is the maximum one that is equivalent to testing whether the current model is adequate along the LARS solution path. We reject all hypotheses up to $\hat{k}_\phi$ to obtain the final model.

3 Numerical Studies

A few related R packages have been available in the R community since 2015. The most important packages are **PoSI** (Berk et al. 2013), **covTest** (Lockhart et al. 2014), and **selectiveInference** (Lee et al. 2016). Among them, packages **PoSI** and **covTest** cannot handle the high-dimensional case of "small n and large p." The functions in **selectiveInference** incorporated the methods from Lockhart et al. (2014), Lee et al. (2016), G'Sell et al. (2016). We term it *LARS-sI* for the methods from **selectiveInference** in the LARS context. We assess the performance of the proposed cosine post-selection inference (termed *cosine PoSI*) method by extensive simulation studies and compare the results with those from *LARS-sI*. The function $\phi = \frac{x}{\sqrt{1-x^2}}$ is used to determine the stop point along the LARS solution path, and the test significance level is set to be 0.01. The package **selectiveInference** uses the *ForwardStop* (G'Sell et al. 2016) to determine the stop point with $\phi(x) = \log(\frac{1}{1-x})$, which is a special case of the *accumulation test*. The selected model size and the selection accuracy of the selection are calculated by the averaged values of a certain number of replications and are denoted as $E(|\mathcal{M}_s|)$ and $P(\mathcal{T} \subset \mathcal{M}_s)$, respectively, where $\mathcal{T}$ is the set of all "true" variables and $\mathcal{M}_s$ is the set of selected variables.

In Theorem 1, the covariate vectors are assumed to be independent. We would like to assess the robustness of the proposed method against this assumption. In general, a strong correlation among the predictors creates difficulty in high-dimensional variable screening/selection. We will specifically evaluate the performance of the proposed method in different degrees of correlation among the predictors.

3.1 Simulation Studies

To assess the performance of the proposed method, we examine two scenarios. In the first scenario, compound symmetry structure of Σ's is used to assess whether the proposed method can overcome issues associated with strong correlation among predictors. In the second scenario, auto-regressive correlation structure of Σ's is used to show that the proposed method is capable of getting parsimonious models. 100 replications of simulation are run for each scenario.

3.1.1 Scenario I: Compound Symmetry Structure of Σ

For the first scenario, we use model (1) with true $\boldsymbol{\beta} = (5, 5, 5, 0, \ldots, 0)^T$. In this model, $\mathbf{X}_1, \ldots, \mathbf{X}_p$ are the p predictors and $\boldsymbol{\epsilon} \sim N(\mathbf{0}, \sigma^2 \mathbf{I}_n)$ is the noise that is independent of the predictors. In this simulation, a sample of $(X_1, \ldots, X_p)$ with size n was drawn from a multivariate normal distribution $N(\mathbf{0}, \Sigma)$ with covariance matrix $\Sigma = (1-\rho)I_p + \rho \mathbf{1}\mathbf{1}^T$, where $\mathbf{1} = (1, \ldots, 1)^T$. 16 settings of the parameter combinations are generated by using $n = 100$ or 200, $p = 100$ or 1000, $\rho =$

Table 1 Selected model size and selection accuracy for Scenario I

n	Method	Result	p = 100				p = 1000			
			$\rho=0$	$\rho = 0.1$	$\rho = 0.5$	$\rho = 0.9$	$\rho=0$	$\rho = 0.1$	$\rho = 0.5$	$\rho = 0.9$
100	cosine PoSI	$E(|\mathcal{M}_s|)$	3.05	3.17	7.77	11.35	3.23	4.83	16.24	23.90
		$P(\mathcal{T} \subset \mathcal{M}_s)$	1.00	1.00	1.00	1.00	1.00	1.00	1.00	1.00
	LARS-sI	$E(|\mathcal{M}_s|)$	1.00	1.04	1.02	1.00	1.02	1.00	1.00	1.00
		$P(\mathcal{T} \subset \mathcal{M}_s)$	0.00	0.00	0.01	0.00	0.00	0.00	0.00	0.00
200	cosine PoSI	$E(|\mathcal{M}_s|)$	3.00	3.00	5.68	10.02	3.00	3.05	10.98	19.94
		$P(\mathcal{T} \subset \mathcal{M}_s)$	1.00	1.00	1.00	1.00	1.00	1.00	1.00	1.00
	LARS-sI	$E(|\mathcal{M}_s|)$	2.94	3.00	3.00	2.96	1.04	1.04	1.00	1.00
		$P(\mathcal{T} \subset \mathcal{M}_s)$	0.93	0.99	0.98	0.98	0.01	0.00	0.00	0.00

0, 0.1, 0.5, or 0.9, respectively. This scenario follows Example I in Fan and Lv (2008) with a fixed $\sigma^2 = 1$.

Table 1 reports the average model sizes and percentage of all the true predictors included in the selected models. It shows that the proposed *cosine PoSI* method works perfectly for the cases of $n = 200$, $p = 100, 1000$, and $\rho = 0$ (independent predictor variables) and works very well for the cases of $n = 100$, $p = 100, 1000$, and $\rho = 0$. The selected model size increases as the value of ρ increases, but the increments are very small. The selection accuracy is perfect for all the cases, which means the selected final model always contains the entire set of true covariates (with non-zero coefficients). The competitor *LARS-sI* also works very well for the low-dimensional case of $n > p$ ($n = 200$, $p = 100$) with an over 90% selection accuracy, but for the high-dimensional cases $p \geq n$, *LARS-sI* is very conservative by only keeping the "strongest" (the first one) variable in the model.

3.1.2 Scenario II: Auto-Regressive Correlation

In this scenario, we use model (1) with $\boldsymbol{\beta} = (3, 1.5, 0, 0, 2, 0, \ldots, 0)^T$. The predictors $\mathbf{X}_1, \ldots, \mathbf{X}_p$ and the noise ϵ are generated the same as in the first scenario, but having different covariance matrices for the predictors. The covariance matrix Σ has entries $\sigma_{ii} = 1$, $i = 1, \ldots, p$ and $\sigma_{ij} = \rho^{|i-j|}$, $i \neq j$. This example is modified from Example 1 of Tibshirani (1996) with ρ being set at $0, 0.5, 0.7$, or 0.9.

The average model sizes and percentage of all the true predictors included in the selected models are reported in Table 2. We see the same pattern as in the first scenario that the proposed post-selection method always selects the true model with an accuracy rate of 100%, even when the predictors are highly correlated as with $\rho = 0.9$, with a small increment of model size. The selected model size increases as the value of ρ increases. The competitor *LARS-sI* works fine for the low-dimensional case ($n > p$) with a bit low accuracy between 50 and 80%. Since it always misses some predictors by only keeping one predictor in the final model for high-dimensional cases ($n < p$), the accuracy is zero.

Table 2 Selected model size and selection accuracy for Scenario II

n	Method	Result	$p = 100$				$p = 1000$			
			$\rho = 0$	$\rho = 0.5$	$\rho = 0.7$	$\rho = 0.9$	$\rho = 0$	$\rho = 0.5$	$\rho = 0.7$	$\rho = 0.9$
100	cosine PoSI	$E(|\mathcal{M}_S|)$	3.03	3.15	3.51	4.24	3.23	3.33	3.79	4.71
		$P(\mathcal{T} \subset \mathcal{M}_S)$	1.00	1.00	1.00	1.00	1.00	1.00	1.00	1.00
	LARS-sI	$E(|\mathcal{M}_S|)$	1.12	1.04	1.00	1.00	1.02	1.00	1.00	1.00
		$P(\mathcal{T} \subset \mathcal{M}_S)$	0.01	0.00	0.00	0.00	0.00	0.00	0.00	0.00
200	cosine PoSI	$E(|\mathcal{M}_S|)$	3.00	3.04	3.39	4.10	3.00	3.04	3.39	4.01
		$P(\mathcal{T} \subset \mathcal{M}_S)$	1.00	1.00	1.00	1.00	1.00	1.00	1.00	1.00
	LARS-sI	$E(|\mathcal{M}_S|)$	2.74	2.73	2.77	2.37	1.00	1.00	1.00	1.00
		$P(\mathcal{T} \subset \mathcal{M}_S)$	0.76	0.80	0.82	0.46	0.00	0.00	0.00	0.00

3.2 A Real-Data Application

We apply the proposed method on the data reported in Scheetz et al. (2006) to illustrate the usage of the proposed method. In this chapter, $F1$ rats were intercrossed, and the eye tissues from 120 twelve-week-old male $F2$ offspring rates were obtained. The microarray technique is then used to obtain the gene expressions of those eye tissues from the rats for over 31042 genes. Among those genes, one gene labeled "$TRIM32$" was recently found causing the Bardet–Biedl syndrome, and it is believed to be linked with a small number of other genes. We are interested in finding those genes that are possibly linked to the "$TRIM32$" using the gene expression data.

A subset of the microarray study can be found in the R package **flare**. The dataset contains two parts:

(1) The gene expression data of 200 genes for the 120 rats are recorded in **X**—an 120 × 200 matrix.
(2) The gene expression data of the gene "$TRIM32$" for the 120 rats are recorded in a vector **Y**.

The relationship of the gene expression of "$TRIM32$" and other genes is postulated using model (1). The Leave-One-Out (LOO) cross-validation technique is used to estimate the model accuracy in the selection process, measured by the total square error $\sum_{i=1}^{n}(Y_i - \hat{Y}_i)^2$. We invoke the methods to obtain the models using the post-selection inference procedures on the training set, then obtain the OLS estimator of those variables via a linear regression, and use the obtained model to predict the gene expression of the "$TRIM32$" gene that was left out. Table 3 reports the mean and the standard deviation (SD) of the total square errors for prediction and the mean and median of model sizes from the n training sets. It can be seen that both the mean total squared error and the standard error from the proposed *cosine PoSI* are much smaller than those from *LARS-sI*, which justifies that the proposed *cosine PoSI* method keeps the useful genes in the post-selection inference procedure, while

Table 3 Data analysis of eye microarray data (LOOCV)

Method	Mean square errors	SD square errors	Model size (mean)	Model size (median)
cosine PoSI	0.3548	0.3523	27.6750	28.0000
LARS-sI	15.5772	1.5019	1.0000	1.0000

Table 4 Final models for eye microarray full data

Method	Model Size	MSE	$Adjusted\ R^2$
cosine PoSI	29	0.0041	0.8009
LARS-sI	1	0.0087	0.5776

LARS sI is too conservative and most likely screens out many relevant genes. The *LARS sI* still only contains the very first entered variable in analysis.

We then apply the *cosine PoSI* method, in contrast to the *LARS-sI* approach, to obtain a final model by applying them to the full data to first select relevant genes and then obtain the final model by estimating the coefficients in the linear regression. Table 4 reports the selected final model size, the mean square error (MSE), and adjusted R^2 for the two approaches. We see the proposed *cosine PoSI* method contains a larger model than that from the *LARS-sI* procedure. The final model from *cosine PoSI* method keeps 29 genes (ID in package **flare**): {153, 55, 99, 87, 42, 85, 180, 177, 109, 90, 199, 112, 36, 185, 62, 136, 200, 155, 187, 146, 188, 134, 141, 172, 127, 11, 54, 181, 164}, while the final model from the *LARS-sI* procedure is too conservative and only includes the first gene. The adjusted R^2 from the proposed model is 0.8009, while it is only 0.5776, which means some useful genes are screened out in the *LARS-sI*. We also note that our own LARS code generates the same solution path as that of the function "lar" in the package **selectiveInference**.

4   Discussion

When using a traditional linear regression model, a fixed hypothesis test is conducted to observe which variables are significant at significance level α and report $(1 - \alpha)$ confidence intervals for the significant variables. The randomness aspect in the high-dimensional context brought confliction between model selection and the inference. In high-dimensional data analysis, the data-driven selection procedure is critically important, and the model should be selected to be adaptive to the data instead of devising a model before collecting data. Hence, a sequence of random hypothesis tests is required to do post-selection inference (also termed selective inference). In this chapter, we proposed a *cosine PoSI* procedure to select variables via least angle regression path, which is a novel post-selection inference method based on a cosine distribution. We discuss the geometric aspect in LARS and apply the *cosine PoSI* in the LARS solution path to make inference regarding the variables to be included in the final model. Comparing with the methods in R package **selectiveInference**, the proposed *cosine PoSI* performs better in the combination of "small n and large p" scenarios than that of the methods in **selectiveInference**. The proposed *cosine PoSI* method has the advantage in providing a parsimony model for independent predictor variables and is robust with predictor "multicollinearity."

Lee et al. (2016)'s "Polyhedral selection" draws inferences about $\eta^T \mu$ conditional on the event $\{M\mathbf{y} \le b\}$ using a truncated normal distribution. $\eta^T \mathbf{y}$ denotes the parameter estimator constrained to a variable in $\mathcal{M}$ and $\eta^T \mathbf{y} \sim N(\eta^T \mu, \eta^T \Sigma \eta)$. Let $\gamma = \Sigma \eta (\eta^T \Sigma \eta)^{-1}$, $\mathbf{d} = \mathbf{y} - \gamma \eta^T \mathbf{y}$, $\mathcal{V}^-(\mathbf{d}) = \max\limits_{j:(M\gamma)_j<0} \frac{b_j-(M\mathbf{d})_j}{(M\gamma)_j}$, $\mathcal{V}^+(\mathbf{d}) = \min\limits_{j:(M\gamma)_j>0} \frac{b_j-(M\mathbf{d})_j}{(M\gamma)_j}$, $\mathcal{V}^0(\mathbf{d}) = \min\limits_{j:(M\gamma)_j=0} \{b_j - (M\mathbf{d})_j\}$ and $\mathcal{V}^-, \mathcal{V}^+, \mathcal{V}^0$ are independent of $\eta^T \mathbf{y}$, $\{M\mathbf{y} \le b\}$ can be rewritten in terms of $\eta^T \mathbf{y}$ and $\mathbf{d}$ as follows:

$$\{M\mathbf{y} \le b\} = \{\mathcal{V}^-(\mathbf{d}) \le \eta^T \mathbf{Y} \le \mathcal{V}^+(\mathbf{d}), \mathcal{V}^0 \ge 0\}, \tag{18}$$

with $e_j^T(\mathbf{X}_{\mathcal{M}}^T \mathbf{X}_{\mathcal{M}})^{-1} \mathbf{X}_{\mathcal{M}}^T \mu = \eta^T \mu$. Hence, $\eta^T \mathbf{y} | \{M\mathbf{y} \le b, \mathbf{d} = \mathbf{d}_0\}$ is a truncated normal between $\mathcal{V}^-(\mathbf{d}_0)$ and $\mathcal{V}^-(\mathbf{d}_0)$ where $\mathbf{d}_0$ is a fixed value of $\mathbf{d}$ and its CDF follows about a standard uniform distribution.

Inspired by the "Polyhedral selection," another cosine distribution can also be constructed to approximate normal distribution based on the angles. The density function and cumulative density function are given by

$$f(\theta) = \begin{cases} \dfrac{1}{2\pi}(1 + \cos\theta) & \text{if } |\theta| \le \pi, \\ \\ 0 & \text{otherwise.} \end{cases} \tag{19}$$

$$F(\theta) = \begin{cases} 0 & \text{if } \theta < -\pi, \\ \dfrac{1}{2\pi}(\pi + \theta + \sin\theta) & \text{if } |\theta| \le \pi, \\ 1 & \text{if } \theta > \pi. \end{cases} \tag{20}$$

We conjecture that some statistics based on this cosine distribution are able to measure how much improvement the kth entering predictor variable X_{j_k} made over the interval $(\hat{C}_{k-1}, \hat{C}_{k+1})$. Then the predictor variables having negligible contribution on this interval can be screened out. We may also combine the results with other post-selection inference methods to refine the candidate predictor selection using LARS in high-dimensional data analysis.

Acknowledgments This research was partially supported by the Natural Sciences and Engineering Research Council of Canada (NSERC).

References

Berk, R., Brown, L., Buja, A., Zhang, K., & Zhao, L. (2013). Valid post-selection inference. *Annals of Statistics, 41*, 802–837.

Efron, B., Hastie, T., Johnstone, I., & Tibshirani, R. (2004). Least angle regression. *Annals of Statistics, 32*, 407–499.

Fan, J., & Lv, J. (2008). Sure independence screening for ultrahigh dimensional feature space. *Journal of the Royal Statistical Society: Series B (Statistical Methodology), 70*, 849–911.

Fan, J., & Lv, J. (2010). A selective overview of variable selection in high dimensional feature space. *Statistica Sinica, 20*, 101–148.

G'Sell, M. G., Wager, S., Chouldechova, A., & Tibshirani, R. (2016). Sequential selection procedures and false discovery rate control. *Journal of the Royal Statistical Society: Series B (Statistical Methodology), 78*, 423–444.

Lee, J. D., Sun, D. L., Sun, Y., & Taylor, J. E. (2016). Exact post-selection inference, with application to the lasso. *Annals of Statistics, 44*, 907–927.

Li, A., & Barber, R. F. (2017). Accumulation tests for FDR control in ordered hypothesis testing. *Journal of the American Statistical Association, 112*, 837–849.

Lockhart, R., Taylor, J., Tibshirani, R. J., & Tibshirani, R. (2014). A significance test for the lasso. *Annals of Statistics, 42*, 413–468.

Scheetz, T. E., Kim, K.-Y. A., Swiderski, R. E., Philp, A. R., Braun, T. A., Knudtson, K. L., Dorrance, A. M., DiBona, G. F., Huang, J., Casavant, T. L., Sheffield, V. C., & Stone, E. M. (2006). Regulation of gene expression in the mammalian eye and its relevance to eye disease. *Proceedings of the National Academy of Sciences, 103*, 14429–14434.

Tibshirani, R. (1996). Regression shrinkage and selection via the lasso. *Journal of the Royal Statistical Society. Series B (Methodological), 58*, 267–288.

Zhao, B., Liu, X., He, W., & Yi, G. Y. (2021). Dynamic tilted current correlation for high-dimensional variable screening. *Journal of Multivariate Analysis, 182*, 104693.

Minimum Wasserstein Distance Estimator Under Finite Location-Scale Mixtures

Qiong Zhang and Jiahua Chen

Abstract When a population exhibits heterogeneity, we often model it via a finite mixture: decompose it into several different but homogeneous subpopulations. Contemporary practice favors learning the mixtures by maximizing the likelihood for statistical efficiency and the convenient EM algorithm for numerical computation. Yet the maximum likelihood estimate (MLE) is not well defined for finite location-scale mixture in general. We hence investigate feasible alternatives to MLE such as minimum distance estimators. Recently, the Wasserstein distance has drawn increased attention in the machine learning community. It has intuitive geometric interpretation and is successfully employed in many new applications. Do we gain anything by learning finite location-scale mixtures via a minimum Wasserstein distance estimator (MWDE)? This chapter investigates this possibility in several respects. We find that the MWDE is consistent and derive a numerical solution under finite location-scale mixtures. We study its robustness against outliers and mild model mis-specifications. Our moderate scaled simulation study shows the MWDE suffers some efficiency loss against a penalized version of MLE in general without noticeable gain in robustness. We reaffirm the general superiority of the likelihood-based learning strategies even for the non-regular finite location-scale mixtures.

Keywords Finite mixture model · Location scale family · Minimum distance estimator · Penalized maximum likelihood estimator · Wasserstein distance.

1 Introduction

Let $\mathcal{F} = \{f(\cdot|\boldsymbol{\theta}) : \boldsymbol{\theta} \in \Theta\}$ be a parametric distribution family with density function $f(\cdot|\boldsymbol{\theta})$ with respect to some σ-finite measure. Denote by $G = \sum_{k=1}^{K} w_k\{\boldsymbol{\theta}_k\}$ a

Q. Zhang · J. Chen (✉)
Department of Statistics, University of British Columbia, Vancouver, BC, Canada
e-mail: qiong.zhang@stat.ubc.ca; jhchen@stat.ubc.ca

© The Author(s), under exclusive license to Springer Nature Switzerland AG 2022
W. He et al. (eds.), *Advances and Innovations in Statistics and Data Science*, ICSA
Book Series in Statistics, https://doi.org/10.1007/978-3-031-08329-7_4

69

distribution assigning probability w_k on $\boldsymbol{\theta}_k \in \Theta$. A distribution with the following density function:

$$f(x|G) = \int f(x|\boldsymbol{\theta})dG(\boldsymbol{\theta}) = \sum_{k=1}^{K} w_k f(x|\boldsymbol{\theta}_k)$$

is called a finite $\mathcal{F}$ mixture. We call $f(x|\boldsymbol{\theta})$ the subpopulation density function, $\boldsymbol{\theta}$ the subpopulation parameter, and w_k the mixing weight of the kth subpopulation. We use $F(x|\boldsymbol{\theta})$ and $F(x|G)$ for the cumulative distribution functions (CDF) of $f(x|\boldsymbol{\theta})$ and $f(x|G)$, respectively. Let

$$\mathbb{G}_K = \Big\{ G : G = \sum_{k=1}^{K} w_k\{\boldsymbol{\theta}_k\}, 0 \leq w_k \leq 1, \sum_{k=1}^{K} w_k = 1, \boldsymbol{\theta}_k \in \Theta \Big\}$$

be a space of mixing distributions with at most K support points. A mixture distribution of (exactly) order K has its mixing distribution G being a member of $\mathbb{G}_K - \mathbb{G}_{K-1}$.

We study the problem of learning the mixing distribution G given a set of independent and identically distributed (IID) observations $\mathcal{X} = \{x_1, x_2, \ldots, x_N\}$ from a mixture $f(x|G)$. Throughout the paper, we assume the order of G is known and $\mathcal{F}$ is a known location-scale family. That is,

$$f(x|\boldsymbol{\theta}) = \frac{1}{\sigma} f_0\Big(\frac{x-\mu}{\sigma}\Big)$$

for some probability density function $f_0(x)$ with $x \in \mathbb{R}$ with respect to Lebesgue measure where $\boldsymbol{\theta} = (\mu, \sigma)$ with $\Theta = \{\mathbb{R} \times \mathbb{R}^+\}$.

Finite mixture models provide a natural representation of heterogeneous population that is believed to be composed of several homogeneous subpopulations (Pearson 1894; Schork et al. 1996). They are also useful for approximating distributions with unknown shapes that are particularly relevant in image generation (Kolouri et al. 2018), image segmentation (Farnoosh & Zarpak 2008), object tracking (Santosh et al. 2013), and signal processing (Plataniotis & Hatzinak 2000).

In statistics, the most fundamental task is to learn the unknown parameters. In early days, the method of moments was the choice for its ease of computation (Pearson 1894) under finite mixture models. Nowadays, the maximum likelihood estimate (MLE) is the first choice due to its statistical efficiency and the availability of an easy-to-use EM algorithm. Under a finite location-scale mixture model, the log-likelihood function of G is given by

$$\ell_N(G|\mathcal{X}) = \sum_{n=1}^{N} \log f(x_n|G) = \sum_{n=1}^{N} \log \Big\{ \sum_{k=1}^{K} \frac{w_k}{\sigma_k} f_0\Big(\frac{x_n - \mu_k}{\sigma_k}\Big) \Big\}. \tag{1}$$

At an arbitrary mixing distribution $G_\epsilon = 0.5\{(x_1, \epsilon)\} + 0.5\{(0, 1)\}$, we have $\ell_N(G_\epsilon | \mathcal{X}) \to \infty$ as $\epsilon \to 0$. Hence, the MLE of G is not well defined or is ill defined. Various remedies, such as penalized maximum likelihood estimate (pMLE), have been proposed to overcome this obstacle (Chen et al. 2008; Chen & Tan 2009). At the same time, MLE can be thought of a special minimum distance estimator. It minimizes a specific Kullback–Leibler divergence between the empirical distribution and the assumed model $\mathcal{F}$. Other divergences and distances have been investigated in the literature as in Choi (1969); Yakowitz (1969); Woodward et al. (1984); Clarke and Heathcote (1994); Cutler and Cordero-Brana (1996); Deely and Kruse (1968). Recently, the Wasserstein distance has drawn increased attention in machine learning community due to its intuitive interpretation and good geometric properties (Evans & Matsen 2012; Arjovsky et al. 2017). The Wasserstein distance-based estimator for learning finite mixture models is absent in the literature.

Are there any benefits to learn finite location-scale mixtures by the minimum Wasserstein distance estimator (MWDE)? This chapter answers this question from several angles. We find that the MWDE is consistent and derive a numerical solution under finite location-scale mixtures. We compare the robustness of the MWDE with pMLE in the presence of outliers and mild model mis-specifications. We conclude that the MWDE suffers some efficiency loss against pMLE in general without obvious gain in robustness. Through this chapter, we better understand the pros and cons of the MWDE under finite location-scale mixtures. We reaffirm the general superiority of the likelihood-based learning strategies even for the non-regular finite location-scale mixtures.

In the next section, we first introduce the Wasserstein distance and some of its properties. This is followed by a formal definition of the MWDE, a discussion of its existence, and consistency under finite location-scale mixtures. In Sect. 2.4, we give some algebraic results that are essential for computing 2-Wasserstein distance between the empirical distribution and the finite location-scale mixtures. We then develop a BFGS algorithm scheme for computing the MWDE of the mixing distribution. In addition, we briefly review the penalized likelihood approach and its numerical issues. In Sect. 3, we characterize the efficiency properties of the MWDE relative to pMLE in various circumstances via simulation. We also study their robustness when the data contains outliers, is contaminated, or when the model is mis-specified. We then apply both methods in an image segmentation example. We conclude the paper with a summary in Sect. 4.

2 Wasserstein Distance and the Minimum Distance Estimator

We introduce the Wasserstein distance and the minimum Wasserstein distance estimator in this section.

2.1 Wasserstein Distance

Wasserstein distance is a distance between probability measures. Let Ω be a Polish space endowed with a ground distance $D(\cdot, \cdot)$ and $\mathcal{P}(\Omega)$ the space of Borel probability measures on Ω. Let $\eta \in \mathcal{P}(\Omega)$ be a probability measure. If for some $p > 0$,

$$\int_\Omega D^p(x, x_0)\eta(dx) < \infty,$$

for some (and thus any) $x_0 \in \Omega$, we say η has finite pth moment. Denote by $\mathcal{P}_p(\Omega) \subset \mathcal{P}(\Omega)$ the space of probability measures with finite pth moment. For any $\eta, \nu \in \mathcal{P}(\Omega)$, we use $\Pi(\eta, \nu)$ to denote the space of the bivariate probability measures on $\Omega \times \Omega$ whose marginals are η and ν. Namely,

$$\Pi(\eta, \nu) = \{\pi \in \mathcal{P}(\Omega^2) : \int_\Omega \pi(x, dy) = \eta(x), \int_\Omega \pi(dx, y) = \nu(y)\}.$$

The p-Wasserstein distance is defined as follows.

Definition 1 (p-Wasserstein Distance) For any $\eta, \nu \in \mathcal{P}_p(\Omega)$ with $p \geq 1$, the pth Wasserstein distance between η and ν is

$$W_p(\eta, \nu) = \left\{ \inf_{\pi \in \Pi(\eta, \nu)} \int_{\Omega^2} D^p(x, y)\pi(dx, dy) \right\}^{1/p}.$$

Suppose X and Y are two random variables whose distributions are F and G and induced probability measures are η and ν. We regard the p-Wasserstein distance between η and ν and also the distance between random variables or distributions: $W_p(X, Y) = W_p(F, G) = W_p(\eta, \nu)$.

The p-Wasserstein distance is a distance on $\mathcal{P}_p(\Omega)$ as shown by Villani (2003, Theorem 7.3). For any $\eta, \nu, \xi \in \mathcal{P}_p(\Omega)$, it has the following properties:

1. Non-negativity: $W_p(\eta, \nu) \geq 0$ and $W_p(\eta, \nu) = 0$ if and only if $\eta = \nu$.
2. Symmetry: $W_p(\eta, \nu) = W_p(\nu, \eta)$.
3. Triangular inequality: $W_p(\eta, \nu) \leq W_p(\eta, \xi) + W_p(\xi, \nu)$.

The Wasserstein distance has many nice properties. Let us denote $\eta_n \xrightarrow{d} \eta$ for convergence in distribution or measure. Villani (2003, Theorem 7.1.2) shows that it has the following properties:

Property 1. For any $q \geq p \geq 1$, $W_q(\eta, \nu) \geq W_p(\eta, \nu)$.
Property 2. $W_p(\eta_n, \eta) \to 0$ as $n \to \infty$ if and only if both:

(i) $\eta_n \xrightarrow{d} \eta$.
(ii) $\int D^p(x, x_0)\eta_n(dx) \to \int D^p(x, x_0)\eta(dx)$ for some (and thus any) $x_0 \in \Omega$.

Computing the Wasserstein distance involves a challenging optimization problem in general but has a simple solution under a special case. Suppose Ω is the space of real numbers, $D(x, y) = |x - y|$, and F and G are univariate distributions. Let $F^{-1}(t) := \inf\{x : F(x) \geq t\}$ and $G^{-1}(t) := \inf\{x : G(x) \geq t\}$ for $t \in [0, 1]$ be their quantile functions. We can easily compute the Wasserstein distance based on the following property:

Property 3. $W_p(F, G) = \left\{ \int_0^1 |F^{-1}(t) - G^{-1}(t)|^p dt \right\}^{1/p}.$

2.2 Minimum Wasserstein Distance Estimator

Let $W_p(\cdot, \cdot)$ be the p-Wasserstein distance with ground distance $D(x, y) = |x - y|$ for univariate random variables. Let $\mathcal{X} = \{x_1, x_2, \ldots, x_N\}$ be a set of IID observations from finite location-scale mixture $f(x|G)$ of order K and $F_N(x) = N^{-1} \sum_{n=1}^N \mathbb{1}(x_n \leq x)$ be the empirical distribution. We introduce the MWDE of the mixing distribution G to be

$$\hat{G}_N^{\text{MWDE}} = \arg\inf_{G \in \mathbb{G}_K} W_p(F_N(\cdot), F(\cdot|G)) = \arg\inf_{G \in \mathbb{G}_K} W_p^p(F_N(\cdot), F(\cdot|G)). \tag{2}$$

As we pointed out earlier, the MLE is not well defined under finite location-scale mixtures. Is the MWDE well defined? We examine the existence or sensibility of the MWDE. We show that the MWDE exists when $f_0(\cdot)$ satisfies certain conditions.

Assume that $f_0(0) > 0$, $f_0(x)$ is bounded, continuous, and has finite pth moment. Under these conditions, we can see

$$0 \leq W_p(F_N(\cdot), F(\cdot|G)) < \infty$$

for any $G \in \mathbb{G}_K$. When $N \leq K$, the solution to (2) merits special attention. Let $G_\epsilon = \sum_{n=1}^N (1/N)\{(x_n, \epsilon)\}$ be a mixing distribution assigning probability $1/N$ on $\boldsymbol{\theta}_n = (x_n, \epsilon)$. When $\epsilon \to 0$, each subpopulation in the mixture $f(x|G_\epsilon)$ degenerates to a point mass at x_n. Hence, as $\epsilon \to 0$,

$$W_p(F_N(\cdot), F(\cdot|G_\epsilon)) \to 0.$$

Since none of $G \in \mathbb{G}_K$ has zero distance from $F_N(\cdot)$, the MWDE does not exist unless we expand $\mathbb{G}_K$ to include $G_0 = \sum_{n=1}^N (1/N)\{(x_n, 0)\} = \lim G_\epsilon$. To remove this technical artifact, in the MWDE definition, we expand the space of σ to $[0, \infty)$. We denote by $F(\cdot|(\theta_0, 0))$ a distribution with point mass at $x = \theta_0$. With this expansion, G_0 is the MWDE when $N \leq K$.

Let $\delta = \inf\{W_p(F_N(\cdot), F(\cdot|G)) : G \in \mathbb{G}_K\}$. Clearly, $0 \leq \delta < \infty$. By definition, there exists a sequence of mixing distributions $G_m \in \mathbb{G}_K$ such that $W_p(F_N(\cdot), F(\cdot|G_m)) \to \delta$ as $m \to \infty$. Suppose one mixing weight of G_m has limit 0. Removing this support point and rescaling, we get a new mixing distribution sequence, and it still satisfies $W_p(F_N(\cdot), F(\cdot|G_m)) \to \delta$. For this reason, we assume that its mixing weights have non-zero limits by selecting converging subsequence if necessary to ensure the limits exist. Further, when the mixing weights of G_m assume their limiting values while keeping subpopulation parameters the same, we still have $W_p(F_N(\cdot), F(\cdot|G_m)) \to \delta$ as $m \to \infty$. In the following discussion, we therefore discuss the sequence of mixing distributions whose mixing weights are fixed.

Suppose the first subpopulation of G_m has its scale parameter $\sigma_1 \to \infty$ as $m \to \infty$. With the boundedness assumption on $f_0(x)$, the mass of this subpopulation will spread thinly over entire $\mathbb{R}$ because $\sigma_1^{-1} f_0((x - \mu_1)/\sigma_1) \to 0$ uniformly. For any fixed finite interval, $[a, b]$, this thinning makes

$$F(b|\boldsymbol{\theta}_1) - F(a|\boldsymbol{\theta}_1) \to 0$$

as $m \to \infty$. It implies that for any given $t \in (0, 0.5)$, we have

$$|F^{-1}(t|\boldsymbol{\theta}_1)| + |F^{-1}(1 - t|\boldsymbol{\theta}_1)| \to \infty.$$

This further implies for any $t \in (0, w_1/2)$, we have

$$|F^{-1}(t|G_m)| + |F^{-1}(1 - t|G_m)| \to \infty$$

as $m \to \infty$. In comparison, the empirical quantile satisfies $x_{(1)} \le F_N^{-1}(t) \le x_{(N)}$ for any t. By Property 3 of $W_p(\cdot, \cdot)$, these lead to $W_p(F_N(\cdot), F(\cdot|G_m)) \to \infty$ as $m \to \infty$. This contradicts the assumption $W_p(F_N(\cdot), F(\cdot|G_m)) \to \delta$. Hence, $\sigma_1 \to \infty$ is not a possible scenario of G_m nor $\sigma_k \to \infty$ for any k.

Can a subpopulation of G_m instead have its location parameter $\mu \to \infty$? For definitiveness, let this subpopulation correspond to $\boldsymbol{\theta}_1$. Note that at least $w_1\{1 - F_0(0)\}$-sized probability mass of $F(x|G_m)$ is contained in the range $[\mu_1, \infty)$. Because of this, when $\mu_1 \to \infty$, we have $F^{-1}(1 - t|G_m) \to \infty$ for $t = w_1\{1 - F_0(0)\}/2$. Therefore, $W_p(F_N(\cdot), F(\cdot|G_m)) \to \infty$ by Property 3. This contradicts $W_p(F_N(\cdot), F(\cdot|G_m)) \to \delta < \infty$. Hence, $\mu_1 \to \infty$ is not a possible scenario of G_m either. For the same reason, we cannot have $\mu_k \to \pm\infty$ for any k.

After ruling out $\mu_k \to \pm\infty$ and $\sigma_k \to \infty$, we find G_m has a converging subsequence whose limit is a proper mixing distribution in $\mathbb{G}_K$. This limit is then an MWDE and the existence is verified.

The MWDE may not be unique, and the mixing distribution may lead to a mixture with degenerate subpopulations. We will show that the MWDE is consistent as the sample size goes to infinity. Thus, having degenerated subpopulations in the learned mixture is a mathematical artifact and also a sensible solution. In contrast, no matter how large the sample size becomes, there are always degenerated mixing distributions with unbounded likelihood values.

2.3   Consistency of MWDE

We consider the problem when $X = \{x_1, \ldots, x_N\}$ are IID observations from a finite location-scale mixture of order K. The true mixing distribution is denoted as G^*. Assume that $f_0(x)$ is bounded, continuous, and has finite pth moment. We say the location-scale mixture is identifiable if

$$F(x|G_1) = F(x|G_2)$$

for all x given $G_1, G_2 \in \mathbb{G}_K$ implies $G_1 = G_2$. We allow subpopulation scale $\sigma = 0$. The most commonly used finite location-scale mixtures, such as the normal mixture, are well known to be identifiable (Teicher 1961). Holzmann et al. (2004) give a sufficient condition for the identifiability of general finite location-scale mixtures. Let $\varphi(\cdot)$ be the characteristic function of $f_0(t)$. The finite location-scale mixture is identifiable if for any $\sigma_1 > \sigma_2 > 0$, $\lim_{t \to \infty} \varphi(\sigma_1 t)/\varphi(\sigma_2 t) = 0$.

We consider the MWDE based on p-Wasserstein distance with ground distance $D(x, y) = |x - y|$ for some $p \geq 1$. The MWDE under finite location-scale mixture model as defined in (2) is asymptotically consistent.

Theorem 1 *With the same conditions on the finite location-scale mixture and same notations above, we have the following conclusions:*

1. *For any sequence $G_m \in \mathbb{G}_K$ and $G^* \in \mathbb{G}_K$, $W_p(F(\cdot|G_m), F(\cdot|G^*)) \to 0$ implies $G_m \xrightarrow{d} G^*$ as $m \to \infty$.*
2. *The MWDE satisfies $W_p(F(\cdot|G^*), F(\cdot|\hat{G}_N^{MWDE})) \to 0$ as $N \to \infty$ almost surely.*
3. *The MWDE is consistent: $W_p(\hat{G}_N^{MWDE}, G^*) \to 0$ as $N \to \infty$ almost surely.*

Proof We present these three conclusions in the current order that is easy to understand. For the sake of proof, a different order is better. For ease presentation, we write $F^* = F(\cdot|G^*)$ and $\hat{G} = \hat{G}_N^{MWDE}$ in this proof.

We first prove the second conclusion. By the triangular inequality and the definition of the minimum distance estimator, we have

$$W_p(F^*, F(\cdot|\hat{G}_N)) \leq W_p(F_N, F^*) + W_p(F_N, F(\cdot|\hat{G}_N)) \leq 2W_p(F_N, F^*).$$

Note that F_N is the empirical distribution and F^* is the true distribution; we have $F_N(x) \to F^*(x)$ uniformly in x almost surely. At the same time, under the assumption that $F_0(x)$ has finite pth moment, $F^*(x)$ also has finite pth moment. The pth moment of $F_N(x)$ converges to that of $F^*(x)$ almost surely. Given the ground distance $D(x, y) = |x - y|$, the pth moment in Wasserstein distance sense is the usual moments in probability theory. By Property 2, we conclude $W_p(F_N, F(\cdot|G^*)) \to 0$ as both conditions there are satisfied.

Conclusion 3 is implied by Conclusions 1 and 2. With Conclusion 2 already established, we only need to prove Conclusion 1 to complete the whole proof. By Helly's lemma (Van der Vaart 2000, Lemma 2.5) again, G_m has a converging subsequence though the limit can be a subprobability measure. Without loss of generality, we assume that G_m itself converges with limit $\tilde{G}$. If $\tilde{G}$ is a subprobability measure, so would be $F(\cdot|\tilde{G})$. This will lead to

$$W_p(F(\cdot|G_m), F(\cdot|G^*)) \to W_p(F(\cdot|\tilde{G}), F(\cdot|G^*)) \neq 0,$$

which violates the theorem condition. If $\tilde{G}$ is a proper distribution in $\mathbb{G}_K$ and

$$W_p(F(\cdot|\tilde{G}), F(\cdot|G^*)) = 0,$$

then by identifiability condition, we have $\tilde{G} = G^*$. This implies $G_m \to G^*$ and completes the proof.   □

The multivariate normal mixture is another type of location-scale mixture. The above consistency result of MWDE can be easily extended to finite multivariate normal mixtures.

Theorem 2 *Consider the problem when $X = \{x_1, \ldots, x_N\}$ are IID observations from a finite multivariate normal mixture distribution of order K and $\hat{G}_N^{MWDE}$ is the minimum Wasserstein distance estimator defined by* (2). *Let the true mixing distribution be G^*. The MWDE is consistent: $W_p(\hat{G}_N^{MWDE}, G^*) \to 0$ as $N \to \infty$ almost surely.*

The rigorous proof is long though the conclusion is obvious. We offer a less formal proof based on several well-known probability theory results:

(I) A multivariate random variable sequence Y_n converges in distribution to Y if and only if $\mathbf{a}^\tau Y_n$ converges to $\mathbf{a}^\tau Y$ for any unit vector $\mathbf{a}$.

(II) If Y is multivariate normal if and only if $\mathbf{a}^\tau Y$ is normal for all $\mathbf{a}$.

(III) The normal distribution has finite moment of any order.

Let X_m be a random vector with distribution $F(\cdot|G_m)$ for some $G_m \in \mathbb{G}_K$, $m = 0, 1, 2, \ldots$, in a general mixture model setting. Suppose as $m \to \infty$, with the notation we introduced previously

$$W_p(X_m, X_0) \to 0.$$

Then for any unit vector $\mathbf{a}$, based on property 2 of the Wasserstein distance and the result (I), we can see that

$$W_p(\mathbf{a}^\tau X_m, \mathbf{a}^\tau X_0) \to 0.$$

Next, we apply this result to normal mixture so that $F(\cdot|G_m)$ becomes $\Phi(\cdot|G_m)$ that stands for a finite multivariate normal mixture with mixing distribution G_m. In this case, X_m is a random vector with distribution $\Phi(\cdot|G_m)$. Let $(\boldsymbol{\mu}_k, \Sigma_k)$ be generic subpopulation parameters. We can see that the distribution of $\mathbf{a}^\tau X_m$, $\Phi_{\mathbf{a}}(\cdot|G_m)$ is a finite normal mixture with subpopulation parameters $(\mathbf{a}^\tau \boldsymbol{\mu}_k, \mathbf{a}^\tau \Sigma_k \mathbf{a})$, and mixing weighs the same as those of G_m. Let the mixing distributions after projection be $G_{m,\mathbf{a}}$ and $G_{0,\mathbf{a}}$.

By the same argument in the proof of Theorem 1,

$$W_p(\Phi(\cdot|\hat{G}_N), \Phi(\cdot|G^*)) \to 0$$

almost surely as $N \to \infty$. This implies

$$W_p(\Phi_{\mathbf{a}}(\cdot|\hat{G}_N), \Phi_{\mathbf{a}}(\cdot|G^*)) \to 0$$

almost surely as $N \to \infty$ for any $\mathbf{a}$. Hence, by Conclusion 1 of Theorem 1, $\hat{G}_{N,\mathbf{a}} \xrightarrow{d} \hat{G}_{\mathbf{a}}^*$ almost surely for any unit vector $\mathbf{a}$. We therefore conclude the consistency result: $\hat{G}_N \xrightarrow{d} \hat{G}^*$ almost surely.

2.4 Numerical Solution to MWDE

Both in applications and in simulation experiments, we need an effective way to compute the MWDE. We develop an algorithm that leverages the explicit form of the Wasserstein distance between two measures on $\mathbb{R}$ for the numerical solution to the MWDE. The strategy works for any p-Wasserstein distance, but we only provide specifics for $p = 2$ as it is the most widely used.

Let Y be a random variable with distribution $f_0(\cdot)$. Denote the mean and variance of Y by $\mu_0 = \mathbb{E}(Y)$ and $\sigma_0^2 = \text{Var}(Y)$. Recall that $G = \sum_{k=1}^{K} w_k\{(\mu_k, \sigma_k)\}$. Let $x_{(1)} \leq x_{(2)} \leq \cdots \leq x_{(N)}$ be the order statistics, $\overline{x^2} = N^{-1}\sum_{n=1}^{N} x_n^2$, and $\xi_n = F^{-1}(n/N|G)$ be the (n/N)th quantile of the mixture for $n = 0, 1, \ldots, N$. Let

$$T(x) = \int_{-\infty}^{x} t f_0(t) dt$$

and define

$$\Delta F_{nk} = F_0\left(\frac{\xi_n - \mu_k}{\sigma_k}\right) - F_0\left(\frac{\xi_{n-1} - \mu_k}{\sigma_k}\right),$$

$$\Delta T_{nk} = T\left(\frac{\xi_n - \mu_k}{\sigma_k}\right) - T\left(\frac{\xi_{n-1} - \mu_k}{\sigma_k}\right).$$

When $p = 2$, we expand the squared W_2 distance, $\mathbb{W}_N$, between the empirical distribution and $F(\cdot|G)$ as follows:

$$\mathbb{W}_N(G) = W_2^2(F_N(\cdot), F(\cdot|G))$$
$$= \int_0^1 \{F_N^{-1}(t) - F^{-1}(t|G)\}^2 dt$$

$$= \overline{x^2} + \sum_{k=1}^{K} w_k \{\mu_k^2 + \sigma_k^2(\mu_0^2 + \sigma_0^2) + 2\mu_k\sigma_k\mu_0\}$$

$$-2\sum_k w_k \Big\{\mu_k \sum_{n=1}^{N} x_{(n)} \Delta F_{nk} + \sigma_k \sum_{n=1}^{N} x_{(n)} \Delta T_{nk}\Big\}.$$

The MWDE minimizes $\mathbb{W}_N(G)$ with respect to G. The mixing weights and subpopulation-scale parameters in this optimization problem have natural constraints. We may replace the optimization problem with an unconstrained one by the following parameter transformation:

$$\sigma_k = \exp(\tau_k),$$

$$w_k = \exp(t_k) / \Big\{ \sum_{j=1}^{K} \exp(t_j) \Big\}$$

for $k = 1, 2, \ldots, K$. We may then minimize $\mathbb{W}_N$ with respect to $\{(\mu_k, \tau_k, t_k) : k = 1, 2, \ldots, K\}$ over the unconstrained space $\mathbb{R}^{3K}$. Furthermore, we adopt the quasi-Newton BFGS algorithm (Nocedal & Wright 2006, Section 6.1). To use this algorithm, it is best to provide the gradients of $\mathbb{W}_N(G)$, which are given as follows:

$$\frac{\partial}{\partial t_j} \mathbb{W}_N = \sum_{k=1}^{K} \Big\{ \frac{\partial w_k}{\partial t_j} \frac{\partial}{\partial w_k} \mathbb{W}_N \Big\} = \sum_k w_j (\delta_{jk} - w_k) \frac{\partial}{\partial w_k} \mathbb{W}_N,$$

$$\frac{\partial}{\partial \mu_j} \mathbb{W}_N = 2w_j \Big\{ \mu_j + \sigma_j\mu_0 - \sum_{n=1}^{N} x_{(n)} \Delta F_{nj} \Big\},$$

$$\frac{\partial}{\partial \tau_j} \mathbb{W}_N = 2w_j \Big\{ \sigma_j(\mu_0^2 + \sigma_0^2) + \mu_j\mu_0 - \sum_{n=1}^{N} x_{(n)} \Delta T_{nj} \Big\} \frac{\partial \sigma_j}{\partial \tau_j},$$

for $j = 1, 2, \ldots, K$, where

$$\frac{\partial}{\partial w_k} \mathbb{W}_N = \{\mu_k^2 + \sigma_k^2(\mu_0^2 + \sigma_0^2) + 2\mu_k\sigma_k\mu_0\} - 2\sum_{n=1}^{N-1} \{x_{(n+1)} - x_{(n)}\}\xi_n F(\xi_n | \mu_k, \sigma_k)$$

$$-2\{\mu_k \sum_{n=1}^{N} x_{(n)} \Delta F_{nk} + \sigma_k \sum_{n=1}^{N} x_{(n)} \Delta T_{nk}\}.$$

Since $\mathbb{W}_N(G)$ is non-convex, the algorithm may find a local minimum of $\mathbb{W}_N(G)$ instead of a global minimum as required for MWDE. We use multiple initial values for the BFGS algorithm and regard the one with the lowest $\mathbb{W}_N(G)$ value as the solution. We leave the algebraic details in the Appendix.

This algorithm involves computing the quantiles ξ_n and ΔT_{nj} repeatedly that may lead to high computational cost. Since ξ_n is between $\min_k F^{-1}(n/N|\theta_k)$ and $\max_k F^{-1}(n/N|\theta_k)]$, it can be found efficiently via a bisection method. Fortunately, $T(x)$ has simple analytical forms under two widely used location-scale mixtures that make the computation of ΔT_{nj} efficient:

1. When $f_0(t) = (2\pi)^{-1/2} \exp(-x^2/2)$, which is the density function of the standard normal, we have $t f_0(t) = -f_0'(t)$. In this case, we find

$$T(x) = -f_0(x).$$

2. For a finite mixture of location-scale logistic distributions, we have

$$f_0(t) = \frac{\exp(-x)}{(1 + \exp(-x))^2}$$

and

$$T(x) = \int_{-\infty}^{x} t f_0(t) dt = \frac{x}{1 + \exp(-x)} - \log(1 + \exp(x)). \tag{3}$$

2.5 Penalized Maximum Likelihood Estimator

A well-investigated inference method under a finite mixture of location-scale families is the pMLE (Tanaka 2009; Chen et al. 2008). Chen et al. (2008) consider this approach for finite normal mixture models. They recommend the following penalized log-likelihood function:

$$p\ell_N(G|\mathcal{X}) = \ell_N(G|\mathcal{X}) - a_N \sum_k \left\{ s_x^2/\sigma_k^2 + \log \sigma_k^2 \right\}$$

for some positive a_N and sample variance s_x^2. The log-likelihood function is given in (1). They suggest us to learn the mixing distribution G via pMLE defined as

$$\hat{G}_N^{\mathrm{pMLE}} = \arg \sup p\ell_N(G|\mathcal{X}).$$

The size of a_N controls the strength of the penalty, and a recommended value is $N^{-1/2}$. Regularizing the likelihood function via a penalty function fixes the problem caused by degenerated subpopulations (i.e., some $\sigma_k = 0$). The pMLE is shown to be strongly consistent when the number of components has a known upper bound under the finite normal mixture model.

The penalized likelihood approach can be easily extended to a finite mixture of location-scale families. Let $f_0(\cdot)$ be the density function in the location-scale family as before. We may replace the sample variance s_x^2 in the penalty function by any scale-invariance statistic such as the sample inter-quartile range. This is applicable even if the variance of $f_0(\cdot)$ is not finite.

We can use the EM algorithm for numerical computation. Let $\mathbf{z}_n = (z_{n1}, \ldots, z_{nK})$ be the membership vector of the nth observation. That is, the kth entry of $\mathbf{z}_n$ is 1 when the response value x_n is an observation from the kth subpopulation and 0 otherwise. When the complete data $\{(\mathbf{z}_n, x_n), n = 1, 2, \ldots, N\}$ are available, the penalized complete data likelihood function of G is given by

$$p\ell_N^c(|\mathcal{X}) = \sum_{n=1}^{N} \sum_{k=1}^{K} z_{nk} \log\left\{ \frac{w_k}{\sigma_k} f_0\left(\frac{x_i - \mu_k}{\sigma_k}\right) \right\} - a_N \sum_k \{s_x^2/\sigma_k^2 + \log(\sigma_k^2)\}.$$

Given the observed data $\mathcal{X}$ and proposed mixing distribution $G^{(t)}$, we have the conditional expectation

$$w_{nk}^{(t)} = \mathbb{E}(z_{nk}|\mathcal{X}, G^{(t)}) = \frac{w_k^{(t)} f(x_n|\mu_k^{(t)}, \sigma_k^{(t)})}{\sum_{j=1}^{K} w_j^{(t)} f(x_n|\mu_j^{(t)}, \sigma_j^{(t)})}.$$

After this E-step, we define

$$Q(G|G^{(t)}) = \sum_{n=1}^{N} \sum_{k=1}^{K} w_{nk}^{(t)} \log\left\{ \frac{w_k}{\sigma_k} f_0\left(\frac{x_n - \mu_k}{\sigma_k}\right) \right\} - a_N \sum_k \{s_x^2/\sigma_k^2 + \log(\sigma_k^2)\}.$$

Note that the subpopulation parameters are separated in $Q(\cdot|\cdot)$. The M-step is to maximize $Q(G|G^{(t)})$ with respect to G. The solution is given by the mixing distribution $G^{(t+1)}$ with mixing weights

$$w_k^{(t+1)} = N^{-1} \sum_{n=1}^{N} w_{nk}^{(t)}$$

and the subpopulation parameters

$$\theta_k^{(t+1)} = \arg\min_{\theta} \left\{ \sum_n w_{nk}^{(t)} \{\log \sigma - f(x_n|\boldsymbol{\theta})\} + a_N\{s_x^2/\sigma^2 + \log \sigma^2\} \right\} \tag{4}$$

with the notational convention $\boldsymbol{\theta} = (\mu, \sigma)$.

For general location-scale mixture, the M-step (4) may not have a closed-form solution, but it is merely a simple two-variable function. There are many effective algorithms in the literature to solve this optimization problem. The EM algorithm for pMLE increases the value of the penalized likelihood after each iteration. Hence, it should converge as long as the penalized likelihood function has an upper bound. We do not give a proof as it is a standard problem.

3   Experiments

We now study the performance of MWDE and pMLE under finite location-scale mixtures. We explore the potential advantages of the MWDE and quantify its efficiency loss, if any, by simulation experiments. Consider the following three location-scale families (Chen et al. 2020):

1. Normal distribution: $f_0(x) = (2\pi)^{-1/2} \exp(-x^2/2)$. Its mean and variance are given by $\mu_0 = 0$ and $\sigma_0^2 = 1$.
2. Logistic distribution: $f_0(x) = \exp(-x)/(1 + \exp(-x))^2$. Its mean and variance are given by $\mu_0 = 0$ and $\sigma_0^2 = \pi^2/3$.
3. Gumbel distribution (type I extreme-value distribution): $f_0(x) = \exp(-x - \exp(-x))$. Its mean and variance are given by $\mu_0 = \gamma$ and $\sigma_0^2 = \pi^2/6$, where γ is the Euler constant.

We will also include a real-data example to compare the image segmentation result of using the MWDE and pMLE.

3.1   Performance Measure

For vector-valued parameters, the commonly used performance metric of their estimators is the mean-squared error (MSE). A mixing distribution with finite and fixed support points can be regarded as a real-valued vector in theory. Yet the mean-squared errors of the mixing weights, the subpopulation means, and the subpopulation scales are not comparable in terms of the learned finite mixture. In this chapter, we use two performance metrics specific for finite mixture models. Let $\hat{G}$ and G^* be the learned mixing distribution and the true mixing distribution. We use L_2 distance between the learned mixture and the true mixture as the first performance metric. The L_2 distance between two mixtures $f(\cdot|G)$ and $f(\cdot|\tilde{G})$ is defined to be

$$L_2(f(\cdot|G), f(\cdot|\tilde{G})) = \{\mathbf{w}^\tau S_{GG}\mathbf{w} - 2\mathbf{w}^\tau S_{G\tilde{G}}\tilde{\mathbf{w}} + \tilde{\mathbf{w}}^\tau S_{\tilde{G}\tilde{G}}\tilde{\mathbf{w}}\}^{1/2},$$

where $S_{GG}, S_{G\tilde{G}}$ and $S_{\tilde{G}\tilde{G}}$ are three square matrices of size $K \times K$ with their (n, m)th elements given by

$$\int f(x|\boldsymbol{\theta}_n)f(x|\boldsymbol{\theta}_m)dx, \quad \int f(x|\boldsymbol{\theta}_n)f(x|\tilde{\boldsymbol{\theta}}_m)dx, \quad \int f(x|\tilde{\boldsymbol{\theta}}_n)f(x|\tilde{\boldsymbol{\theta}}_m)dx.$$

Given an observed value x of a unit from the true mixture population, by Bayes' theorem, the most probable membership of this unit is given by

$$k^*(x) = \arg\max_k \{w_k^* f^*(x|\boldsymbol{\theta}_k^*)\}.$$

Following the same rule, if $\hat{G}$ is the learned mixing distribution, then the most likely membership of the unit with observed value x is

$$\hat{k}(x) = \arg\max_k \{\hat{w}_k f(x|\hat{\boldsymbol{\theta}}_k)\}.$$

We cannot directly compare $k^*(x)$ and $\hat{k}(x)$ because the subpopulation themselves is not labeled. Instead, the adjusted Rand index (ARI) is a good performance metric for clustering accuracy. Suppose the observations in a dataset are divided into K clusters $A_1, A_2, \ldots, A_K$ by one approach, and K' clusters $B_1, B_2, \ldots, B_{K'}$ by another. Let $N_i = \#(A_i)$, $M_j = \#(B_j)$, $N_{ij} = \#(A_i B_j)$ for $i, j = 1, 2, \ldots, K$, where $\#(A)$ is the number of units in set A. The ARI between these two clustering outcomes is defined to be

$$\text{ARI} = \frac{\sum_{i,j}\binom{N_{ij}}{2} - \binom{N}{2}^{-1}\sum_{i,j}\binom{N_i}{2}\binom{M_j}{2}}{\frac{1}{2}\sum_i\binom{N_i}{2} + \frac{1}{2}\sum_j\binom{M_j}{2} - \binom{N}{2}^{-1}\sum_{i,j}\binom{N_i}{2}\binom{M_j}{2}}.$$

When the two clustering approaches completely agree with each other, the ARI value is 1. When data are assigned to clusters randomly, the expected ARI value is 0. ARI values close to 1 indicate a high degree of agreement. We compute ARI based on clusters formed by $k^*(x)$ and $\hat{k}(x)$.

For each simulation, we choose or generate a mixing distribution $G^{*(r)}$ and then generate a random sample from mixture $f(x|G^{*(r)})$. This is repeated R times. Let $\hat{G}^{(r)}$ be the learned G based on the rth dataset. We obtain the two performance metrics as follows:

1. Mean L_2 distance:

$$\text{ML2} = R^{-1}\sum_{r=1}^{R} L_2(f(\cdot|\hat{G}^{(r)}), f(\cdot|G^{*(r)})).$$

2. Mean-adjusted Rand index:

$$\text{MARI} = R^{-1}\sum_{r=1}^{R} \text{ARI}(\hat{G}^{(r)}, G^{*(r)}).$$

The lower the ML2 and the higher the MARI, the better the estimator performs.

3.2 Performance Under Homogeneous Model

The homogeneous location-scale model is a special mixture model with a single subpopulation $K = 1$. Both MWDE and MLE are applicable for parameter estimation. There have been no studies of MWDE in this special case in the literature. It is therefore of interest to see how MWDE performs under this model.

Under three location-scale models given earlier, the MWDE has closed analytical forms. Using the same notation introduced, their analytical forms are as follows:

1. Normal distribution:

$$\hat{\mu}^{\text{MWDE}} = \bar{x}, \quad \hat{\sigma}^{\text{MWDE}} = \sum_{n=1}^{N} x_{(n)} \left\{ f_0(\xi_{n-1}) - f_0(\xi_n) \right\}.$$

2. Logistic distribution:

$$\hat{\mu}^{\text{MWDE}} = \bar{x}, \quad \hat{\sigma}^{\text{MWDE}} = \frac{3}{\pi^2} \sum_{n=1}^{N} x_{(n)} \left\{ T(\xi_n) - T(\xi_{n-1}) \right\},$$

where $T(x)$ is given in (3).
3. Gumbel distribution:

$$\hat{\mu}^{\text{MWDE}} = \{1 - \gamma r\}^{-1} \{\bar{x} - \gamma T\}, \quad \hat{\sigma}^{\text{MWDE}} = T - r \hat{\mu}^{\text{MWDE}},$$

where

$$T = \{\gamma^2 + \pi^2/6\}^{-1} \sum_{n=1}^{N} x_{(n)} \int_{\xi_{n-1}}^{\xi_n} t f_0(t) dt$$

and $r = \gamma/(\gamma^2 + \pi^2/6)$.

The MLEs under the logistic and Gumbel distributions do not have an easy-to-use analytical form. We employ a numerical optimization program to solve for MLE. We generate samples of sizes between $N = 10$ and $N = 100,000$ with $R = 1000$ repetitions. Under the homogeneous model, it is most convenient to compute the MSE of the location and scale parameters separately. Due to the invariance property, we generate data from distributions with $\mu = 0$ and $\sigma = 1$. The simulation results are summarized as plots in Fig. 1. Both the x and y axes in these plots are in logarithm scale. For both MLE and MWDE, their log-MSE and $\log(N)$ values are close to the straight lines with slope -1. This phenomenon indicates that both estimators have the expected convergence rates $O(N^{-1/2})$ as the sample size $N \to \infty$.

The performances of the estimators for the location parameter and scale parameter are different. For the location parameter under all three models, the lines formed by MLE and MWDE are nearly indistinguishable though the MLE is always below

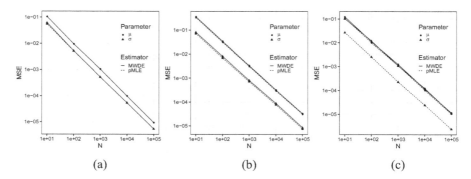

Fig. 1 The MSEs of the MWDE and MLE for location and scale parameters versus sample size N under different homogeneous models. (**a**) Normal. (**b**) Logistic. (**c**) Gumbel

the MWDE. For the scale parameter σ, the MLE is also more efficient than the MWDE, but the difference is negligible under the normal and logistic models. Under the Gumbel model, the MWDE is less efficient.

In summary, using MWDE under a homogeneous model may not be preferred but may be acceptable under the normal and logistic models. We do not investigate the performance of MWDE under Gumbel mixture due to its efficiency loss under the homogeneous model. With these observations, we move to its performance under finite location-scale mixtures.

3.3 Efficiency and Robustness Under Finite Location-Scale Mixtures

We next study the efficiency and robustness of the MWDE for learning finite location-scale mixtures. Since the MLE is not well defined, we compare the performance of MWDE with the pMLE (Chen & Tan 2009) instead. We compare their performances when the mixture model is correctly specified, when the data is contaminated, or when the model is mildly mis-specified.

3.3.1 Efficiency

A widely employed two-component mixture model (Cutler & Cordero-Brana 1996; Zhu 2016) has a density function in the following form:

$$f(x|G) = pf(x|0, a) + (1 - p)f(x|b, 1) \tag{5}$$

for some density function $f(\cdot|\theta)$ from a location-scale family. Namely, we have $K = 2$ is known, the mixing weights be $w_1 = p$, $w_2 = 1 - p$, and subpopulation parameters be $\theta_1 = (0, a)$ and $\theta_2 = (b, 1)$. By choosing different combinations of p, a, and b, we obtain mixtures with different properties. Due to the invariance property, we need to consider only the case where one of the location parameters is 0 and one of the scale parameters is 1.

We generate samples from $f(x|G)$ according to the following scheme: generate an observation Y from distribution with density function $f_0(x)$, and let

$$X = \begin{cases} aY, & \text{with probability } p; \\ Y + b, & \text{otherwise.} \end{cases} \tag{6}$$

We can easily see that the distribution of X is $f(x|G)$ specified earlier.

The level of difficulty to precisely estimate the mixture largely depends on the degree of overlap between the subpopulations. Let

$$o_{j|i} = \mathbb{P}\big(w_i f(X|\mu_i, \sigma_i) < w_j f(X|\mu_j, \sigma_j)|X \sim f(x|\mu_i, \sigma_i)\big).$$

This is the probability of a unit from subpopulation i misclassified as a unit in subpopulation j by the maximum posterior rule. The degree of overlap between the ith and jth subpopulations is therefore

$$o_{ij} = o_{j|i} + o_{i|j}. \tag{7}$$

We employ the following a, b, and p values in our simulation experiments:

1. Mixing proportion $p = 0.15, 0.25, 0.5, 0.75, 0.85$.
2. Scale of the first subpopulation $a^2 = 1, 2$.
3. Location parameter b values such that $o_{12} = 0.03, 0.1$.

The combination of these choices leads to 24 mixtures with various shapes. The sample size N in our experiments is chosen to be 100, 500, and 1000, respectively.

We obtain the average L_2 distance (ML2) and adjusted Rand index (MARI) based on $R = 1000$ repetitions on data generated from normal and logistic mixture distributions as specified by (6). Figures 2 and 3, respectively, contain plots of ML2 and MARI of the WMDE and pMLE estimators against sample size N under these two models. We can see that when the sample size increases, ML2 of both estimators decreases and MARI of both estimators increases, supporting the theory that both WMDE and pMLE are consistent. Under the normal mixture, these two estimators have nearly equal L_2 distances. The MWDE slightly outperforms pMLE in terms of the MARI, when the degree of overlap is large ($o_{12} = 0.1$) and the two subpopulations have both equal scale and highly unbalanced weights. Under logistic mixture, as shown in plots (a) and (b) of Fig. 3, the pMLE always outperforms the MWDE in terms of the L_2 distance. In terms of the MARI, the MWDE is better when the scale parameters are equal and weights are highly unbalanced. When the scale parameters are different, the pMLE is better than MWDE when $p > 0.5$ and worse than MWDE when $p < 0.5$.

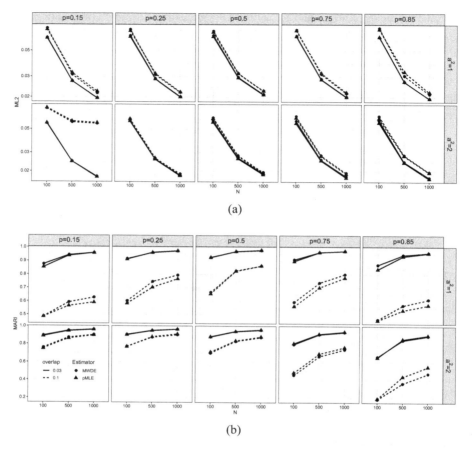

Fig. 2 Performances of pMLE and MWDE under 2-component normal mixture. (**a**) L_2 distance. (**b**) Adjusted Rand index

We next investigate the performance of the MWDE and pMLE for learning 3-component normal mixtures. We come up with 8 such distributions with different configurations. The three subpopulations have the same or different weights and same or different scale parameter values. They lead to different degrees of overlap as defined by

$$\texttt{MeanOmega} = \text{mean}_{1 \leq i < j \leq 3}\{o_{ij}\},$$

where o_{ij} is the degree of overlap between subpopulations i and j in (7). See Table 1 for detailed parameter values.

Figure 4 contains plots of the ML2 and MARI values of two estimators. It is seen that the pMLE consistently outperforms MWDE in terms of ML2 but the difference

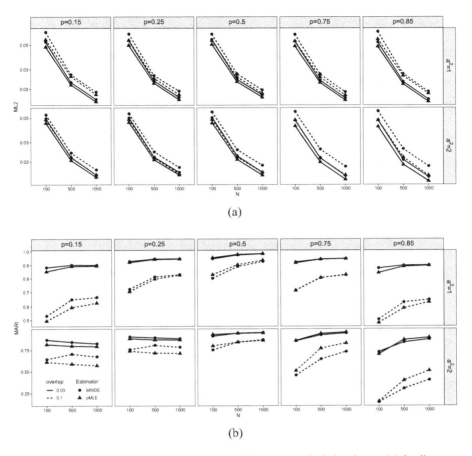

Fig. 3 Performances of pMLE and MWDE under 2-component logistic mixture. (**a**) L_2 distance. (**b**) Adjusted Rand index

Table 1 Parameter values of 3-component normal mixtures

	MeanOmega	w_1	w_2	w_3	μ_1	μ_2	μ_3	σ_1	σ_2	σ_3
I	0.288 (low)	0.4	0.5	0.1	-2	0	1	0.3	2	0.4
II	0.367 (high)	0.4	0.5	0.1	-2	0	1	0.3	1	0.4
III	0.097 (low)	0.3	0.5	0.2	-3	0	3	1	1	1
IV	0.249 (high)	0.3	0.5	0.2	-2	0	2	1	1	1
V	0.148 (low)	1/3	1/3	1/3	-1	0	1	1.5	0.1	0.5
VI	0.267 (high)	1/3	1/3	1/3	-0.5	0	0.5	1.5	0.1	0.5
VII	0.091 (low)	1/3	1/3	1/3	-3	0	3	1	1	1
VIII	0.226 (high)	1/3	1/3	1/3	-2	0	2	1	1	1

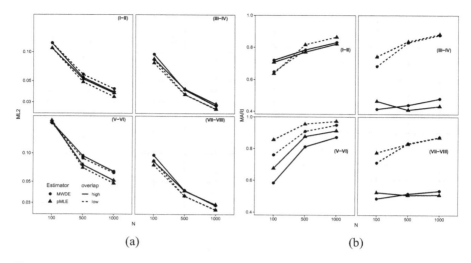

Fig. 4 Performances of pMLE and MWDE under 3-component normal mixture. (**a**) L_2 distance.
(**b**) Adjusted Rand index

is small. The performances of the MWDE and pMLE are mixed in terms of MARI
and the differences are small. The pMLE is clearly better under I and II.

3.3.2 Robustness

Robustness is another important property of estimators. Sample mean is the most
efficient unbiased estimator of the population mean in terms of variance under
normality or some other well-known parametric models. However, the value of
the sample mean changes dramatically even if the dataset contains merely a single
extreme value. Sample median offers a respectable alternative and still has high
efficiency across a broader range of parametric models.

In the context of learning finite location-scale mixture models, both pMLE and
MWDE rely on a parametric distribution family assumption through $f_0(x)$. How
important is to have $f_0(x)$ correctly specified? We shed some light into this problem
by simulation experiments in this section. We learn finite normal mixtures assuming
$K = 2$ but generate data from the following distributions:

1. Mixture with outliers: $(1 - \alpha)\{p\phi(x|0, a) + (1 - p)\phi(x|b, 1)\} + \alpha\phi(x|8, 1)$ with
   $\alpha = 0.01$ and $\phi(x|\mu, \sigma) = \exp(-(x - \mu)^2/2\sigma^2)/\sqrt{2\pi\sigma^2}$.
2. Mixture contaminated: $(1 - \alpha)\{p\phi(x|0, a) + (1 - p)\phi(x|b, 1)\} + \alpha\phi(x|b/2, 7)$ with
   $\alpha = 0.01$.
3. Mixture mis-specified I: $pf_0(x|0, a) + (1 - p)f_0(x|b, 1)$ with $f_0(x)$ being Student-t
   with 4 degrees of freedom.

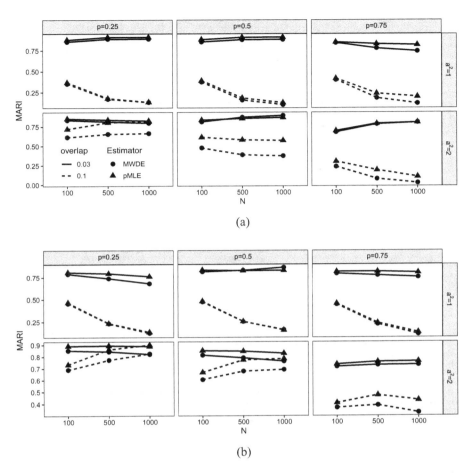

Fig. 5 Adjusted Rand index based on pMLE and MWDE when data contains outliers or is contaminated. (**a**) Mixture with outliers. (**b**) Mixture contaminated

4. Mixture mis-specified II: $pf_1(x|0, a) + (1 - p)f_2(x|b, 1)$ with $f_1(x)$ and $f_2(x)$ being Student-t with 2 and 4 degrees of freedom.

In every case, we use the combinations of the a, b, and p values the same as before. We regard $(1 - \alpha)\{p\phi(x|0, a) + (1 - p)\phi(x|b, 1)\}$ as the true distribution in all cases and computed the MARI accordingly.

We obtain the MARI values based on $R = 1000$ repetitions with sample sizes $N = 100$, 500, and 1000, see Figs. 5 and 6. We see that when the degree of overlap is low, MWDE and pMLE have similar performances. When the subpopulation variance is larger ($a^2 = 2$), the performance of pMLE is generally better. In general, we conclude that pMLE is preferred.

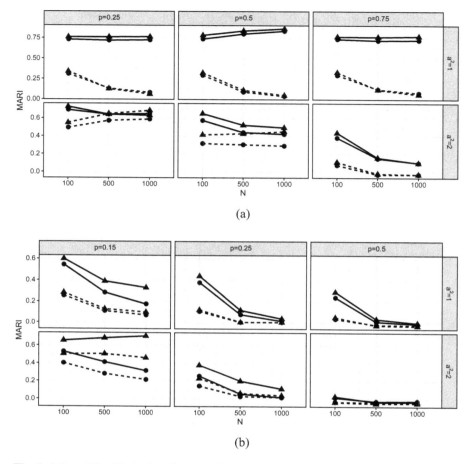

Fig. 6 Adjusted Rand index based on pMLE and MWDE when subpopulation distributions are mis-specified. (**a**) Mixture mis-specified I. (**b**) Mixture mis-specified II

Statistical inference usually becomes more accurate when the sample size increases. This is not the case in this simulation experiment. We can see that MARI often decreases (becomes less accurate) when the sample size increases. This is not caused by simulation error. When the model is mis-specified, the learned model does not converge to the "true model" as $N \to \infty$. Hence, the inference does not necessarily improve. The moral of this simulation study is that the MWDE is not more robust than the pMLE, against our intuition.

3.4 Image Segmentation

Image segmentation aims to partition an image into regions, each with a reasonably homogeneous visual appearance or corresponds to objects or parts of objects (Bishop 2006, Chapter 9). In this section, we perform image segmentation with finite normal mixtures, a common practice in the machine learning community.

Each pixel in an image is represented by three numbers within the range of $[0, 1]$ that corresponds to the intensities of the Red, Green, and Blue (RGB) channels. Since the intensity values are always between 0 and 1, unlike the common practice in the literature, we feel obliged to transform the intensity values to ensure the normal mixture model fits better. Let $y = \Phi^{-1}((x + 1/N)/(1 + 2/N))$ with x being the intensity and N the total number of pixels in the image. We then learn a two-component normal mixture on y values from each channel. Namely, we learn three normal mixtures on red, green, and blue channels, respectively.

We use the maximum posterior probability rule to assign each pixel to one of two clusters. We then form an image segment by pixels assigned to the same cluster. We visualize the segregated images channel by channel by re-drawing the image with the original intensity value replaced by the average intensity of the pixels assigned to the specific cluster.

The segregated images depend heavily on the fitted mixture distributions. We compare the segregated images obtained by the normal mixtures learned via the pMLE and MWDE. We retrieved an image from Pexels[1] as shown in Fig. 7a. Clark (2015) resized the original high-resolution image to 433×650 grids using Lanczos filter. We learn a normal mixture of order $K = 2$ for each channel based on resized datasets and evaluated its utility of segregating the foreground and the background.

We present the specifications of the learned mixing distributions by pMLE and MWDE in Table 2. Plots (d), (g), and (j) in Fig. 7 are histograms of the transformed intensity values of RGB channels, together with the mixture densities learned via pMLE and MWDE. The corresponding segmented images are shown as plots (e), (h), and (k) for pMLE and (f), (i), and (l) for MWDE. The estimated parameter values and the fitted density on the red and green channels based on these two approaches are very similar. For the blue channel, the fitted densities and the segmentation results are very similar although the estimated parameter values of the second component are quite different. Both approaches can produce images with meaningful structures segregating foreground from background.

There are two clusters in each of 3 channels leading to 8 refined clusters. We may paint each pixel with the average RGB intensity triplet according to these 8 refined clusters. The re-created images via pMLE and MWDE, respectively, are shown in (b) and (c). We note these two images are very similar, showing that both learning strategies are effective.

---

[1] https://www.pinterest.se/pin/761952830692007143/.

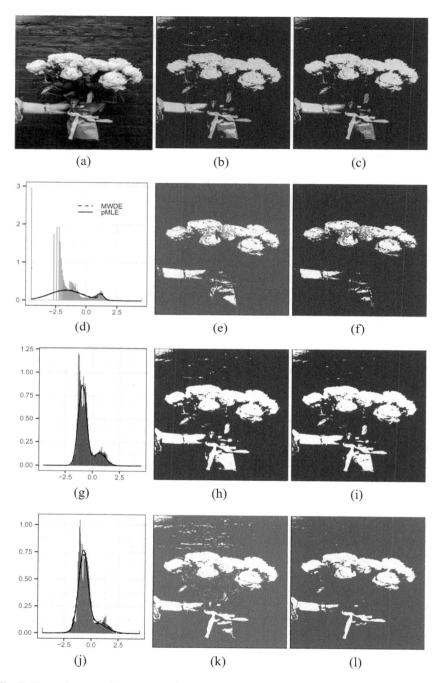

Fig. 7 Flower image and its segmentation outcomes. (**a**), (**b**) and (**c**): original image; aggregated images based on segmentation outcomes via pMLE and MWDE. (**d**), (**g**) and (**j**): histograms of pixel intensity of Red, Green, and Blue channels together with the fitted mixtures. (**e**), (**h**) and (**k**): segregated images via PMLE in RGB channels. (**f**), (**i**) and (**l**): segregated images via MWDE in RGB channels

Table 2 Estimated mixing distributions of the flower image by pMLE and MWDE.

Channel	Estimator	w_1	w_2	μ_1	μ_2	σ_1	σ_2
Red	pMLE	0.896	0.104	−1.668	1.139	1.321	0.277
	MWDE	0.915	0.085	−1.617	1.220	1.316	0.213
Green	pMLE	0.804	0.196	−0.935	0.637	0.373	0.595
	MWDE	0.819	0.181	−0.926	0.724	0.378	0.510
Blue	pMLE	0.735	0.265	−0.753	0.268	0.414	1.034
	MWDE	0.862	0.138	−0.722	1.019	0.473	0.592

4 Conclusion

The MWDE provides another approach for learning finite location-scale mixtures. We have shown the MWDE is well defined and consistent. Our moderate scaled simulation study shows it suffers some efficiency loss against a penalized version of MLE in general without noticeable gain in robustness. We gain the knowledge on the benefits and drawbacks of the MWDE under finite location-scale mixtures. We reaffirm the general superiority of the likelihood-based learning strategies even for non-regular models.

Acknowledgments The authors would like to thank Richard Schonberg for proofreading the manuscript.

Appendix

Numerically Friendly Expression of $W_2(F_N, F(\cdot|G))$

To learn the finite mixture distribution through MWDE, we must compute

$$\mathbb{W}_N(G) = W_2^2(F_N(\cdot), F(\cdot|G)) = \int_0^1 \{F_N^{-1}(t) - F^{-1}(t|G)\}^2 dt$$

for finite location-scale mixture

$$F(\cdot|G) = \sum_{k=1}^K \pi_k F(\cdot|\boldsymbol{\theta}_k) = \sum_{k=1}^K \pi_k \sigma_k^{-1} F_0((x - \mu_k)/\sigma_k).$$

We write $\mathbb{E}_k(\cdot)$ as expectation under distribution $F(\cdot|\boldsymbol{\theta}_k)$. For instance,

$$\mathbb{E}_k\{X^2\} = \mu_k^2 + \sigma_k^2(\mu_0^2 + \sigma_0^2) + 2\mu_k\sigma_k\mu_0.$$

Let $I_n = ((n-1)/N, n/N]$ for $n = 1, 2, \ldots, N$ so that $F_N^{-1}(t) = x_{(n)}$ when $t \in I_n$, where $x_{(n)}$ is the nth order statistic. For ease of notation, we write $x_{(n)}$ as x_n. Over this interval, we have

$$\int_{I_n} \{F_N^{-1}(t) - F^{-1}(t|G)\}^2 dt = \int_{I_n} [x_n^2 - 2x_n F^{-1}(t|G) + \{F^{-1}(t|G)\}^2] dt. \qquad (8)$$

The integration of the first term in (8), after summing over n, is given by

$$\sum_{n=1}^{N} \int_{I_n} x_n^2 dt = N^{-1} \sum_n x_n^2 = \overline{x^2}.$$

The integration of the third term in (8) is

$$\sum_{n=1}^{N} \int_{I_n} \{F^{-1}(t|G)\}^2 dt = \int_{-\infty}^{\infty} x^2 f(x|G) dx = \sum_{k=1}^{K} w_k \mathbb{E}_k\{X^2\}.$$

Let $\xi_0 = -\infty$, $\xi_{N+1} = \infty$, and $\xi_n = F^{-1}(n/N|G)$ for $n = 1, \ldots, N$. Denote

$$\Delta F_{nk} = F(\xi_n|\boldsymbol{\theta}_k) - F(\xi_{n-1}|\boldsymbol{\theta}_k)$$

and

$$T(x) = \int_{-\infty}^{x} t f_0(t) dt, \quad \Delta T_{nk} = T((\xi_n - \mu_k)/\sigma_k) - T((\xi_{n-1} - \mu_k)/\sigma_k).$$

Then

$$\int_{I_n} F^{-1}(t|G) dt = \sum_k w_k \int_{\xi_{n-1}}^{\xi_n} x f(x|\mu_k, \sigma_k) dx$$

$$= \sum_k w_k \{\mu_k \Delta F_{nk} + \sigma_k \Delta T_{nk}\}.$$

These lead to numerically convenient expression

$$\mathbb{W}_N(G) = \overline{x^2} + \sum_k w_k \mathbb{E}_k\{X^2\} - 2 \sum_k w_k \{\mu_k \Delta F_{nk} + \sigma_k \Delta T_{nk}\}.$$

To most effectively use BFGS algorithm, it is best to provide gradients of the objective function. Here are some numerically friendly expressions of some partial derivatives.

Lemma 1 *Let* $\delta_{jk} = 1$ *when* $j = k$ *and* $\delta_{jk} = 0$ *when* $j \neq k$. *For* $n = 1, \ldots, N$ *and* $j = 1, 2, \ldots, K$, *we have*

$$\frac{\partial}{\partial w_j} F(\xi_n | \boldsymbol{\theta}_k) = f(\xi_n | \boldsymbol{\theta}_k) \frac{\partial \xi_n}{\partial w_j},$$

$$\frac{\partial}{\partial \mu_j} F(\xi_n | \boldsymbol{\theta}_k) = f(\xi_n | \boldsymbol{\theta}_k) \left(\frac{\partial \xi_n}{\partial \mu_j} - \delta_{jk} \right),$$

$$\frac{\partial}{\partial \sigma_j} F(\xi_n | \boldsymbol{\theta}_k) = f(\xi_n | \boldsymbol{\theta}_k) \left(\frac{\partial \xi_n}{\partial \sigma_j} - \left\{ \frac{\xi_n - \mu_k}{\sigma_k} \right\} \delta_{jk} \right),$$

and

$$\frac{\partial}{\partial w_j} T \left(\frac{\xi_n - \mu_k}{\sigma_k} \right) = f(\xi_n | \boldsymbol{\theta}_k) \left(\frac{\xi_n - \mu_k}{\sigma_k} \right) \frac{\partial \xi_i}{\partial w_j},$$

$$\frac{\partial}{\partial \mu_j} T \left(\frac{\xi_n - \mu_k}{\sigma_k} \right) = f(\xi_n | \boldsymbol{\theta}_k) \left(\frac{\xi_n - \mu_k}{\sigma_k} \right) \left(\frac{\partial \xi_n}{\partial \mu_j} - \delta_{jk} \right),$$

$$\frac{\partial}{\partial \sigma_j} T \left(\frac{\xi_n - \mu_k}{\sigma_k} \right) = f(\xi_n | \boldsymbol{\theta}_k) \left(\frac{\xi_n - \mu_k}{\sigma_k} \right) \left\{ \frac{\partial \xi_i}{\partial \sigma_j} - \left(\frac{\xi_n - \mu_k}{\sigma_k} \right) \delta_{jk} \right\}.$$

Furthermore, we have

$$\frac{\partial \xi_n}{\partial \mu_k} = \frac{w_k f(\xi_i | \boldsymbol{\theta}_k)}{f(\xi_n | G)},$$

$$\frac{\partial \xi_n}{\partial \sigma_k} = \frac{w_k f(\xi_n | \boldsymbol{\theta}_k)}{f(\xi_i | G)} \left(\frac{\xi_n - \mu_k}{\sigma_k} \right),$$

$$\frac{\partial \xi_n}{\partial w_k} = -\frac{F(\xi_n | \boldsymbol{\theta}_k)}{f(\xi_n | G)}.$$

Based on this lemma, it is seen that

$$\frac{\partial}{\partial \mu_j} \mathbb{W}_N = 2 w_j (\mu_j + \sigma_j \mu_0) - 2 w_j \sum_{n=1}^{N} x_{(n)} \Delta F_{nj}$$

$$-2 \sum_{n=1}^{N} \sum_{k} w_k \mu_k x_{(n)} \left\{ \frac{\partial F_0(\xi_n | \boldsymbol{\theta}_k)}{\partial \mu_j} - \frac{\partial F_0(\xi_{n-1} | \boldsymbol{\theta}_k)}{\partial \mu_j} \right\}$$

$$-2 \sum_{n=1}^{N} \sum_{k} w_k \sigma_k x_{(n)} \frac{\partial}{\partial \mu_j} \left\{ T \left(\frac{\xi_n - \mu_k}{\sigma_k} \right) - T \left(\frac{\xi_{n-1} - \mu_k}{\sigma_k} \right) \right\}$$

with $F_0(\xi_0 | \boldsymbol{\theta}_k) = 0$, $F_0(\xi_{N+1} | \boldsymbol{\theta}_k) = 1$, $T \left(\frac{\xi_0 - \mu_k}{\sigma_k} \right) = 0$, and $T \left(\frac{\xi_{N+1} - \mu_k}{\sigma_k} \right) = \int_{-\infty}^{\infty} t f_0(t) dt$ is a constant that does not depend on any parameters. Substituting the partial derivatives in Lemma 1, we then get

$$\frac{\partial}{\partial \mu_j} \mathbb{W}_N = 2 w_j (\mu_j + \sigma_j \mu_0) - 2 w_j \sum_{n=1}^{N} x_{(n)} \Delta F_{nj}$$

$$-2 \sum_{n=1}^{N-1} x_{(n)} \xi_n \sum_k w_k f(\xi_n | \mu_k, \sigma_k) \left(\frac{\partial \xi_n}{\partial \mu_j} - \delta_{jk} \right)$$

$$+2 \sum_{n=1}^{N-1} x_{(n)} \xi_{n-1} \sum_k w_k f(\xi_{n-1} | \mu_k, \sigma_k) \left(\frac{\partial \xi_{n-1}}{\partial \mu_j} - \delta_{jk} \right)$$

$$= 2 w_j \left\{ \mu_j + \sigma_j \mu_0 - \sum_{n=1}^{N} x_{(n)} \Delta F_{nj} \right\}.$$

Similarly, we have

$$\frac{\partial}{\partial \sigma_j} \mathbb{W}_N = 2 w_j \{ \sigma_j (\mu_0^2 + \sigma_0^2) + \mu_j \mu_0 - \sum_{n=1}^{N} x_{(n)} \Delta \mu_{nj} \},$$

$$\frac{\partial}{\partial w_k} \mathbb{W}_N = \{ \mu_k^2 + \sigma_k^2 (\mu_0^2 + \sigma_0^2) + 2 \mu_k \sigma_k \mu_0 \} - 2 \sum_{n=1}^{N-1} \{ x_{(n+1)} - x_{(n)} \} \xi_i F(\xi_n | \theta_k)$$

$$-2 \left\{ \mu_k \sum_{n=1}^{N} x_{(n)} \Delta F_{nk} + \sigma_k \sum_{n=1}^{N} x_{(n)} \Delta T_{nk} \right\}.$$

Computing the quantiles of the mixture distribution $F(\cdot | G)$ for each G is one of the most demanding tasks. The property stated in the following lemma allows us to develop a bi-section algorithm.

Lemma 2 *Let* $F(x | G) = \sum_{k=1}^{K} F(x | \mu_k, \sigma_k)$ *be a* K-*component mixture, and* $\xi(t) = F^{-1}(t | G)$ *and* $\xi_k(t) = F^{-1}(t | \theta_k)$, *respectively, the* t-*quantile of the mixture and its* kth *subpopulation. For any* $t \in (0, 1)$,

$$\min_k \xi_k(t) \le \xi(t) \le \max_k \xi_k(t). \tag{9}$$

Proof Since $F(x | \theta)$ has a continuous CDF, we must have $F(\xi_k(t) | \theta_k) = t$. By the monotonicity of the CDF $F(\cdot | \theta_k)$, we have

$$F(\min_k \xi_k(t) | \theta_k) \le F(\xi_k(t) | \theta_k) \le F(\max_k \xi_k(t) | \theta_k).$$

Multiplying by w_k and summing over k lead to

$$F(\min_k \xi_k(t) | G) \le t \le F(\max_k \xi_k(t) | G).$$

This implies (9) and completes the proof.   □

In view of this lemma, we can easily find the quantiles of $F(\cdot|\theta_k)$ to form an interval containing the targeting quantile of $F(\cdot|G)$. We can quickly find $F^{-1}(t|G)$ value through a bi-section algorithm.

References

Arjovsky, M., Chintala, S., & Bottou, L. (2017). Wasserstein GAN. Preprint. arXiv:1701.07875.

Bishop, C. M. (2006). *Pattern recognition and machine learning*. Springer.

Chen, J., & Tan, X. (2009). Inference for multivariate normal mixtures. *Journal of Multivariate Analysis, 100*(7), 1367–1383.

Chen, J., Tan, X., & Zhang, R. (2008). Inference for normal mixtures in mean and variance. *Statistica Sinica, 18*(2), 443–465.

Chen, J., Li, P., & Liu, G. (2020). Homogeneity testing under finite location-scale mixtures. *Canadian Journal of Statistics, 48*(4), 670–684.

Choi, K. (1969). Estimators for the parameters of a finite mixture of distributions. *Annals of the Institute of Statistical Mathematics, 21*(1), 107–116.

Clark, A. (2015). Pillow (PIL Fork) documentation.

Clarke, B., & Heathcote, C. (1994). Robust estimation of k-component univariate normal mixtures. *Annals of the Institute of Statistical Mathematics, 46*(1), 83–93.

Cutler, A., & Cordero-Brana, O. I. (1996). Minimum Hellinger distance estimation for finite mixture models. *Journal of the American Statistical Association, 91*(436), 1716–1723.

Deely, J., & Kruse, R. (1968). Construction of sequences estimating the mixing distribution. *The Annals of Mathematical Statistics, 39*(1), 286–288.

Evans, S. N., & Matsen, F. A. (2012). The phylogenetic Kantorovich–Rubinstein metric for environmental sequence samples. *Journal of the Royal Statistical Society: Series B (Methodological), 74*(3), 569–592.

Farnoosh, R., & Zarpak, B. (2008). Image segmentation using Gaussian mixture model. *IUST International Journal of Engineering Science, 19*(1–2), 29–32.

Holzmann, H., Munk, A., & Stratmann, B. (2004). Identifiability of finite mixtures-with applications to circular distributions. *Sankhyā: The Indian Journal of Statistics, 66*(3), 440–449.

Kolouri, S., Rohde, G. K., & Hoffmann, H. (2018). Sliced Wasserstein distance for learning Gaussian mixture models. In *Proceedings of the IEEE Conference on Computer Vision and Pattern Recognition* (pp. 3427–3436).

Nocedal, J., & Wright, S. (2006). *Numerical optimization*. Springer Science & Business Media.

Pearson, K. (1894). Contributions to the mathematical theory of evolution. *Philosophical Transactions of the Royal Society of London. A, 185*(326-330), 71–110.

Plataniotis, K. N., & Hatzinak, D. (2000). Gaussian mixtures and their applications to signal processing. In S. Stergiopoulos (Ed.), *Advanced signal processing handbook: theory and implementation for radar, sonar, and medical imaging real time systems* (vol. 25, chapter 3, pp. 3-1–3-35, 1st edn). Boca Raton: CRC Press.

Santosh, D. H. H., Venkatesh, P., Poornesh, P., Rao, L. N., & Kumar, N. A. (2013). Tracking multiple moving objects using Gaussian mixture model. *International Journal of Soft Computing and Engineering (IJSCE), 3*(2), 114–119.

Schork, N. J., Allison, D. B., & Thiel, B. (1996). Mixture distributions in human genetics research. *Statistical Methods in Medical Research, 5*(2), 155–178.

Tanaka, K. (2009). Strong consistency of the maximum likelihood estimator for finite mixtures of location–scale distributions when penalty is imposed on the ratios of the scale parameters. *Scandinavian Journal of Statistics, 36*(1), 171–184.

Teicher, H. (1961). Identifiability of mixtures. *The Annals of Mathematical Statistics, 32*(1), 244–248.

Van der Vaart, A. W. (2000). *Asymptotic statistics* (vol. 3). Cambridge University Press.

Villani, C. (2003). *Topics in optimal transportation* (vol. 58). American Mathematical Society.

Woodward, W. A., Parr, W. C., Schucany, W. R., & Lindsey, H. (1984). A comparison of minimum distance and maximum likelihood estimation of a mixture proportion. *Journal of the American Statistical Association, 79*(387), 590–598.

Yakowitz, S. (1969). A consistent estimator for the identification of finite mixtures. *The Annals of Mathematical Statistics, 40*(5), 1728–1735.

Zhu, D. (2016). A two-component mixture model for density estimation and classification. *Journal of Interdisciplinary Mathematics, 19*(2), 311–319.

An Entropy-Based Comment Ranking Method with Word Embedding Clustering

Yuyang Zhang and Hao Yu

Abstract Automatically ranking comments by their relevance plays an important role in text mining. In this chapter, we introduce a new text digitization method: the bag-of-word clusters model, i.e., grouping semantic-related words as clusters using pre-trained word2vec word embeddings and representing each comment as a distribution of word clusters. This method extracts both semantic and statistical information from texts. Next, we propose an unsupervised ranking algorithm that identifies relevant comments by their distance to the "ideal" comment. This "ideal" comment is the maximum general entropy comment with respect to the global word cluster distribution. The intuition is that the "ideal" comment highlights aspects of a product that many other comments frequently mention. Therefore, it is regarded as a standard to judge a comment's relevance to this product. At last, we analyze our algorithm's performance on a real Amazon product.

Keywords Bag-of-word clusters · Comment ranking · Cosine similarity · General entropy · K-L divergence · Word2vec

1 Introduction

Online shopping has become popular all over the world. The most obvious benefit of online shopping is convenience, and shoppers can simply access online stores from their computers whenever they have free time available, in particularly, during current pandemic time. Another benefit is that online shopping provides a greater diversity of products. This means you can choose goods that suit your requirements

Y. Zhang · H. Yu (✉)
Department of Statistical and Actuarial Sciences, University of Western Ontario, London, ON, Canada
e-mail: yyzhang9603@gmail.com; hyu@uwo.ca

© The Author(s), under exclusive license to Springer Nature Switzerland AG 2022
W. He et al. (eds.), *Advances and Innovations in Statistics and Data Science*, ICSA
Book Series in Statistics, https://doi.org/10.1007/978-3-031-08329-7_5

and budget the most. However, there are also disadvantages of online shopping. One of the most obvious ones is the lack of interactivity. You cannot touch and feel the product you want to buy. Besides, the lack of touch and feel creates concerns over the quality of the product. With a large variety of goods and websites, people tend to do a lot of research before making a purchasing decision when doing online shopping. They will browse web pages about product details and, more importantly, check other buyer's comments on the product site.

Gathering information based on other people's opinions is an essential part of the purchasing decision process (Chevalier & Mayzlin 2006). With the rapid growth of the Internet, these conversations in online markets provide a large amount of product information. So when doing online shopping, consumers rely on online product comments, posted by other consumers, for their purchase decisions.

However, a large number of comments for a single product may make it harder for people to evaluate the true underlying quality of a product. In this situation, consumers tend to focus on the average rating of a product, like the number of stars on Amazon.com. But in reality, some products can easily obtain high average ratings by cheating, while some other products may get unfair low ratings. Therefore, it is very important to extract these relevant and high-quality comments from the product site, which help consumers obtain accurate information about this product.

1.1 How to Judge a Comment's Quality?

Before we start to construct a comment ranking algorithm, the fundamental question is how to judge a comment's quality. Most online business sites evaluate their comments' quality using criteria such as overall rating or helpfulness. Helpfulness is typically a score measured as the total votes given by consumers, which is an interesting way of defining a comment's relevance and quality. Many researches in comments ranking area also use this type of helpfulness score as their comments' evaluation score (Zhang & Varadarajan 2006). However, this method fails to identify these most recent comments with few votes. For example, we may always observe that only a few comments published a long time ago have a high helpfulness score in a product site, and most other comments have no votes. The reason for the phenomenon is that most people only read the first few pages of comments before making their purchase decisions. A new comment that has just appeared on the product site and has not received any votes until recently may remain at the bottom of the comment list. This comment may contain important information about this product and thus has the potential to rise to the top of the list.

1.2 Ranking Comments Using Entropy

Ranking comments is a very important task, and there is no doubt that there are many studies in this field. Some researches treat this ranking task as a supervised learning task, such as Hsu et al. (2009) and Alberto et al. (2015). Most of them used the consumers' votes, such as helpfulness scores, as their training target. Then they adopted or designed several statistical or machine-learning models based on training data. As mentioned before, the reliability of this training data is hard to be assured; some high-quality comments may have relatively low votes. Moreover, these supervised ranking models cannot be used on multiple products simultaneously since they have to be retrained for different products.

In this situation, we propose a comment ranking algorithm that is **unsupervised**, which means we do not require any human-annotated training set. Besides, as we mentioned before, in most cases, online business sites may not be able to provide some information, such as the reviewer's reputation. We prefer to develop an algorithm that ranks comments based on their contents. To construct this ranking algorithm, we need to solve these two problems below.

1. How to define a metric that can evaluate both comments' relevance and text complexity?

2. How to effectively retrieve information from comments' content?

Let us take a look at the first question first. When it comes to text complexity or information richness, we naturally think of **Shannon's entropy** (Shannon 1948). However, **Shannon's entropy** does not measure comment's relevance to the product. So how to redefine entropy and take comment's relevance into account? Zhang (2019) defined a new entropy value called **the general entropy**. In his thesis, he developed an unsupervised ranking method on Amazon's dataset and used the general entropy to measure the answer's information quality. The general entropy is defined as follows:

$$E(\mathbf{P}) = -\sum_{i=0}^{n} Q_i \cdot P_i \cdot \log P_i, \tag{1}$$

where $\mathbf{P} = [P_0, ..., P_n]$ is the words' distribution of an individual comment and $\mathbf{Q} = [Q_0, ..., Q_n]$ is the distribution of the words of all comments combined under the same product, which is called global distribution. So general entropy assigns weight on each self-information of word where the weight is the corresponding word probability in the global comment set. Since we want to measure the information richness and the relevance of a comment, we give higher weight to these words that other comments also mentioned and lower weight to words that other comments hardly mentioned.

The general entropy seems a good ranking metric that measures both relevance and text complexity. However, comment with high complexity (e.g., very long comment with many different kinds of words) and almost no relevance to this product may get very high general entropy. These comments may have high ranks since most comments' entropy scores are close to each other. So instead of calculating scores for every comment, we first find an "ideal" comment and then judge comment by how far or how different it is from our "ideal" comment. Naturally, we define a comment with maximum general entropy as our "ideal" comment, and we call this "ideal" comment the **Maximum General Entropy**

Comment. Since this "ideal" comment has the maximum general entropy, it keeps a good balance of relevance and information richness. We define the **Maximum General Entropy Comment** as follows:

$$\mathbf{B} = \arg \max_{\mathbf{P}} E(\mathbf{P}). \tag{2}$$

Note that the maximum entropy comment is a comment with the maximum general entropy within all possible comments. This comment may not exist in the existing comment set. Now, the question is how to measure each comment's "distance" to this "ideal" comment. Since we treat each comment as a distribution, we use **Kullback–Leibler (K-L) divergence** defined as follows:

$$D_{KL}(\mathbf{P}|\mathbf{B}) = \sum_{i=0}^{n} P_i \cdot \log\left(\frac{P_i}{B_i}\right). \tag{3}$$

Notice that this is a divergence, not a "distance." Actually, K-L divergence is used to measure how one probability distribution is different from others. In our application, we need to compare how each comment is different from the maximum general entropy comment. If a comment is similar to the maximum general entropy comment, it gets low divergence. Otherwise, if a comment is very different from the maximum general entropy comment, it may get high divergence. Compared to the method purely using the general entropy, this method achieved better performance in our experiment since it is more sensitive to comments' relevance to the product.

1.3 Text Representation

Let us consider the second problem described before: **How to retrieve information from comments' content effectively?** As we discussed in the previous subsection, in order to use entropy as our comments' ranking metric, we need to treat each comment as a distribution of words $\mathbf{P} = [P_1, ..., P_n]$. $\mathbf{P}$ is a numerical vector where each dimension indicates the frequency of a word that appeared in the comment, and n indicates the number of unique words in the whole collection of comments. This is actually called the bag-of-words (BOW) model. A bag-of-words is a representation of text that describes the occurrence of words within a document. Despite the simplicity of this representation method, it has two significant disadvantages:

(1) The number of unique words in comments data is about 10,000, while each comment has only 10–200 words, and using the BOW model leads to high-dimensional and sparse vectors.
(2) BOW representation does not consider the semantic relation between words, and it assumes all the words are independent. This assumption may have some problems, for example, "used bicycle" and "old bike" will be considered entirely different phrases because they have no words in common.

In this chapter, we construct an entirely different method to solve both the BOW model's sparsity and the semantic problem. We called our model: the bag-of-word clusters model. Unlike the traditional bag-of-words model that treats each word as an independent item, we group semantic-related words as clusters using pre-trained word2vec word embeddings (see Mikolov et al. 2013a,b). For example, consider the "used bike" and "old bicycle" example, and we have four unique words: "old," "bike," "used," and "bicycle." By using the traditional BOW model, we represent "old bike" as vector $[\frac{1}{2}, \frac{1}{2}, 0, 0]$ and represent "used bicycle" as $[0, 0, \frac{1}{2}, \frac{1}{2}]$. It turns out that these two vectors are orthogonal, and two vectors have no elements in common. But in reality "used bicycle" and "old bike" are semantic-related. Using our methods, we first group similar words such as "bicycle" and "bike" into the same cluster and treat them as the same item. For example, we have two groups: cluster #1: "used," "old"; cluster #2: "bike," "bicycle." Then we represent "old bike" as $[\frac{1}{2}, \frac{1}{2}]$, where each dimension indicates one cluster, and then the bag-of-word clusters representation of "used bicycle" is also $[\frac{1}{2}, \frac{1}{2}]$. Using this example, our method solves the BOW model's sparsity problem, and the number of clusters is significantly smaller than the number of unique words. Also, we retrieve semantic information from text, and similar phrases "old bike" and "used bicycle" are represented as the same vector in our model. Besides, unlike Zhang's method, which only considers keywords and treats all other words as noise, our method keeps most words and treats related words as the same item. We believe our method can extract more information from text and thus has a better ranking performance. More detail about the bag-of-word clusters model is introduced in the next section.

The rest of this chapter is organized as follows. In Sect. 2, we propose a new text representation method: the bag-of-word clusters model. In Sect. 3, we give a detailed description of our ranking algorithm. Section 4 introduces our experiment with a real Amazon product using the Amazon product dataset (see He and McAuley 2016; McAuley et al. 2015).

2 Bag-of-Words Model with Word Embedding Clusters

In most text mining or text analytics applications, the first and fundamental problem is how we represent text as input to our model or algorithm. More specifically, how do we represent the text documents to make them mathematically computable? Various text representation methods were proposed during the last few years, and the most commonly used text representation model in the area of text mining is called the vector space model (VSM) (Manning et al. 2008), which aims to represent a text document as numerical vectors. One main advantage of VSM is that it is straightforward to compute the similarity between each vector (document), for example, by using cosine similarity.

One of the commonly used VSMs is the BOW. A bag-of-words is a representation of text that describes the occurrence of words within a document. And to build a BOW model, people need to provide two things: the vocabulary of known words and a measure of the presence of known words. Given the document collection $D = \{d_i, \ i = 1, 2, 3...n\}$ and m unique words in these documents, mathematically, each document d_i is represented by an $m \times 1$ vector $v_i \in R^{m \times 1}$. For instance, consider there are three documents in this collection D:

d_1: I like learning text mining.
d_2: What is text mining?
d_3: Apple tastes good.

Now we make a list of all words in our model's vocabulary. The unique words here (ignoring case and punctuation) are: {*I, like, learning, text, mining, what, is, apple, taste, good*}. Thus we have 10 unique words and 12 words in total within this collection D.

Next step is to score each word in the document. There are many methods of scoring. Let us consider the simple Boolean first. If a word appears in a document, its corresponding weight is 1; otherwise, it is 0. Since our vocabulary has 10 words, we use a fixed-length vector representation, with each position in the vector to score a word. Then the vector representations of these three documents are like this

$$v_1 = [1, 1, 1, 1, 1, 0, 0, 0, 0, 0],$$

$$v_2 = [0, 0, 0, 1, 1, 1, 1, 0, 0, 0],$$

$$v_3 = [0, 0, 0, 0, 0, 0, 0, 1, 1, 1].$$

Notice that the order of word index is the same as the unique word list above.

The intuition of this model is that the information within a document is from its content, which are words in this case. Documents are similar if they have similar words. Since each of the three vectors has a fixed length, we use cosine similarity to measure their similarity. Consider two vectors **A** and **B** with a fixed length N, and cosine similarity is defined as follows:

$$Cosine\ Similarity = \frac{\mathbf{A} \cdot \mathbf{B}}{||\mathbf{A}||\,||\mathbf{B}||} = \frac{\sum_{i=1}^{i=N} A_i B_i}{\sqrt{\sum_{i=1}^{i=N} A_i^2}\sqrt{\sum_{i=1}^{i=N} B_i^2}}, \tag{4}$$

where A_i and B_i are components of vectors **A** and **B**, respectively.

The cosine value ranges between $[-1, 1]$, 1 for vectors pointing at the same direction, 0 for orthogonal, and -1 for vectors pointing in the opposite direction. For documents, the term values are usually non-negative, so the cosine similarity ranges between $[0, 1]$, and the higher the value is, the more similar two documents are.

Now we calculate the similarity between documents d_1, d_2 and d_3 using this formula,

$$\cos(d_1, d_2) = 0.4472; \ \cos(d_1, d_3) = 0; \ \cos(d_2, d_3) = 0.$$

We believe that this result is consistent with our observation, d_1 and d_2 are similar to each other because they are both talking about text mining, d_3 has no relation with d_1 and d_2, and thus their cosine similarity is zero.

The BOW model is very straightforward and is easy to implement. For the word weight in the BOW model, besides the simple Boolean model, we also use counts of words, frequency, or term frequency-inverse document frequency (tf-idf) as word weight, and more information about this is referred to Salton and Buckley (1988).

Despite the simplicity of this representation method, we face two significant disadvantages if we want to adapt this method on our comments data: (1) The vocabulary size in comments data is about 10,000, while each comment has only 10–200 words, and using the BOW model will lead to high-dimensional and sparse vectors. (2) BOW representation does not consider the semantic relation between words, and it assumes all the words are independent. This assumption may have some problems, for example, "used bicycle" and "old bike" will be considered as entirely different phrases because they have no words in common.

Next we develop a new text representation method based on the BOW model to overcome these disadvantages. First, we introduce word embeddings, a learned representation of words where words with the same meaning will have similar representations (Manning et al. 2008). Word2vec (see Mikolov et al. 2013a,b) is a very effective algorithm to train word embeddings based on the local documents. With these word embeddings, we group similar words as a cluster using the clustering method. Finally, instead of representing document (comment) as "bag of words," we represent them as "bag of word clusters." In this way, we retrieve semantic information from the text, for example, "bike" and "bicycle" are grouped together because they have the same or similar meaning. Moreover, the BOW model's sparsity problem is handled since the number of clusters is significantly smaller than the vocabulary size.

Word2vec was created and published in 2013 by a team of researchers led by Tomas Mikolov at Google (Mikolov et al. 2013a,b). Word2vec is a group of related models used to produce word vectors (also called word embeddings). Usually, word2vec is referred to two model architectures and two related training techniques:

- **2 model architectures**: continuous bag-of-words (CBOW) and skip-gram (SG). CBOW aims to predict a center word from the surrounding context in terms of word vectors. Skip-gram does the opposite and predicts the probability of context words from a center word.
- **2 training techniques**: negative sampling and hierarchical softmax. Negative sampling defines an objective by sampling negative examples, while hierarchical softmax defines an objective using an efficient tree structure to compute probabilities of appearance for all the vocabulary.

In our application, the skip-gram model with negative sampling is used. The detailed steps are given in the first author's master thesis. For a detailed explanation of other models in word2vec, one refers to Rong (2014). Moreover, since skip-gram is a neural network model, if you are not familiar with the neural network model, you can refer to Goodfellow et al. (2016).

```
w2v_model.wv.most_similar('baby')          w2v_model.wv.most_similar('apple')

[('child', 0.6217172145843506),           [('carrot', 0.5864819288253784),
 ('babe', 0.5719802379608154),             ('banana', 0.5851048231124878),
 ('infant', 0.5226951241493225),           ('fruit', 0.5847668051719666),
 ('little_guy', 0.5223316550254822),       ('veggie', 0.5716378688812256),
 ('son', 0.5125443935394287),              ('grape', 0.5633351802825928),
 ('kid', 0.5019221305847168),              ('pear', 0.5447382926940918),
 ('kiddo', 0.4887546896934509),            ('strawberry', 0.5204207897186279),
 ('daughter', 0.47309964895248413),        ('pea', 0.4928736686706543),
 ('newborn', 0.4703175127506256),          ('avocado', 0.4899260997772217),
 ('him', 0.4476194977760315)]              ('fruit_veggie', 0.48924189805984497)]

               w2v_model.wv.most_similar('well') # :

               [('nicely', 0.6807569265365601),
                ('beautifully', 0.6258641481399536),
                ('wonderfully', 0.5551607608795166),
                ('fine', 0.5284466743469238),
                ('amazingly', 0.5153716802597046),
                ('too', 0.5069817304611206),
                ('perfectly', 0.5052441358566284),
                ('decently', 0.48130089044570923),
                ('sturdily', 0.46339577436447144),
                ('fabulously', 0.4559105634689331)]
```

Fig. 1 Word2vec example

Training using word2vec model produces N-dimensional vectors for each word in our vocabulary. These word embeddings have many good properties. Since each word embeddings have the same size N, it is easy to measure the distance between a pair of word embeddings. Another property of these pre-trained word embeddings is that semantically related words usually have a close distance. Here we use the cosine similarity defined by (4), and the more similar two words are the higher cosine similarity of their word embeddings. Figure 1 shows three examples of words "baby," "apple," and "well" with their top 10 most similar words in the whole vocabulary with around 10^4 words. More detail about how these word embeddings trained is described in Sect. 4.

In our method, we adopt the K-means algorithm (Hartigan & Wong 1979) to perform word embeddings clustering. K-means is a straightforward and efficient algorithm for general clustering. We introduce how K-means are applied in our method, and let us review this algorithm first.

In this clustering problem, we are given n word embeddings as our training set $\{w^{(1)}, w^{(2)}, ..., w^{(n)}\}$ and $w^{(i)} \in \mathbb{R}^N$. The number of clusters is a pre-set parameter K, and the K-means algorithm is as follows:

1. Initialize cluster centroids $\mu_1, \mu_2, ..., \mu_K \in \mathbb{R}^N$ randomly.
2. Repeat until convergence: {
        for every $i \in \{1, ..., n\}$, set

$$c^{(i)} := \arg\min_{j} ||w^{(i)} - \mu_j||^2; \tag{5}$$

for every $j \in \{1, ..., K\}$, set

$$\mu_j = \frac{\sum_{i=1}^{n} 1\{c^{(i)} = j\} w^{(i)}}{\sum_{i=1}^{n} 1\{c^{(i)} = j\}}. \tag{6}$$

}

For every repetition, there are two steps, first is to assign each training sample $w^{(i)}$ to its nearest cluster μ_j and update its assigned cluster index c^i. Then, update the cluster μ_j to the mean of the points assigned to it. The K-means algorithm is also regarded as a coordinate descent on the distortion function J,

$$J(c, \mu) = \sum_{i=1}^{n} ||w^{(i)} - \mu_{c^{(i)}}||^2. \tag{7}$$

Clearly, the distortion function is a non-convex function, so the K-means algorithm is easily got stuck in local minima. One common solution to this problem is to run K-means many times with a different random initialization of μ, and out of all different clusters founded, use the one with the lowest distortion J as our final solution.

Normally, we use cosine similarity to measure the distance between word embeddings as we mentioned before, but K-means use only Euclidean distance as the distance measure. Although other clustering methods use cosine as a distance measure like K-medoids (Kaufmann 1987), we still use K-means due to its much higher computational efficiency. And we justify that for normalized vectors, cosine similarity and Euclidean distance are linearly connected. For two normalized vectors $A = \{A_i\}$, $B = \{B_i\}$ $(\sum A_i^2 = \sum B_i^2 = 1)$, the Euclidean distance between A and B is

$$\begin{aligned}
||A - B||^2 &= \sum (A_i - B_i)^2 \\
&= \sum (A_i^2 + B_i^2 - 2A_i B_i) \\
&= \sum A_i^2 + \sum B_i^2 - 2 \sum A_i B_i \\
&= 1 + 1 - 2\cos(A, B) \\
&= 2(1 - \cos(A, B)).
\end{aligned} \tag{8}$$

Note that for normalized vectors $\cos(A, B) = \frac{\sum A_i B_i}{\sqrt{\sum A_i^2}\sqrt{\sum B_i^2}} = \sum A_i B_i$. The higher two word embeddings' cosine similarity is, the closer their Euclidean distance is, which is consistent with our objective. Thus in our application, we perform K-means on the normalized pre-trained word embeddings.

So instead of representing text documents as "bag of words," we represent them as "bag of word clusters." Now we have our pre-trained word embeddings, and then we perform K-means algorithm, which assigns each word a unique cluster index. Then constructing bag-of-word clusters representation of text document is summarized as the following steps:

1. Preprocess and tokenize the text, and then each text is represented as a list of words.
2. Given pre-trained K word cluster, replace each word in the list as its cluster index, if there are unknown words, replace them with $K + 1$, so this vector is transformed to numerical lists with the number 1 to $K + 1$.
3. Calculate each cluster's frequency in the text list, and construct a vector with length k+1 where each term will be the calculated frequency of clusters with the corresponding index number. And this new vector is our "bag of clusters" representation of text.

With the above steps, we transform each text into a $K + 1$-dimensional vector. For example, we have a short text:

```
"I love eating apples, they are delicious"
```

and we have four pre-trained word clusters: $C_1 = \{$"I," "they," "you"$\}$, $C_2 = \{$"apple," "pear," "banana"$\}$, $C_3 = \{$"is," "are," "was"$\}$, and $C_4 = \{$"delicious," "good," "tasty"$\}$. First, we tokenize this text as a vector $v = [$"I," "love," "eating," "apples," "they," "are," "delicious"$]$, then replace these words with the corresponding clusters $v = [1, 5, 5, 2, 1, 3, 4]$, and remember to replace unknown words with "k+1" that is 5 here. Next we calculate each cluster's relative frequency: $f_1 = \frac{2}{7}$, $f_2 = \frac{1}{7}$, $f_3 = \frac{1}{7}$, $f_4 = \frac{1}{7}$, $f_5 = \frac{2}{7}$, and represent this text with new vector $v' = [f_1, f_2, f_3, f_4, f_5] = [\frac{2}{7}, \frac{1}{7}, \frac{1}{7}, \frac{1}{7}, \frac{2}{7}]$.

Text digitalization or representing text as numerical vectors is an essential part of every text mining application. Our "bag of word clusters" model can extract not only statistical information but also part of semantic information from text.

3   Ranking Comments with General Entropy

In this section, we use **General Entropy** (Zhang 2019) to rank comments based on the entropy value. First we define the **Maximum Entropy Comment**. By treating the maximum entropy comment as an "ideal" comment, we measure each comments distance to the "ideal" comment by using K-L divergence and rank comments based on its value. Moreover, there are two features of our comment ranking algorithm:

(1) Our method is unsupervised, which means there is no human-labeled training set to learn from, and all we have is a group of comments without any order. In other words, our method does not depend on an annotated training set.

(2) Judging the quality of a comment is subjective, and we cannot just create a judgment standard from nothing. So the objective of our method is not to distinguish these top-ranked comments but to make sure those unrelated or "fake" comments have as lower ranks as possible. In general, one of the objectives of our method is to filter out "bad" comments.

After the pre-trained word embedding clustering, given n clusters of words and m comments under a product, we regard the collection of all m comments together as the **Global Comments Set**. Then we calculate the number of each word cluster appears in the global comments set, which is represented as $\{Num_0^G, Num_1^G, Num_2^G, ..., Num_n^G\}$, and notice that Num_0^G is the number of unknown words that appear in the collection. Now we define the **global probability** of word cluster i in the global comments set as

$$Q_i = \frac{Num_i^G}{Num_0^G + Num_1^G + Num_2^G + ... + Num_n^G}, i = 0, 1, \ldots, n. \tag{9}$$

And for all global probabilities, we have

$$\sum_{i=0}^{n} Q_i = 1. \tag{10}$$

Since word2vec model has to be trained on a large corpus with around 10^4–10^5 unique words, we group these words into n word clusters. One feature of our bag-of-word clusters model is that these pre-trained word clusters are used for many products at the same time. So for one product, it is possible that no word within its global comments set falls into the word cluster i^*. In other words, it is possible that global probability $Q_{i*} = 0$ for this product.

In our comments ranking method, we tend to treat each text or comment as a distribution of word clusters. If two comments have similar distributions, they probably expressed similar meanings. And as an unsupervised method, without any training set, the global comments set's distribution can be an essential reference for determining each individual comment's relevance to others. We believe that under a product, most comments will focus on some specific aspects of this product, which tend to have similar distributions of words, and if a comment has a completely different word distribution with the others, it might be a "fake comment."

Similarly, for an individual comment with index j, we have the number of each word cluster in the comment as $\{Num_0^j, Num_1^j, Num_2^j, ..., Num_n^j\}$, the probability of word cluster i in the jth comment is defined as

$$P_i^j = \frac{Num_i^j}{Num_0^j + Num_1^j + Num_2^j + ... + Num_n^j}, i = 0, 1 ..., n, \tag{11}$$

where

$$\sum_{i=0}^{n} P_i^j = 1, \tag{12}$$

and note that if $Q_i = 0$, then $P_i^j = 0$.

Thus with our new definition, for global comment set, the vector is $[Q_0, Q_1, Q_2, ..., Q_n]$, and for individual comment j is $[P_0^j, P_1^j, P_2^j, ..., P_n^j]$. By treating each comment as a distribution, we assess each comment's information quality by calculating entropy based on these probabilities.

In terms of comments, we treat each comment as a multinomial distribution of word clusters with probability $\mathbf{P}^j = [P_0^j, P_1^j, P_2^j, ..., P_n^j]$, that is, if we randomly sample a word from this comment, this word should have this probability distribution. For the worst scenario, if a comment only has one type of word in it like "good good good...good," then this comment has a distribution with $P(good) = 1$, and the entropy of this comment is zero. For the best scenario, without any constraint, the uniform distribution is the maximum entropy probability distribution for a random variable. The reason is that the entropy score is the "expected information gain," and the hardest distribution to predict is the uniform distribution when using a binomial score. For example, if a comment has an equal probability of every word cluster in it, it would have the maximum entropy. However, if we use entropy defined at (11) as our ranking score, a comment with uniform distribution would rank highest under any product, which cannot be used in our application. That is why we have to consider each comment relevance to the others, so we define the **General Entropy** as follows:

Definition 1 (General Entropy) Given global probability $\mathbf{Q} = \{Q_0, Q_1, ..., Q_n\}$ and a comment with probability $\mathbf{P}^j = \{P_0^j, P_1^j, ..., P_n^j\}$, the general entropy of this comment is

$$E(\mathbf{P}^j) = - \sum_{i=0, P_i^j \neq 0}^{n} Q_i \cdot P_i^j \cdot \log P_i^j.$$

Notice that P_i^j can be 0 since a comment may not include all word clusters. The general entropy measures the average information rate for an individual comment j with respect to the global probability. From the entropy definition given by (1), it assigns weight on each self-information of word cluster where the weight is the corresponding global probability. As we mentioned before, the global probability is regarded as a high-level abstraction of the topic in the comments under this product. Since we want to measure the information richness and the relevance of a comment, we give higher weight to these words that other comments also mentioned and lower weight to words that other comments hardly mentioned.

At last, we summarize our general entropy ranking algorithm as follows:

Algorithm 1 Ranking comments based on the general entropy

Input:
    Input: The set of n word clusters;
    The set of m comments under a product;
Output:
    Output Ranking results of all comments;
1: Covert all comments into their bag-of-word clusters representations;
2: Calculate the global probability $\mathbf{Q} = [Q_0, Q_1, Q_2, ..., Q_n]$;
3: Calculate each comment's probability: $\mathbf{P}^j = [P_0^j, P_1^j, P_2^j, ..., P_n^j]$, $j = 1, 2...m$;
4: Calculate each comment's general entropy $E(\mathbf{P}^j)$;
5: Rank comments based on their general entropy, comment with higher general entropy is ranked higher;
6: **return** Ranking results;

In our experiment, comment with high complexity (e.g., very long comment with many different kinds of words) and almost no relevance to this product can get pretty high general entropy. These comments may have high ranks since most comments' entropy scores are close to each other. So instead of calculating scores for every comment, we first find an "ideal" comment and then judge comment by how far or how different it is from our "ideal" comment. Naturally, can define a comment with maximum general entropy as our "ideal" comment, and we call this "ideal" comment the **Maximum General Entropy Comment**. Since the maximum general entropy comment has the maximum general entropy, it keeps a good balance of relevance and information richness. We define the **Maximum General Entropy Comment** as follows:

Definition 2 (Maximum General Entropy Comment) Given global probability $\mathbf{Q} = \{Q_0, Q_1, \ldots, Q_n\}$, the maximum general entropy comment $\mathbf{B} := \{B_0, B_1, ..., B_n\}$ is defined as

$$\mathbf{B} = \arg\max_{\mathbf{P}} E(\mathbf{P}),$$

where $\mathbf{P} := \{P_0, P_1, ..., P_n\}$ and $\sum_{i=0}^{n} P_i = 1$. □

Note that the maximum entropy comment is a comment with the maximum general entropy within all possible comments. This comment may not exist in the existing comment set. However, it is regarded as a standard to judge each comment's relevance to the product. The following theorem shows that the maximum entropy comment exists and is unique, given a collection of comments. Its proof can be found in the first author's master thesis.

Theorem 1 *Given global probability* $\mathbf{Q} = \{Q_0, Q_1, ..., Q_n\}$ *and an index set* C *that* $i \in C$ *if* $Q_i \neq 0$ *and* $i \notin C$ *otherwise. Then there exists a unique maximum general entropy answer* $\mathbf{B} = \{B_0, B_1, ..., B_n\}$ *so that* $\mathbf{B} = \arg\max_{\mathbf{P}} E(\mathbf{P})$ *and* $B_i =$
$$\begin{cases} e^{-1-\frac{\lambda}{Q_i}} & i \in C \\ 0 & i \notin C, \end{cases}$$
where λ *is a unique value and* $\sum_{i=0}^{n} B_i = 1$.

After the definition of the "ideal" comment, now we need a method to measure each comment's distance to the maximum general entropy comment. As we mentioned before, we treat each comment as a multinomial distribution with probability $\{P_0^j, P_1^j, ..., P_n^j\}$, that is, if we randomly sample a word from this comment, this word belongs to word cluster i with probability P_i^j. We treat the maximum general entropy answer the same way as it is a multinomial distribution with $\{B_0^j, B_1^j, ..., B_n^j\}$. To measure how one probability distribution is different from others, we use **K-L divergence** defined as follows:

Definition 3 (K-L Divergence) Given jth comment probability $\mathbf{P}^j = \{P_0^j, P_1^j, ..., P_n^j\}$ and the maximum general entropy comment $\mathbf{B} = \{B_0, B_1, ..., B_n\}$, the Kullback–Leibler divergence from the maximum general entropy comment $\mathbf{B}$ to jth comment $\mathbf{P}^j$ is defined to be

$$D_{KL}(\mathbf{P}^j | \mathbf{B}) = \sum_{i=0, P_i^j \neq 0}^{n} P_i^j \cdot \log\left(\frac{P_i^j}{B_i}\right).$$

In statistics, we call $\mathbf{B}$ the prior probability distribution and $\mathbf{P}^j$ the posterior probability distribution, and the K-L divergence from $\mathbf{B}$ to $\mathbf{P}^j$ is

$$D_{KL}(\mathbf{P}^j | \mathbf{B}) = \sum_{i=0, P_i^j \neq 0}^{n} P_i^j \cdot \log\left(\frac{P_i^j}{B_i}\right)$$

$$= -\sum_{i=1, P_i^j \neq 0}^{n} P_i^j \cdot \log(B_i) - \left(-\sum_{i=1, P_i^j \neq 0}^{n} P_i^j \cdot \log(P_i^j)\right) \quad (13)$$

$$= -\sum_{i=1, P_i^j \neq 0}^{n} P_i^j \cdot \log(B_i) - H(\mathbf{P}^j).$$

$D_{KL}(\mathbf{P}^j | \mathbf{B})$ is actually the information gain if we use distribution $\mathbf{B}$ to approximate $\mathbf{P}^j$. When two distributions are close to each other, this value is relatively small, and otherwise, it is large if two distributions are very different. The first item $-\sum_{i=1, P_i^j \neq 0}^{n} P_i^j \cdot \log(B_i)$ in (13) is called **cross-entropy**, which is a very popular loss function of classification problem in machine-learning area.

Finally, we summarize our ranking process as follows:

Algorithm 2 Ranking comments based on K-L divergence to the maximum general entropy comment

---

Input:
    The set of n word clusters;
    The set of m comments under a product;
Output:
    Output Ranking results of all comments;
1: Covert all comments into their bag-of-word clusters representations;
2: Calculate the global probability: $\mathbf{Q} = [Q_0, Q_1, Q_2, ..., Q_n]$;
3: Calculate each comment's probability: $\mathbf{P}^j = [P_0^j, P_1^j, P_2^j, ..., P_n^j]$, $j = 1, 2...m$;
4: Based on the global probability $\mathbf{Q}$, find the maximum general entropy comment: $\mathbf{B} = \{B_0, B_1, ..., B_n\}$;
5: Calculate each comment's K-L divergence to the maximum general entropy comment $\mathbf{B}$;
6: Rank comments based on their K-L divergence, comment with lower divergence is ranked higher;
7: **return** Ranking results.

The next step is to assess this algorithm by evaluating the ranking quality. Here we introduce **normalized Discounted Cumulative Gain (nDCG)** (Järvelin & Kekäläinen 2002); it is often used to measure the effectiveness of web search engine algorithms, but it can also be applied to text ranking application. Many researches mentioned before (Hsu et al. 2009; Woloszyn et al. 2017) adapt this method to assess their ranking algorithm. First, let us define **Discounted Cumulative Gain (DCG)**.

Definition 4 (DCG) Given a ranked list with m comments, and rel_i is graded relevance of the result at position i, discounted cumulative gain is defined as

$$DCG_m = \sum_{i=1}^{m} \frac{rel_i}{\log_2(i+1)}.$$

According to this definition, if a comment with high graded relevance appears lower in the ranking result, it will be penalized as the graded relevance value is reduced logarithmically proportional to the position of the ranking result. To achieve high DCG value, the algorithm should rank a high relevance comment higher than low relevance one. Notice that in our application, graded relevance rel_i is a manually annotated comment quality score that will not be used as an input in our algorithm, and more detail about our experiment is described in Sect. 4.

While DCG is already a valid measure of ranking quality, it does not have a proper upper and lower bound to let people better compare the performance of different ranking results, and then **nDCG** is defined as follows:

Definition 5 (nDCG) Given a ranked list with m comments and its DCG value, the normalized discounted cumulative gain is computed as

$$nDCG_m = \frac{DCG_m}{IDCG_m},$$

where $IDCG_m$ is the ideal discounted cumulative gain.

$IDCG_m$ is straightforward to compute where the ideal ranking result is to rank these comments directly based on their graded relevance. nDCG ranges from 0 to 1, while 0 will not be able to achieve, and the closer our nDCG is to 1, the better quality our result has.

4 Experiment with Amazon Review Data

In this section, we conduct our experiment based on the Amazon product dataset (see He and McAuley 2016; McAuley et al. 2015), which contains users' reviews on Amazon website spanning 1996–2014. We choose one of the Amazon products and rank its comments using both pure general entropy and K-L divergence to "ideal comment." By comparing these two methods on a real dataset, we understand each method's characteristics and how they distinguish "fake" comments from actual comments. Moreover, we also analyze the relationship between general entropy and K-L divergence.

Amazon product data contain more than one hundred million reviews over millions of products, and these reviews were grouped into different categories. In our experiment, we chose the category "baby," which includes 160,782 comments of 7701 products. Notice that the dataset is titled "5-core," which means each of the users and products has at least 5 comments. In that case, we assume that most of the comments in this dataset are reasonable.

As described in Sect. 2, in order to keep our word embedding's quality, we need a large amount of data to train our word2vec model. In that case, we combine all comment text in "baby" category as our corpus, which is used as an input to our word2vec model. The first step is data cleaning that is an essential part of every text mining application. We need to carefully remove all noise or unnecessary words in the text and keep as much information as possible. We performed our data cleaning process using a Python package called Gensim (Řehůřek & Sojka 2010). After cleaning the dataset, we feed the corpus to our word2vec model with K-means clustering. The detailed steps are described in the first author's master thesis.

Table 1 shows part of the results of our word clusters; notice that the "Semantic category" titles are manually assigned and not used in the ranking algorithm. We observe that in cluster #133, word "she" is in the same cluster as "baby." That is an interesting feature of the word2vec model; remember our dataset is the collection of all products' comments under the "baby" category. In these comments, "she" always indicates a "baby," where these two words have similar context words and thus have similar word embeddings. That is also why word "poorly" and "perfectly" are in the same cluster; despite the two words are antonyms, they have similar context words in the corpus. This property does not affect our application since we only care about each comment's relevance, and criticism and praise of a product are both information-rich comments.

Assigning similar words with the same cluster number enables us to distinguish comments more accurately. With our word embedding clusters, we transform each comment into its "bag of word clusters" digital representation. Now we apply our ranking algorithm on a real product. We used a product called "OXO Tot Waterproof Silicone Roll Up Bib with Comfort-Fit Fabric Neck" (ASIN: B00D3TPGAO) (Oxo tot waterproof silicone roll up bib with comfort-fit fabric neck 2014). This product also belongs to the "baby" category, which means we will have no difficulties transforming comments into their bag-of-word clusters representation. The details of this product are shown in Fig. 2.

This product has 95 comments in total. We checked all comments and made sure that they are all related to the products. Let us first take a look at the word cluster distribution of all comments, which we also called global probability in Sect. 3. Figure 3 is the histogram of global word distribution, where the horizontal axis represents the cluster index, and the vertical axis represents frequency. The word clusters distribution is not very uniform, and some clusters have significantly higher frequencies than the others. Tables 2 and 3 show the top 3 most frequent and least frequent word clusters in the whole collection of comments. Obviously, one of the most frequent words under this product should be "bib," and its corresponding

Table 1 Examples of the word embedding clusters

Cluster#	Semantic category	Examples of clustered words
133	Baby	Baby, son, daughter, child, kid, she, little_guy, kiddo, babe,...
11	Automobile	Car, trunk, vehicle, drive, SUV, truck, Sedan, van, Ford,...
248	Food	Banana, apple, veggie, pea, chicken, meat, pasta, avocado,...
116	Adverb	Well, fine, perfectly, nicely, properly, beautifully, poorly,...
104	Media	Picture, movie, video, image, show, pic, visual, television,...

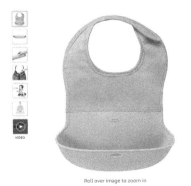

OXO Tot Waterproof Silicone Roll Up Bib with Comfort-Fit Fabric Neck, Aqua
by OXO Tot
★★★★☆ ∨   234 ratings | 6 answered questions

Price: $25.44 + No Import Fees Deposit & $7.34 Shipping to Canada Details

- Bib features unique combination of comfortable fabric and durable silicone which are easy to wipe clean and are machine washable
- Wide, soft, food safe silicone pocket effectively catches crumbs and bib length is designed so soft pocket does not interfere with high chair tray or table
- Soft fabric conforms to the body and is comfortable around baby's neck
- Strong neck closure keeps bib secure and is adjustable for comfort as baby grows; great for children 6+ months
- Fabric neatly rolls into pocket and secures closed for easy transport
> See more product details

Compare with similar items

Roll over image to zoom in

Fig. 2 Product detail (Oxo tot waterproof silicone roll up bib with comfort-fit fabric neck 2014)

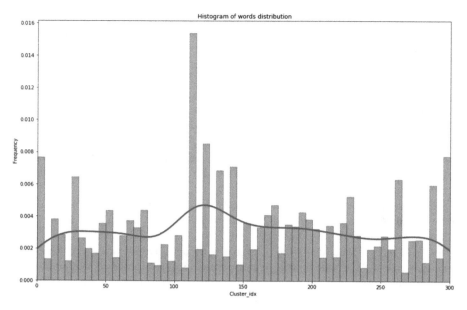

Fig. 3 Global word distribution

Table 2 Top 3 most frequent word clusters

Cluster#	Frequency	Examples of clustered words
112	0.0701	Bib, spoon, bowl, plate, dish, fork, catch_food...
133	0.0299	Baby, son, daughter, child, kid, little_guy, kiddo...
1	0.0216	Easy, easier, simple, useful, handy, make_easier...

word clusters have the highest frequency. It is not just because this cluster includes the word "bib," it also includes many related words such as "spoon," "fork," "catch_food," which may also appear a lot in the comments. The second most frequent cluster includes "baby" related words; these words appear a lot in the comments as this is a baby product. The third cluster is "easy" related words; many users describe this product using these adjectives. If these clusters have high frequency appearing in a comment, this comment is likely related to our product. After analyzing the global word cluster distribution, we find that global probabilities contain a lot of information regarding our product and are capable of judging the relevance of a comment to this product, which partially proves our methods' feasibility.

In the following, we apply our two ranking methods on our dataset: general entropy and K-L divergence to the maximum general entropy comment. In the dataset, we have one product with 95 comments, and these comments are considered as **relevant comment**. Since we do not judge these 95 comments' quality, we arbitrarily select 5 sets of comments that are not related to this product. Each set

Table 3 Top 3 least frequent word clusters

Cluster#	Frequency	Examples of clustered words
20	0	Phone, iPhone, tablet, computer, laptop, smartphone...
259	0	Brush, hair, bristle, toothbrush, nail_cliper, scalp...
263	0.0047	Sleep, sleeping, fall_asleep, cozy, snuggle, cuddle...

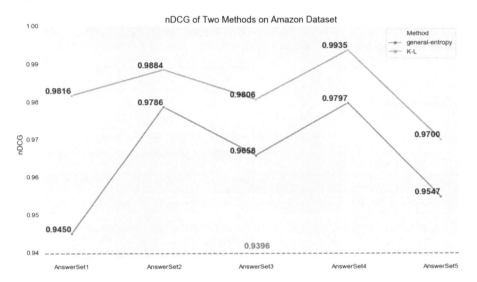

Fig. 4 nDCG of two methods on Amazon dataset

contains 10 comments. We called these comments **fake comment**, and they are all real comments under other Amazon products. It is worth mentioning that during the experiment, we are not aware of which comment is fake. We calculate global distribution and the maximum general entropy comment based on all comments, including fake comments.

To assess the ranking performance, we used the evaluation metric nDCG given in Sect. 3. According to the definition, we need to assign each comment a relevance score rel_i. In our experiment, we assigned the 95 original comments with relevance score **10** and fake comments with relevance score **−10**. To achieve higher nDCG value, the original comments should rank higher than fake comments. Moreover, in the best scenario, fake comments happen to have the lowest ranks, and we can calculate our ideal DCG (iDCG) based on this case.

Figure 4 shows the nDCG values of two methods on 5 different fake answer sets. Remember that nDCG ranges from 0 to 1, where a higher score indicates better performance. The red dashed line at the bottom of this figure is the baseline of our application. To construct the baseline, we generate 100,000 random sequences as the ranking results and calculate the mean of their nDCG values, which is 0.9396. Both of the two methods have better performance than the baseline, which shows our methods' effectiveness. The K-L method generally outperforms the general entropy method, and they have the same trend. We observe that when the K-L achieves higher nDCG scores, the general entropy always has a higher score as well. The reason for this phenomenon is that they both rank comments based on their relevance to the global distribution. K-L method is more sensitive to each comment word distribution, and the variation of comments' K-L score is bigger than that of the general entropy method, so it has better discrimination power. In conclusion, the K-L method is more sensitive to the word distribution, while the general entropy puts more weight on the text complexity.

References

Alberto, T. C., Lochter, J. V., & Almeida, T. A. (2015). TubeSpam: Comment spam filtering on YouTube. In *2015 IEEE 14th international conference on machine learning and applications (ICMLA)* (pp. 138–143)

Chevalier, J. A., & Mayzlin, D. (2006). The effect of word of mouth on sales: Online book reviews. *Journal of Marketing Research, 43*(3), 345–354.

Goodfellow, I., Bengio, Y., & Courville, A. (2016). *Deep learning.* MIT Press. http://www.deeplearningbook.org.

Hartigan, J. A., & Wong, M. A. (1979). Algorithm as 136: A k-means clustering algorithm. *Journal of the Royal Statistical Society. Series C (Applied Statistics), 28*(1), 100–108.

He, R., & McAuley, J. (2016). Ups and downs: Modeling the visual evolution of fashion trends with one-class collaborative filtering. In *Proceedings of the 25th international conference on world wide web* (pp. 507–517).

Hsu, C., Khabiri, E., & Caverlee, J. (2009). Ranking comments on the social web. In *2009 International Conference on Computational Science and Engineering*, (vol. 4 , pp. 90–97).

Järvelin, K., & Kekäläinen, J. (2002). Cumulated gain-based evaluation of IR techniques. *ACM Transactions on Information Systems, 20*(4), 422–446.

Kaufmann, L. (1987). Clustering by means of medoids. *Proceedings Statistical Data Analysis Based on the L1 Norm Conference, Neuchatel, 1987*, 405–416.

Manning, C. D., Schütze, H., & Raghavan, P. (2008). *Introduction to information retrieval.* USA: Cambridge University Press.

McAuley, J., Targett, C., Shi, Q., & Van Den Hengel, A. (2015). Image-based recommendations on styles and substitutes. In *Proceedings of the 38th international ACM SIGIR conference on research and development in information retrieval* (pp. 43–52)

Mikolov, T., Chen, K., Corrado, G. S., & Dean, J. (2013a). Efficient estimation of word representations in vector space. *CoRR abs/1301.3781.*

Mikolov, T., Sutskever, I., Chen, K., Corrado, G. S., & Dean, J. (2013b). Distributed representations of words and phrases and their compositionality. In *Advances in neural information processing systems 26.* Curran Associates, Inc. (pp. 3111–3119).

OXO tot waterproof silicone roll up bib with comfort-fit fabric neck. https://www.amazon.com/dp/B00D3TPGAO, 2014. Accessed: 2020-03-02.

Řehůřek, R., & Sojka, P. (2010). Software framework for topic modelling with large corpora. In *Proceedings of the LREC 2010 workshop on new challenges for NLP frameworks* (Valletta, Malta, May 2010). ELRA (pp. 45–50). http://is.muni.cz/publication/884893/en.

Rong, X. (2014). word2vec parameter learning explained. *CoRR abs/1411.2738.*

Salton, G., & Buckley, C. (1988). Term-weighting approaches in automatic text retrieval. *Information Processing & Management 24*(5), 513–523.

Shannon, C. E. (1948). A mathematical theory of communication. *The Bell System Technical Journal 27*(3), 379–423 (1948).

Woloszyn, V., dos Santos, H. D. P., Wives, L. K., & Becker, K. (2017). MRR: An unsupervised algorithm to rank reviews by relevance. In *Proceedings of the international conference on web intelligence*, WI'17 (pp. 877–883). New York, NY, USA: Association for Computing Machinery.

Zhang, G. (2019). How to rank answers in text mining. *Electronic Thesis and Dissertation Repository, 6250*. PHD Thesis, Western University.

Zhang, Z., & Varadarajan, B. (2006). Utility scoring of product reviews. In *Proceedings of the 15th ACM international conference on information and knowledge management*, CIKM '06 (pp. 51–57). New York, NY, USA: Association for Computing Machinery.

A Robust Approach to Statistical Quality Control for High-Dimensional Non-Normal Data

M. Rauf Ahmad and S. Ejaz Ahmed

Abstract A recently proposed modification to the limit of the Hotelling's T^2-statistic for statistical control under high-dimensional settings is evaluated for its robustness to the normality assumption. The limit, evaluated for high-dimensional asymptotics, is shown to be robust under a few mild assumptions and a general multivariate model covering normality as a special case. Further, the limit holds without any dimension reduction or preprocessing. The validity of the limit is demonstrated through simulations.

Keywords High-dimensional theory · Profile monitoring · Robust statistics

1 Introduction

Let $\mathbf{X}_i = (X_{i1}, \ldots, X_{ip})' \in \mathbb{R}^p$, $i = 1, \ldots, n$, be iid random vectors from certain non-degenerate multivariate distribution, $\mathcal{F}$, with $E(\mathbf{x}_i) = \boldsymbol{\mu} \in \mathbb{R}^p$ and $Cov(\mathbf{X}_i) = \boldsymbol{\Sigma} \in \mathbb{R}^{p \times p}$. Assuming $\mathcal{F}$ to be multivariate normal, $\mathcal{N}_p(\boldsymbol{\mu}, \boldsymbol{\Sigma})$, Ahmad and Ahmed (2020) proposed a modification to the Hotelling's T^2 statistic used in statistical monitoring when the data are high-dimensional, i.e., $p \gg n$. The modified statistic is shown to follow a scaled χ^2 or, alternatively, a normal distribution, as $n, p \to \infty$. Using the results of simulations under several parameter settings, the validity of the proposed limit is demonstrated, particularly for high-dimensional data settings.

The T^2 chart is the most commonly used multivariate control chart and, under the normality assumption, has several optimality properties. For general references, see Johnson and Wichern (2007), Montgomery (2013), and Qiu (2014). As high-

M. R. Ahmad
Department of Statistics, Uppsala University, St. Uppsala, Sweden
e-mail: rauf.ahmad@statistik.uu.se

S. E. Ahmed (✉)
Department of Mathematics and Statistics, Brock University, St. Catharines, ON, Canada
e-mail: sahmed5@brocku.ca

© The Author(s), under exclusive license to Springer Nature Switzerland AG 2022
W. He et al. (eds.), *Advances and Innovations in Statistics and Data Science*, ICSA
Book Series in Statistics, https://doi.org/10.1007/978-3-031-08329-7_6

dimensional theory is getting inroads in all classical multivariate methods, the improvement of process monitoring for such data has also become the need of the day, due to the availability of large data sets and associated questions that cannot be addressed by classical theory. The modification proposed in Ahmad and Ahmed (2020) addresses this issue for T^2 chart, which cannot be used for high-dimensional data.

The present note aims to evaluate and extend the aforementioned modification, in a high-dimensional setting, but relaxing the normality assumption. The normality assumption is replaced with a general multivariate model often used in high-dimensional, non-normal inference. The extended modified limit is shown, theoretically and via simulations using a variety of parameter settings, to be valid for $p \gg n$. As many practical applications involve data which is far from normal, this robust extension, along with the original modification in Ahmad and Ahmed (2020), provides a substantial alternative for high-dimensional statistical process monitoring, where the proposed modification can be used for a wide spectrum of multivariate distributions.

Most of the attempts in the literature on statistical monitoring, including for high-dimensional data, have investigated the theory only under normality; see the references discussed in Ahmad and Ahmed (2020). However, a few attempts have also been made by relaxing the normality assumption, or even purely non-parametrically; see, for example, Chen et al. (2016), Capizzi and Masarotto (2017), Qiu (2008, 2018), Qiu and Hawkins (2001), and Zou et al. (2008). An interesting case for statistical monitoring as an important tool to deal with large data is argued in Qiu (2019).

After a brief notational set up in Sect. 2, a robust extension of the modification is presented in Sect. 3. The simulation based evaluation of the accuracy of robustness is the subject of Sects. 4 and 5 summarizes the main points. All technical results are collected in the appendix.

2 Notations and Preliminaries

We briefly recap the classical T^2 charts here for further reference. For further details, see Johnson and Wichern (2007) and Ahmad and Ahmed (2020). For the data set up in Sect. 1, let

$$\overline{\mathbf{X}} = \frac{1}{n} \sum_{i=1}^{n} \mathbf{X}_i, \qquad \widehat{\boldsymbol{\Sigma}} = \frac{1}{n-1} \sum_{i=1}^{n} \widetilde{\mathbf{X}}_i \widetilde{\mathbf{X}}_i^T \qquad (1)$$

be unbiased estimators of $\boldsymbol{\mu}$ and $\boldsymbol{\Sigma}$, respectively, where $\widetilde{\mathbf{X}}_i = \mathbf{X}_i - \overline{\mathbf{X}}$. Assuming $n > p$ and $\mathbf{X}_i \sim \mathcal{N}_p(\boldsymbol{\mu}, \boldsymbol{\Sigma})$, so that $\overline{\mathbf{X}} \sim \mathcal{N}_p(\boldsymbol{\mu}, \boldsymbol{\Sigma}/n)$ and $(n-1)\widehat{\boldsymbol{\Sigma}} \sim \mathcal{W}_p(n-1, \boldsymbol{\Sigma})$, where $\mathcal{W}_p(\cdot)$ denotes the Wishart distribution, the phase I chart in statistical monitoring consists of plotting (i, T_i^2) where

$$T_i^2 = \widetilde{\mathbf{X}}_i^T \widehat{\boldsymbol{\Sigma}}^{-1} \widetilde{\mathbf{X}}_i, \ i = 1, \dots, n. \tag{2}$$

The criterion to declare an observation as outlier is based on the upper control limit (UCL), i.e., $[(n-1)^2/n]\text{beta}[\alpha; p/2, (n-p-1)/2]$, where beta($\cdot$) denotes $100\alpha\%$ quantile of beta distribution (Johnson and Wichern 2007). After discarding outliers, the cleaned data in phase I provides final estimates of parameters to be used in phase II, where a similar decision can be made for future observations, assuming the process is still in control. The T^2 statistic for future observation, $\mathbf{X}_0$, computed as

$$T_0^2 = \widetilde{\mathbf{X}}_0^T \widehat{\boldsymbol{\Sigma}}^{-1} \widetilde{\mathbf{X}}_0 \tag{3}$$

is compared to the upper bound $[p(n^2 - 1)/(n(n - p))]F_{p,n-p}^\alpha$, where $F_{p,n-p}^\alpha$ denotes a $100(1 - \alpha)\%$ quantile of the F distribution with parameters p and $n - p$, $\widetilde{\mathbf{X}}_0 = \mathbf{X}_0 - \overline{\mathbf{X}}$, and $\overline{\mathbf{X}}$, $\widehat{\boldsymbol{\Sigma}}$ are the final estimates obtained in phase I. A similar procedure holds for subgroup-means charts when multiple observations are available for each unit i. Although, the aforementioned modification and its robust alternative, presented below, apply to all these charts; for brevity, we shall skip further details of subgroup-means charts; see Ahmad and Ahmed (2020, Sec. 2).

3 Modification and Robustness

3.1 Model and Assumptions

Given $\mathbf{X}_i$, let $\mathbf{Y}_i = \mathbf{X}_i - \boldsymbol{\mu}$ with $E(\mathbf{Y}_i) = \mathbf{0}$, $Cov(\mathbf{Y}_i) = \boldsymbol{\Sigma}$. Having relaxed normality, our robustness evaluation will be based on the following general multivariate model:

$$\mathbf{Y}_i = \boldsymbol{\Gamma}\mathbf{U}_i, \tag{4}$$

where $\mathbf{U}_i \in \mathbb{R}^p$ with $E(\mathbf{U}_i) = \mathbf{0}$, $Cov(\mathbf{U}_i) = \mathbf{I}$, and $\boldsymbol{\Gamma} \in \mathbb{R}^{p \times p}$ is a known constant matrix with $\boldsymbol{\Gamma}^T \boldsymbol{\Gamma} = \mathbf{A}$, $\boldsymbol{\Gamma}\boldsymbol{\Gamma}^T = \boldsymbol{\Sigma} > 0$, where $\mathbf{A}$ is any positive semi-definite matrix. Model (4) contains multivariate normality as a special case and is often used for general multivariate inference; see Ahmad (2017) for details and references.

The normality-based modification in Ahmad and Ahmed (2020) is essentially based on a single extra assumption, stated as Assumption 3.1 below, whereas, for the present case under Model (4), we additionally need Assumptions 1–3. Let λ_j, $j = 1, \dots, p$ denote the eigenvalues of $\boldsymbol{\Sigma}$, so that $v_1, \dots, v_p$, $v_j = \lambda_j/p$, denote those of $\boldsymbol{\Lambda} = \boldsymbol{\Sigma}/p$. Further, let $E(U_{ij}^3) = \gamma_1 \in \mathbb{R}$ and $E(U_{ij}^4) = \gamma_2 + 3$, $\gamma_2 \in \mathbb{R}^+$, be the third and fourth moments of the elements of $\mathbf{U}$, respectively.

Assumption 1 $\lim_{p \to \infty} \sum_{j=1}^p v_j = O(1)$.
Assumption 2 Let $\gamma_1, \gamma_2 < \infty$, where γ_1, γ_2 are defined above.

Assumption 3 $\lim_{p \to \infty} tr(\mathbf{A} \odot \mathbf{A})/tr(\mathbf{A} \otimes \mathbf{A}) = 0$ with $\mathbf{A}$ a positive semi-definite matrix, where $\odot$ and $\otimes$ denote Hadamard and Kronecker products, respectively.

Assumption 1 is inevitably needed under Model (4), since the computations involve second moments of quadratic forms. Assumption 2 puts a bound on the average of the scaled eigenvalues, v_j. It is simple, effective, and commonly used in high-dimensional inference; moreover, it has an interesting consequence, $\lim_{p \to \infty} \sum_{s=1}^{p} v_j^2 = O(1)$ which will be referred to in the sequel. To see practical applicability of Assumption 2 and its consequence, let $\mathbf{\Sigma}$ be compound symmetric, which belongs to the group of spiked covariance structures, i.e., $\mathbf{\Sigma} = (1 - \rho)\mathbf{I} + \rho\mathbf{J}$ with $\mathbf{I}$ as identity matrix, $\mathbf{J} = \mathbf{11}'$, $\mathbf{1}$ a vectors of 1s, and $\rho \in \mathbb{R}$, $-1/(p-1) \leq \rho \leq 1$. It can be easily shown that $tr(\mathbf{\Sigma}^i) = O(p^i)$, $i = 1, 2$, which satisfies the assumption and its consequence. Finally, Assumption 3 is mild, because the numerator is a much smaller term, in terms of p, than the denominator.

Note that, in the computations below, $\mathbf{\Gamma}$ in Model (4) will essentially appear as $\mathbf{\Sigma}^{1/2}$, so that $\mathbf{A}$ will be representing $\mathbf{\Sigma}$. For example, the traces in Assumption 3 can be considered for $\mathbf{A}$ as well as for $\mathbf{\Sigma}$. In this context, with normality relaxed, Assumption 3 controls the behavior of the moments of estimators that compose the modified statistic; see Theorem 1 below.

3.2   Statistic, Its Limit, and Robustness

For brevity, we only focus on the charts for an individual observations case. The case of subgroup-means follows similarly. The statistic for an individual observations case, T_i^2, is given in Eq. (2), which, under the normality assumption and for fixed p, follows a beta distribution which provides the upper limit given after Eq. (2). Alternatively, as an approximation for fixed p and $n \to \infty$, a χ_p^2 limit can also be used. These limits, however, are not applicable for a high-dimensional setup, i.e., when p is large, and particularly for $p \gg n$, mainly due to the singularity of $\widehat{\mathbf{\Sigma}}$ in T_i^2. The modified form of T_i^2 in Ahmad and Ahmed (2020), valid for the $p \gg n$ case, is defined as

$$W_i = \frac{n}{n-1} \frac{\|\mathbf{d}_i\|^2}{tr(\widehat{\mathbf{\Lambda}})}, \tag{5}$$

where $\widehat{\mathbf{\Lambda}} = \widehat{\mathbf{\Sigma}}/p$, $\mathbf{d}_i = \widetilde{\mathbf{X}}_i/\sqrt{p}$, $i = 1, \ldots, n$, $\|\cdot\|$ denotes the Euclidean vector norm and $tr(\cdot)$ is the trace operator. It is shown that, under normality and Assumption 2,

$$\frac{W_i - E(W_i)}{\widehat{\sigma}_{W_i}} \xrightarrow{\mathcal{D}} N(0, 1), \tag{6}$$

as $n, p \to \infty$, where $E(W_i) = 1 + o_P(1)$ and $\widehat{\sigma}_{W_i}^2$, a consistent estimator of $\sigma_{W_i}^2$, is defined below; see also Theorem 2 and Corollary 4 in the reference mentioned above. To motivate the evaluation of W_i in (5) for robustness under the general multivariate model, (4), we first note that the limit of W_i in Ahmad and Ahmed (2020) is obtained by using the consistency of $tr(\widehat{\Lambda})$ for $n, p \to \infty$ and showing that W_i has the same limit as that of

$$A_i = \frac{n}{n-1} \frac{\|\mathbf{d}_i\|^2}{tr(\Lambda)}. \tag{7}$$

Under normality assumption, $E(A_i) = 1$, $Var(A_i) = 2/f$, where $f = [tr(\Lambda)]^2/tr(\Lambda^2)$. This helps determine the limit of A_i, and thus that of W_i, as χ_f^2/f whose first two moments coincide with those of A_i.

When we replace normality with Model (4), $E(A_i) = 1$ remains same, using $E(\|\mathbf{d}_i\|^2) = [(n-1)/n]tr(\Lambda)$, but $Var(\|\mathbf{d}_i\|^2)$ differs. The following lemma, the proof of which follows easily using Theorem 3, collects the moments of $\|\mathbf{d}_i\|^2$ under Model (4):

Lemma 1 *For $\|\mathbf{d}_i\|^2$ defined above, we have, under Model (4),*

$$E(\|\mathbf{d}_i\|^2) = \frac{n-1}{n} tr(\Lambda)$$

$$Var(\|\mathbf{d}_i\|^2) = \left(\frac{n-1}{n}\right)^2 \left[2tr(\Lambda^2) + \frac{M_1}{p^2}\right]$$

$$Cov(\|\mathbf{d}_i\|^2, \|\mathbf{d}_j\|^2) = \frac{1}{n^2}\left[2tr(\Lambda^2) + \frac{M_1}{p^2}\right],$$

$\forall\, i \neq j, i, j = 1, \ldots, n,$ *where M_1 is defined in Theorem 3.*

Note that, the moments in Lemma 1 reduce to those in Ahmad and Ahmed (2020) under normality when $\gamma_2 = 0 \Rightarrow M_1 = 0$. Further, these moments help us define the moments of the traces involved in the limit of W_i, and particularly f given above, which in turn justifies the use of Assumption 3 involving the trace operator with Hadamard product. In this context, we exploit the equivalence of the limits of A_i and W_i and consider $\|\mathbf{d}_i\|^2/tr(\Lambda)$, where the scaling trace factor will make the terms involving Hadamard product vanish under the assumption. Finally, this last point will further help us, using the covariance part in Lemma 1, obtain the multivariate limit of the vector of $\|\mathbf{d}_i\|^2$. To approach this multivariate limit, write A_i in (7) as

$$A_i = \frac{n}{n-1} a_i, \tag{8}$$

where $a_i = \|\mathbf{d}_i\|^2/tr(\Lambda)$, $i = 1, \ldots, n$. As a_i are correlated, we are essentially seeking the distribution of the vector $\mathbf{a} = (a_1, \ldots, a_n)^T$. From Lemma 1, it follows that $E(a_i) = [n/(n-1)]$ and it holds without Model (4) or any assumption. Further, for $n \to \infty$ and fixed p, $E(a_i) \to \infty$, $Var(a_i) \to 2/f$ and $Cov(a_i, a_j) \to 0$, without needing any assumptions. Now, when we let $n, p \to \infty$, the so-called high-dimensional setup, then, under Assumption 2 and its consequence, f is uniformly bounded in p (using the moments in Theorem 1 below) so that, under Assumptions 1–3, the convergence for a_i, and therefore also that of A_i, or the vector $\mathbf{A} = (A_1, \ldots, A_n)'$, may hold conveniently. For this, we use Lemma 1 for Eq. (8) and note, for $i \neq j, i, j = 1, \ldots, n$, that

$$E(A_i) = 1$$

$$Var(A_i) = \frac{2}{f}\left[1 + \frac{M_1}{[tr(\mathbf{\Lambda})]^2}\sum_{s=1}^{p} v_j^2\right]$$

$$Cov(A_i, A_j) = \frac{2}{f} \cdot \frac{1}{(n-1)^2}\left[1 + \frac{M_1}{[tr(\mathbf{\Lambda})]^2}\sum_{s=1}^{p} v_j^2\right],$$

where v_j are the eigenvalues of $\mathbf{\Lambda}$; see the assumptions above. Now, under the consequence of Assumption 2 discussed above, $\lim_{p\to\infty}\sum_{s=1}^{p} v_j^2$ in $Var(A_i)$ and $Cov(A_i, A_j)$ is uniformly bounded where the fractional term involving M_1 vanishes under Assumption 3. Note that, this vanishing limit can also be obtained by replacing Assumption 3 with $tr(\mathbf{A} \odot \mathbf{A})/p^2 \to 0$ as $p \to \infty$. But, we also need to assume a simultaneous rate of convergence of p and n, i.e., $p/n \to c \in (0, \infty)$ as $n, p \to \infty$. Assumption 3, for which the denominator implies $tr(\mathbf{A} \otimes \mathbf{A}) = tr(\mathbf{\Lambda} \otimes \mathbf{\Lambda}) = [tr(\mathbf{\Lambda})]^2$, helps us avoid any such (n, p)-relationships.

This argument implies that, even under Model (4), moments of A_i, and later of W_i, behave similarly as under normality so that a limit similar to that in Ahmad and Ahmed (2020) may be obtained. For the entire vector $\mathbf{A}$, we can now write

$$E(\mathbf{A}) = 1, \quad Cov(\mathbf{A}) = \frac{2}{f}\mathbf{I}_n[1 + O(1)] + [(\mathbf{J}_n - \mathbf{I}_n)O(n^{-2})], \tag{9}$$

where $\mathbf{I}_n$ is identity matrix, $\mathbf{J}_n = \mathbf{1}_n\mathbf{1}_n^T$ with $\mathbf{1}_n$ a vector of 1s, so that, using the limits for A_i,

$$\lim_{n,p\to\infty} Cov(\mathbf{A}) = \frac{2}{f}\mathbf{I}_n[1 + o(1)], \tag{10}$$

under the assumptions. As $Cov(\mathbf{A})$ is a diagonal (in fact, a spherical) matrix in the limit, A_i are asymptotically independent and a limit of $\mathbf{A}$ follows by the central limit theorem. Note that, for such vectors with correlated elements, the essential requirement for multivariate limit is that the covariances, $Cov(A_i, A_j)$, or more precisely, the corresponding correlations, converge to the same fixed constant. This limit, in our case, is 0, making $Cov(\mathbf{A})$ a diagonal matrix.

It follows from the above arguments that a limit of W_i under Model (4), similar to (6), follows if consistent and efficient estimators of the traces involved in f are defined for Model (4) under a high-dimensional asymptotic setup. The estimators in Ahmad and Ahmed (2020) are indeed non-parametrically defined and hence applicable under Model (4) as well. These estimators, of $tr(\boldsymbol{\Sigma})$, $tr(\boldsymbol{\Sigma}^2)$ and $[tr(\boldsymbol{\Sigma})]^2$, respectively, are defined as

$$E_1 = tr(\widehat{\boldsymbol{\Sigma}}) \tag{11}$$

$$E_2 = \eta\{(n-1)(n-2)tr(\widehat{\boldsymbol{\Sigma}}^2) + [tr(\widehat{\boldsymbol{\Sigma}})]^2 - nQ\} \tag{12}$$

$$E_3 = \eta\{2tr(\widehat{\boldsymbol{\Sigma}}^2) + (n^2 - 3n + 1)[tr(\widehat{\boldsymbol{\Sigma}})]^2 - nQ\}, \tag{13}$$

where $\eta = (n-1)/[n(n-2)(n-3)]$ and $Q = \sum_{i=1}^n q_i^2/(n-1)$ with $q_i = \|\mathbf{d}_i\|^2$. For an equivalent U-statistics formulation of the estimators, justifying their non-parametric nature, see Sect. 8. Thus, to use them in the present context of robustness, we need efficient and consistent moments of these estimators under Model (4). They are given in the following theorem, proved in Sect. 8, which reduce to Theorem 3 in Ahmad and Ahmed (2020) under normality.

Theorem 1 *The estimators, E_1, E_2, and E_3, defined in Eqs. (11)–(13), are unbiased for $tr(\boldsymbol{\Sigma})$, $tr(\boldsymbol{\Sigma}^2)$ and $[tr(\boldsymbol{\Sigma})]^2$, respectively, with*

$$Var(E_1) = \frac{2}{n-1}tr(\boldsymbol{\Sigma}^2) + M_1$$

$$Var(E_2) = \frac{4}{P(n)}\Big[a(n)tr(\boldsymbol{\Sigma}^4) + b(n)[tr(\boldsymbol{\Sigma}^2)]^2 + 2c(n)M_1 + d(n)\{6M_2 + M_3\}$$

$$-2e(n)M_4\Big]$$

$$Var(E_3) = \frac{4}{P(n)}\Big[4tr(\boldsymbol{\Sigma}^4) + f(n)[tr(\boldsymbol{\Sigma}^2)]^2 + g(n)tr(\boldsymbol{\Sigma}^2)[tr(\boldsymbol{\Sigma})]^2 + d(n)M_1^2$$

$$+h(n)M_1tr(\boldsymbol{\Sigma}^2) + k(n)M_1[tr(\boldsymbol{\Sigma})]^2 - 2e(n)[M_5 + M_4]\Big],$$

where $a(n) = 2n^3 - 12n^2 + 21n - 5$, $b(n) = n^2 - 6n + 11$, $c(n) = (n-1)(n-3)^2$, $d(n) = (n-2)(n-3)/2$, $e(n) = n-3$, $f(n) = n^2 - 6n + 10$, $g(n) = (n-2)(n-3)(2n-3)$, $h(n) = (n-3)(2n-5)$, $k(n) = (n-1)(n-2)(n-3)$, $M_1 = \gamma_1 tr(\mathbf{A} \odot \mathbf{A})$, $M_2 = \gamma_1 tr(\mathbf{A}^2 \odot \mathbf{A}^2)$, $M_3 = \gamma_1^2 tr(\mathbf{A} \odot \mathbf{A})^2$, $M_4 = \gamma_2 tr[(\mathbf{A} \odot \mathbf{A})\mathbf{A}^2]$, $M_5 = \gamma_2 tr(\mathbf{A} \odot \mathbf{A} \odot \mathbf{A}^2)$. Further, $Var(E_i)$ and likewise $Cov(E_i, E_j)$ are uniformly bounded by $O(1/n)$, $i, j = 1, 2, 3,, i \neq j$.

From Theorem 1, the variances and covariances are uniformly bounded in p where the bounds only depend on n. This important consequence will help us arrive at the limit of the test statistic conveniently, which in turn ensures $\widehat{f} = E_3/E_2$ as a consistent estimator of f, implying a consistent estimator of the test statistic, i.e.,

$2/f$. In summary, we have the following theorem, the proof of which is sketched in Sect. 9. Note that, following the arguments around Eqs. (6) and (8), using the consistency of $tr(\widehat{\mathbf{\Lambda}})$, it immediately follows that $E(W_i) = 1 + o_P(1) \to 1$ for $n, p \to \infty$, same as under normality.

Theorem 2 *Given W_i in Eq. (5), Model (4) and Assumptions 2–3. Then, as $n, p \to \infty$*

$$\frac{W_i - E(W_i)}{\widehat{\sigma}_{W_i}} \xrightarrow{\mathcal{D}} N(0, 1),$$

where $E(W_i) = 1$, $\widehat{\sigma}^2_{W_i} = 2/\widehat{f}$ with $\widehat{f} = E_3/E_2$ a consistent estimator of $f = [tr(\mathbf{\Lambda})]^2/tr(\mathbf{\Lambda}^2)$.

Although, Theorem 2 deals with a univariate limit, it follows from the moments of $\mathbf{a}$ in Eq. (9) and the arguments around it that the multivariate limit of the vector $\mathbf{W} = (W_1, \ldots, W_n)'$ can also be conveniently obtained, through a similar limit of $\mathbf{A} = (A_1, \ldots, A_n)$, so that the required limit in Theorem 2 follows simply as a marginal projection. In fact, $Cov(\mathbf{A})$, for $n, p \to \infty$, has the same limit, $[2/f]\mathbf{I}[1 + o(1)]$, as that of $\mathbf{a}$ in Eq. (10). With $Cov(A_i, A_j) = 0$, making A_i's asymptotically independent and the variances uniformly bounded in p, the limit of $\mathbf{a}$, eventually of $\mathbf{A}$, follows as

$$\sqrt{f/2}(\mathbf{A} - E(\mathbf{A})) \xrightarrow{\mathcal{D}} N_n(\mathbf{0}, \mathbf{I}),$$

as $n, p \to \infty$. Likewise, the limit of $\mathbf{W}$ follows by replacing f with its (n, p)-consistent estimator, E_2/E_3. Theorem 2 extends the use of modified T^2 statistic for statistical control to a general model covering normality as a special case.

A very similar approach, with precisely the same limit, holds for the phase II chart of future observation and also for both types of charts for subgroup-means as well. In fact, as shown in Ahmad and Ahmed (2020), the convergence of the limit in case of subgroup-means is relatively better because the statistics are composed of averages. To avoid repetition, we shall not discuss these cases here, but they can be approached following the same steps as above.

4 Simulations

We evaluate the performance of the proposed extension of the modified statistic for robustness to normality for high-dimensional data, using three non-normal distributions, exponential, uniform and t_{10}. For each distribution, we generate n iid vectors each of dimension p, where $n \in \{20, 50, 100\}$ and $p \in \{50, 100, 300, 500, 1000\}$, assuming the distribution has mean vector zero and covariance matrix either compound symmetry (CS) or fist-order autoregressive, AR(1), defined, respectively,

Table 1 Estimated size and Power of W_i for two Distributions

		Size						Power			
		Exponential		Uniform		T		Exponential			
n	p	CS	AR	CS	AR	CS	AR	CS	AR	Uniform	T
20	50	0.051	0.044	0.060	0.063	0.068	0.063	0.488	0.155	0.551	0.197	0.473	0.358
	100	0.053	0.046	0.058	0.061	0.057	0.058	0.663	0.298	0.702	0.303	0.608	0.482
	300	0.049	0.046	0.055	0.058	0.058	0.060	0.774	0.472	0.893	0.598	0.711	0.602
	500	0.052	0.047	0.053	0.056	0.054	0.055	0.936	0.788	1.000	0.806	0.898	0.724
	1000	0.055	0.047	0.054	0.052	0.055	0.057	0.992	0.882	1.000	0.902	0.941	0.875
50	50	0.045	0.048	0.054	0.055	0.062	0.066	0.795	0.403	0.899	0.455	0.885	0.538
	100	0.055	0.051	0.051	0.052	0.055	0.058	0.899	0.571	0.995	0.660	0.942	0.771
	300	0.042	0.045	0.048	0.053	0.054	0.057	0.914	0.889	1.000	0.905	0.991	0.848
	500	0.052	0.049	0.057	0.049	0.049	0.052	0.942	0.915	1.000	1.000	1.000	0.962
	1000	0.044	0.047	0.051	0.046	0.050	0.053	1.000	0.999	1.000	1.000	1.000	1.000
100	50	0.053	0.052	0.054	0.054	0.053	0.051	0.898	0.735	0.993	0.883	0.954	0.821
	100	0.047	0.051	0.057	0.052	0.056	0.052	0.994	0.896	1.000	0.958	1.000	0.990
	300	0.049	0.048	0.054	0.053	0.052	0.047	1.000	0.989	1.000	1.000	1.000	1.000
	500	0.050	0.051	0.058	0.055	0.051	0.048	1.000	1.000	1.000	1.000	1.000	1.000
	1000	0.052	0.046	0.055	0.052	0.047	0.052	1.000	1.000	1.000	1.000	1.000	1.000

as $\kappa \mathbf{I} + \rho \mathbf{J}$ and $\mathrm{Cov}(X_k, X_l) = \kappa \rho^{|k-l|}$, $\forall\, k, l$, where $\mathbf{I}$ is an identity matrix and $\mathbf{J}$ is a matrix of 1s. We use $\rho = 0.5$ and $\kappa = 1$ for both structures. Finally, we set $\alpha = 0.05$ for both test size and power and estimate them as an average over 1000 simulations.

The estimated size and power of the statistic are reported, respectively, in the left and right panels of Table 1. The statistic seems to perform accurately for both criteria, under all distributions, and for both covariance patterns. In particular, we notice an improvement in the accuracy for increasing n, although the accuracy also remains intact for increasing p for any given n. The power shows a similar pattern with discernible improvement for increasing sample sizes. We also note slightly less accuracy and slower improvement, for both size and power, under exponential distribution, which, however, get better with only a small increase in the sample size.

From sample size perspective, the robustness of the modification seems to work well even for a moderate n like 50, where it shows a drastic increase in accuracy for $n = 100$. As this holds for p, and since the test statistic is based on estimators uniformly bounded in dimension, combined with the fact that we do not need to assume any simultaneous rate of increase for n and p, it can be concluded that the robustness holds valid for any reasonable sample size and large dimension.

In summary, the proposed modification seems to work well for high-dimensional data and is robust to normality assumption, so that it can be used as an alternative to the classical T^2 statistic which collapses for large dimensions.

5   Discussion

A modification to the limit of T^2 statistic used in multivariate process control, originally proposed in Ahmad and Ahmed (2020) for high-dimensional normal data, is further extended for its robustness to normality. Replacing normality with a more general multivariate model, requiring only moments up to order four bounded, it is shown that the same normality-based modified limit can also be used for high-dimensional, non-normal data. Simulations are used to demonstrate the accuracy of the proposed limit. This robustness extension provides a useful practical tool for statistical monitoring to deal with large, not necessarily normal, data.

The practical worth of the proposed modification and its robust version follow from certain distinguishing features it offers. It has a simple structure, is based on only a few, very mild, assumptions, particularly not requiring any higher moment assumptions on the unknown covariance matrix or its eigenvalues and no relationship between the growth of sample size and dimension, and it is valid for any moderate sample size and large dimension. It thus provides a valid alternative option to the classical T^2 statistic for multivariate process control.

6   Basic Moments

Following theorem summarizes some important moments of quadratic and bilinear forms under Model (4) which are needed to prove the main results. These moments reduce to those under normality when (4) reduces to the same.

Theorem 3 *Given Model (4) with $E(\mathbf{Y}_i) = 0$, $Cov(\mathbf{Y}_i) = \boldsymbol{\Sigma} \; \forall \; i$, let $Q_i = \mathbf{Y}_i^T \mathbf{Y}_i$ $= \mathbf{X}_i^T \mathbf{A} \mathbf{Y}_i$ and $Q_{ij} = \mathbf{Y}_i \mathbf{Y}_j = \mathbf{X}_i^T \mathbf{A} \mathbf{X}_j$, $K_{ij} = \mathbf{X}_i^T \mathbf{A}^2 \mathbf{X}_j$, $i \neq j$, be quadratic and bilinear forms, respectively. Then*

$$E(Q_i) = tr(\boldsymbol{\Sigma})$$

$$E(Q_{ij}) = 0$$

$$E\left(Q_i^2\right) = 2tr(\boldsymbol{\Sigma}^2) + [tr(\boldsymbol{\Sigma})]^2 + M_1$$

$$E\left(Q_{ij}^2\right) = tr(\boldsymbol{\Sigma}^2)$$

$$E\left(Q_{ij}^3\right) = 0$$

$$E\left(Q_{ij}^4\right) = 6tr(\boldsymbol{\Sigma}^4) + 3[tr(\boldsymbol{\Sigma}^2)]^2 + 6M_2 + M_3$$

$$E(Q_i Q_{ij}) = 0$$

$$E\left(Q_{ij}^2 K_{ij}\right) = M_4$$

$$E(Q_i Q_j K_{ij}) = M_4 + M_5$$

$$E\left(Q_{ij}^2 K_{ii}\right) = 2tr(\boldsymbol{\Sigma}^4) + [tr(\boldsymbol{\Sigma}^2)]^2 + M_2$$

$$E\left(Q_{ij}^2 Q_{ik}^2\right) = 2tr(\boldsymbol{\Sigma}^4) + [tr(\boldsymbol{\Sigma}^2)]^2 + M_2$$

$$E(Q_{ij} Q_{ik} K_{jk}) = tr(\boldsymbol{\Sigma}^4)$$

$$E(Q_{ij} Q_{kj} Q_{ir} Q_{kr}) = tr(\boldsymbol{\Sigma}^4),$$

where $M_1 = \gamma_2 tr(\mathbf{A} \odot \mathbf{A})$, $M_2 = \gamma_2 tr(\mathbf{A}^2 \odot \mathbf{A}^2)$, $M_3 = \gamma_2^2 tr(\mathbf{A} \odot \mathbf{A})^2$, $M_4 = \gamma_1^2 tr[(\mathbf{A} \odot \mathbf{A})\mathbf{A}^2]$, $M_5 = \gamma_1^2 tr(\mathbf{A} \odot \mathbf{A} \odot \mathbf{A}^2)$. Furthermore, $E[A_{ij}^3 A_{ik}]$, $E(A_{ij} A_{ik} K_{ii})$, $E(A_{ij} A_{ik} K_{ij})$, $E(A_{ij}^2 K_{ij})$ and $E(A_{ij}^2 A_{ik} A_{jk})$ all vanish.

Lemma 2 (Jiang 2010, p 183) *Let $Y_1, Y_2, \ldots$ be iid random variables with $E(Y_i) = 0$, $Var(Y_i) = 1$, and b_{ni}, $i = 1, \ldots, n$, be a sequence of constants such that $\max_i b_{ni}^2 \to 0$, as $n \to \infty$. Then $\sum_{i=1}^{n} b_{ni} Y_i \xrightarrow{\mathcal{D}} N(0, 1)$.*

7 Proof of Lemma 1

Given $\mathbf{d}_i = (\mathbf{X}_i - \overline{\mathbf{X}})/p$, with $E(\mathbf{d}_i) = 0$ and $Cov(\mathbf{d}_i) = [(n-1)/n]\boldsymbol{\Lambda}$. Then, $E(\|\mathbf{d}_i\|^2)$ and $Var(\|\mathbf{d}_i\|^2)$ in Lemma 1 follow, using, respectively, $E(Q_i)$ and $E(Q_{ij}^2)$ in Theorem 3. Finally, using the same moments, and the fact that $Cov(\mathbf{d}_i, \mathbf{d}_j) = -\boldsymbol{\Lambda}/n$, gives $Cov(\|\mathbf{d}_i\|^2, \|\mathbf{d}_j\|^2)$. Note that, all these moments hold under Model (4), which includes normality. In particular, under normality, $E(\|\mathbf{d}_i\|^2)$ remains unchanged, where $Var(\|\mathbf{d}_i\|^2)$ and $Cov(\|\mathbf{d}_i\|^2, \|\mathbf{d}_j\|^2)$ reduce, by substituting $M_1 = 0$ (since $\gamma_2 = 0$), to $2(1 - 1/n)^2 tr(\boldsymbol{\Lambda})^2$ and $2tr(\boldsymbol{\Lambda})^2/n^2$, respectively.

8 Proof of Theorem 1

The theoretical properties of estimators can be studied more conveniently by using their alternative forms as U-statistics, as given in Ahmad and Ahmed (2020), i.e.,

$$E_1 = \frac{1}{Q(n)} \sum_{\substack{\pi(\cdot) \\ *}} \frac{1}{2} A_{ij}, \quad E_2 = \frac{1}{P(n)} \sum_{\substack{\pi(\cdot) \\ *}} \frac{1}{12} B_{ijkl}, \quad E_3 = \frac{1}{P(n)} \sum_{\substack{\pi(\cdot) \\ *}} \frac{1}{12} C_{ijkl} \tag{14}$$

with $A_{ij} = \|\mathbf{D}_{ij}\|^2$, $B_{ijkl} = A_{ijkl}^2 + A_{ikjl}^2 + A_{iljk}^2$, $C_{ijkl} = A_{ij} A_{kl} + A_{ik} A_{jl} + A_{il} A_{jk}$, where $\mathbf{D}_{ij} = \mathbf{X}_i - \mathbf{X}_j$, $i \neq j$, with $E(\mathbf{D}_{ij}) = 0$, $Cov(\mathbf{D}_{ij}) = 2\boldsymbol{\Sigma}$, $A_{ijkl}^2 = (\mathbf{D}_{ij}^T \mathbf{D}_{kl})^2$,

$Q(n) = n(n-1)$, $P(n) = n(n-1)(n-2)(n-3)$, and $\sum_*$ indicates sum over all indices and $\pi(\cdot)$ means all indices pairwise unequal. The U-statistics form of E_1, E_2, E_3 in (14) is equivalent to their computational forms in (11)–(13) and is based on symmetric kernels $A_{ij}/2$, $B_{ijkl}/12$, $C_{ijkl}/12$, respectively.

The unbiasedness of E_1, E_2, E_3 follows by noting, for their kernels, that $E(A_{ij}) = tr(\mathbf{\Sigma})$, $E(A_{ijkl}^2) = 4\|\mathbf{\Sigma}\|^2$ and $E(A_{ij}A_{kl}) = 4[tr(\mathbf{\Sigma})]^2$, respectively. For variances, first note that, without loss of generality, $\mathbf{D}_{ij} = \mathbf{X}_i - \mathbf{X}_j = \mathbf{Y}_i - \mathbf{Y}_j$, $\mathbf{Y}_i = \mathbf{X}_i - \boldsymbol{\mu}$. Then, for $Var(E_1)$, we can write its kernel, $h(\mathbf{X}_i, \mathbf{X}_j) = h(\cdot) = A_{ij}$, ignoring 2, as $A_{ij} = \mathbf{Y}_i^T \mathbf{Y}_i - 2\mathbf{Y}_i^T \mathbf{Y}_j + \mathbf{Y}_j^T \mathbf{Y}_j$, so that its projections (conditional expectations) and their variances, ξ_r, $r = 1, 2$, by Theorem 3, are, respectively, $h_1(\mathbf{Y}_i) = \mathbf{Y}_i^T \mathbf{Y}_i + tr(\mathbf{\Sigma}^2) \Rightarrow \xi_1 = 2tr(\mathbf{\Sigma}^2) + M_1$, $h_2(\mathbf{Y}_i, \mathbf{Y}_j) = A_{ikr} \Rightarrow 4\xi_2 = 2tr(\mathbf{\Sigma}^2) + M_1/2$.

Using the variance formula of a U-statistic (see, e.g., Serfling 1980; Ahmad 2017), we get $Var(E_1)$ in Theorem 1. For $Var(E_2)$, similarly write its 4th order kernel, $h(\mathbf{Y}_i, \mathbf{Y}_j, \mathbf{Y}_k, \mathbf{Y}_l) = h(\cdot)$, as

$$h(\cdot) = \left(\mathbf{Y}_k^T \mathbf{Y}_l - \mathbf{Y}_k^T \mathbf{Y}_s - \mathbf{Y}_r^T \mathbf{Y}_l + \mathbf{Y}_r^T \mathbf{Y}_s\right)^2 + \left(\mathbf{Y}_k^T \mathbf{Y}_r - \mathbf{Y}_k^T \mathbf{Y}_s - \mathbf{Y}_l^T \mathbf{Y}_r + \mathbf{Y}_l^T \mathbf{Y}_s\right)^2$$

$$+ \left(\mathbf{Y}_k^T \mathbf{Y}_l - \mathbf{Y}_k^T \mathbf{Y}_r - \mathbf{Y}_s^T \mathbf{Y}_l + \mathbf{Y}_s^T \mathbf{Y}_r\right)^2$$

ignoring 12, with corresponding projections computed as

$$h_1(\cdot) = 6\mathbf{Y}_i^T \mathbf{\Sigma} \mathbf{Y}_i + 6tr(\mathbf{\Sigma}^2)$$

$$h_2(\cdot) = E[h(\cdot)|\mathbf{x}_i, \mathbf{x}_k] = 4\mathbf{Y}_i^T \mathbf{\Sigma} \mathbf{Y}_i + 4\mathbf{Y}_k^T \mathbf{\Sigma} \mathbf{Y}_k + 2(\mathbf{Y}_i^T \mathbf{Y}_k)^2 - 4\mathbf{Y}_i^T \mathbf{\Sigma} \mathbf{Y}_k + 2tr(\mathbf{\Sigma}^2)$$

$$h_3(\cdot) = E[h(\cdot)|\mathbf{x}_i, \mathbf{x}_k, \mathbf{x}_j] = 2\left[\left(\mathbf{Y}_i^T \mathbf{Y}_j\right)^2 + \mathbf{Y}_i^T \mathbf{\Sigma} \mathbf{Y}_i + \left(\mathbf{Y}_k^T \mathbf{Y}_j\right)^2 + \mathbf{Y}_k^T \mathbf{\Sigma} \mathbf{Y}_k - \mathbf{Y}_i^T \mathbf{Y}_j \mathbf{Y}_k^T \mathbf{Y}_j\right.$$

$$\left. - \mathbf{Y}_i^T \mathbf{Y}_k \mathbf{Y}_j^T \mathbf{Y}_k - \mathbf{Y}_i^T \mathbf{Y}_j \mathbf{Y}_i^T \mathbf{Y}_k - \mathbf{Y}_i^T \mathbf{\Sigma} \mathbf{Y}_k + \left(\mathbf{Y}_i^T \mathbf{Y}_k\right)^2 + \mathbf{Y}_j^T \mathbf{\Sigma} \mathbf{Y}_j - \mathbf{Y}_i^T \mathbf{\Sigma} \mathbf{Y}_j - \mathbf{Y}_j^T \mathbf{\Sigma} \mathbf{Y}_k\right]$$

and $h_4(\cdot) = h(\cdot)$. The variances of these projections, ξ_m, $r = 1, \ldots, 4$, using moments from Theorem 3, follow after long and tedious computations which, substituting into the variance formula of a U-statistic, give $Var(E_2)$. $Var(E_3)$ follows the same way, with the projections of its kernel $h(\cdot) = A_{kr}A_{ls} + A_{kl}A_{rs} + A_{ks}A_{lr}$, computed as

$$h_1(\cdot) = 6\mathbf{Y}_k^T \mathbf{Y}_k + 6[tr(\mathbf{\Sigma})]^2$$

$$h_2(\cdot) = 2tr(\mathbf{\Sigma})A_{kr} + 2\left(\mathbf{Y}_k^T \mathbf{Y}_k + tr(\mathbf{\Sigma})\right)\left(\mathbf{Y}_r^T \mathbf{Y}_r + tr(\mathbf{\Sigma})\right)$$

$$h_3(\cdot) = A_{kr}\left(\mathbf{Y}_l^T \mathbf{Y}_l + tr(\mathbf{\Sigma})\right) + A_{kl}\left(\mathbf{Y}_r^T \mathbf{Y}_r + tr(\mathbf{\Sigma})\right) + A_{lr}\left(\mathbf{Y}_k^T \mathbf{Y}_k + tr(\mathbf{\Sigma})\right)$$

and $h_4(\cdot) = h(\cdot)$. Finally, the covariance bounds follow by the Cauchy-Schwarz inequality.

9 Proof of Theorem 2

As argued around Eqs. (5) and (7), the distribution of W_i follows from that of A_i using the consistency of $tr(\widehat{\Lambda})$. We thus focus on the limit of A_i first. From the moments of a_i in Eq. (9), it immediately follows that

$$E(A_i) = \frac{n}{n-1}$$

$$Var(A_i) = \frac{2}{f}\left(\frac{n}{n-1}\right) + \left[O\left(\frac{1}{p^2}\right) + O\left(\frac{1}{np^2}\right)\right]\frac{M_1}{[tr(\Lambda)]^2}$$

$$Cov(A_i, A_j) = \frac{2}{f}\cdot\frac{1}{(n-1)^2} + \left[O\left(\frac{1}{n^2 p^2}\right) + O\left(\frac{1}{n^3 p^2}\right)\right]\frac{M_1}{[tr(\Lambda)]^2},$$

which converge to 1, $2/f$ and 0, respectively, same as those of a_i. Having relaxed normality, and working under Model (4), we proceed as follows: Since $Cov(\mathbf{d}_i) = (n-1)\Sigma/n$, let $\mathbf{u}_i = [\sqrt{n/(n-1)}]\mathbf{d}_i$, so that $Cov(\mathbf{u}_i) = \Sigma$. First, assume p is fixed. Then, with $E(\mathbf{d}_i) = \mathbf{0}$, by the multivariate central limit theorem,

$$\mathbf{u}_i = [\sqrt{n/(n-1)}]\mathbf{d}_i \xrightarrow{\mathcal{D}} N_p(\mathbf{0}, \Sigma),$$

as $n \to \infty$, which further implies, for $[(n-1)/n]\|\mathbf{d}_i\|^2 = \mathbf{u}_i^T \mathbf{u}_i$, that

$$\mathbf{u}_i^T \mathbf{u}_i \xrightarrow{\mathcal{D}} \sum_{s=1}^{p} v_s Z_{is}^2, \tag{15}$$

where Z_{is} are iid $N(0, 1)$ and λ_s are constants. Note that, since $\Sigma > 0 \Rightarrow rank(bs\,\Sigma) = p$ which ensures the sum in the above limit for all p components, although the limit also holds if $\Sigma \geq 0$ with $rank(\Sigma) = r \leq p$, so that the sum in the limit is over r non-zero terms.

From Eq. (15), the limiting moments of A_i, with $tr(\Lambda) = \sum_{s=1}^{p} v_s$ as denominator, are 1 and $2/f$, $f = (\sum_{s=1}^{p} v_s)^2 / \sum_{s=1}^{p} v_s^2 = [tr(\Lambda)]^2/tr(\Lambda^2)$, so that the limit of W_i follows by replacing $tr(\Lambda)$ with E_1, which is consistent under the high-dimensional setup, i.e., $n, p \to \infty$. We, however, use another, direct, approach to obtain the required normal limit in Theorem 2 under the high-dimensional setup. For this, using the limit in (15) for $n \to \infty$, we write as

$$A_i - E(A_i) \xrightarrow{\mathcal{D}} \sum_{s=1}^{p} \omega_s \left(Z_{is}^2 - 1\right)$$

with $\omega_s = v_s / \sum_s v_s$, where $E(A_i - E(A_i)) = 0$ and $Var(A_i - E(A_i)) = 2/f$. Since, Z_{is}^2 are independent, we use Lemma 2, which is a special case of Lindeberg-Feller central limit theorem, with Z_{is}^2's as Y_i's and ω_s as b_{ni}. Letting $p \to \infty$

and assuming $\max \omega_s^2 \to 0$, the required normal limit follows immediately. The consistency of estimators from Theorem 1, implying the consistency of $\widehat{f} = E_3/E_2$, extends the limit to W_i, as required.

Acknowledgments The authors are thankful to the editors and a referee for their useful comments on the original draft. Prof. Ejaz Ahmed's research is supported by the Natural Sciences and the Engineering Research Council of Canada (NSERC).

References

Ahmad, R. (2017). Location-invariant multi-sample U-tests for covariance matrices with large dimension. *Scandinavian Journal of Statistics, 44*, 500–523.

Ahmad, R., & Ahmed, E. (2020). On the distribution of the T^2 statistic, used in statistical process monitoring, for high-dimensional data. *Statistics & Probability Letters, 168*, 108919.

Capizzi, G., & Masarotto, G. (2017). Phase I distribution-free analysis of multivariate data. *Technometrics, 59*, 484–495.

Chen, N., Zi, X., & Zou, C. (2016). A distribution-free multivariate control chart. *Technometrics, 58*, 448–459.

Jiang, J. (2010). *Large sample techniques for statistics*. New York: Springer.

Johnson, R. A., & Wichern, D. W. (2007). *Applied multivariate statistical analysis* (6th ed.). Englewood: Prentice Hall.

Montgomery, D. C. (2013). *Statistical quality control: A modern introduction*. New York: Wiley.

Qiu, P. (2008). Distribution-free multivariate process control based on log-linear modeling. *IIE Transactions, 40*, 664–677.

Qiu, P. (2014). *Introduction to statistical process control*. Boca Raton: CRC.

Qiu, P. (2018). Some perspectives on nonparametric statistical process control. *Journal of Quality Technology, 50*, 49–65.

Qiu, P. (2019). Big data? Statistical process control can help! *The American Statistician, 74*(4), 329–344.

Qiu, P., & Hawkins, D. M. (2001). A rank based multivariate CUSUM procedure. *Technometrics, 43*, 120–132.

Serfling, R.J. (1980). *Approximation theorems of mathematical statistics*. Weinheim: Wiley.

Zou, C., Tsung, F., & Wang, Z. (2008). Monitoring profiles based on nonparametric regression methods. *Technometrics, 50*, 512–526.

Part II
Challenges in Statistical Analysis

Functional Linear Regression for Partially Observed Functional Data

Yafei Wang, Tingyu Lai, Bei Jiang, Linglong Kong, and Zhongzhan Zhang

Abstract In functional linear regression model, many methods have been proposed and studied to estimate the slope function while the functional predictor was observed in the entire domain. However, works on functional linear regression model with partially observed trajectories have received less attention. In this paper, to fill the literature gap we consider the scenario where individual functional predictor maybe observed only on part of the domain. Depending on whether measurement error is presented in functional predictors, two methods are developed, one is based on linear functionals of the observed part of the trajectory and the other one uses conditional principal component scores. We establish the asymptotic properties of the two proposed methods. Finite sample simulations are conducted to verify their performance. Diffusion tensor imaging (DTI) data from Alzheimer's Disease Neuroimaging Initiative (ADNI) study is analyzed.

Keywords ADNI · Functional linear model · Measurement error · Partially observed functional data · Principal components

Y. Wang
Department of Statistics and Data Science, Faculty of Science, Beijing University of Technology, Beijing, China

Department of Mathematical and Statistical Sciences, Faculty of Science, University of Alberta, Edmonton, AB, Canada
e-mail: yafei2@ualberta.ca

T. Lai
College of Mathematics and Statistics, Guangxi Normal University, Guilin, China
e-mail: statisticslai@163.com

B. Jiang · L. Kong (✉)
Department of Mathematical and Statistical Sciences, Faculty of Science, University of Alberta, Edmonton, AB, Canada
e-mail: bei1@ualberta.ca; lkong@ualberta.ca

Z. Zhang (✉)
Department of Statistics and Data Science, Faculty of Science, Beijing University of Technology, Beijing, China
e-mail: zzhang@bjut.edu.cn

© The Author(s), under exclusive license to Springer Nature Switzerland AG 2022
W. He et al. (eds.), *Advances and Innovations in Statistics and Data Science*, ICSA Book Series in Statistics, https://doi.org/10.1007/978-3-031-08329-7_7

137

1 Introduction

With the advance in technology, it is increasingly common to encounter data that are functions or curves in nature (see Ramsay 2005). Functional linear regression models provide a framework for modeling the dynamic relationship between response and functional predictors, which was first introduced by Ramsay and Dalzell (1991). One of the primary goals for functional linear model (FLM) is to get an estimator of functional coefficient. And many procedures have been proposed to approximate functional coefficient, for example, functional principal component analysis (FPCA) based approaches (Cardot et al. 1999; Hall and Horowitz 2007; Yao et al. 2005b), spline-based approaches (Crambes et al. 2009; Marx and Eilers 1999)), wavelet-based approaches (Zhao et al. 2012; Wang et al. 2019)), and others. We refer to Morris (2015) and Reiss et al. (2017) for more informative and extensive reviews on such functional linear models.

Among the different based methods in functional data analysis, FPCA based approaches for capturing the information of covariates are popular (Hall et al. 2006; Che et al. 2017). In the setting where trajectories are observed on dense and regular grid on the entire domain, the existing works can be found in Besse and Ramsay (1986), Rice and Silverman (1991), Cardot et al. (1999), Shin (2009), Horváth and Kokoszka (2012), to name a few. Yao et al. (2005a) emphasize the case where the functional predictors are observed with irregularly sparse measurements which is often referred to as sparse functional data and proposes a nonparametric method to perform FPCA. For general review on FPCA, see Shang (2014). In this paper, we prefer to use FPCA method to get an estimator of the functional coefficient.

Sparse functional data addresses the case where each trajectory is observed at a small number of points that are distributed randomly on the domain which is different from the partially observed functional data (or incomplete or fragmentary functional data) which was first introduced in Liebl (2013). Partially observed functional data addresses each trajectory is observed at points that cover a subset of the domain in such a way that trajectories can be reasonably treated as fragments of curves (Delaigle and Hall 2016) that has great implication in applications, such as in biomedicine, economics (see Kraus 2015; Kneip and Liebl 2020). Considering the partially observed functional data can be treated as missing data for functional curves over the domain, two missing mechanisms are introduced in the existing works: one is missing completely at random (MCAR), that is, the missing data mechanism is independent from other stochastic components (Delaigle and Hall 2016; Goldberg et al. 2014); the other one is the missing mechanism in which depends on systematic strategies, such as missing parts of the trajectories only occur at the upper interval of the domain (see Liebl and Rameseder 2019). In the setting of MCAR, Delaigle and Hall (2016), Goldberg et al. (2014) and Kraus (2015) address the problem for recovering the missing parts of trajectories. Kraus (2015) and Kneip and Liebl (2020) model the functional principal (FPC) scores of an incomplete trajectory. In the scenario where missing data mechanism depends on systematic strategies, Liebl and Rameseder (2019) establishes estimators for the mean and the covariance function of the incomplete functional data via the fundamental theorem of calculus. To the best of our knowledge, no work exists focusing on estimating functional coefficient of FLM with partially observed trajectories.

In this paper, we address the problem of getting an estimator of functional coefficient for the case of partially observed functional data without and with measurement error. In the scenario that trajectories observed without measurement error, instead of deleting the incomplete trajectories, we get estimators of FPC scores for each incomplete trajectory by modeling it as linear functionals of the observed parts of that trajectory. In the setting where trajectories observed with measurement error, we use local linear smoother methods to estimate mean and covariance function of the functional predictor, followed by getting FPC scores via conditional expectation.

The contributions of this paper are as follows. First, we extend FLM approach to partially observed functional data without measurement error, which leads to an improved estimator for functional coefficient comparing with the one obtained through deleting the incomplete trajectories for given dataset. Second, we develop an estimate method for functional coefficient in FLM for incomplete trajectories with measurement error. We illustrate its usefulness by comparing with another two methods: one is based on integration method to get the FPC scores of the functional predictor instead of using conditional expectations; the other estimator is obtained by ignoring the measurement error of the trajectories in the dataset. Third, in both scenarios, we obtain the rate of convergence for the proposed estimators. Overall, the methodological and numerical developments in this paper can provide a practically useful way in analyzing FLM with partially observed functional data.

The rest of this paper is organized as follows. In Sect. 2, we introduce functional linear models. In Sect. 3.1, we develop an estimator for functional coefficient with incomplete trajectories observed without measurement error and establish theoretical properties for the proposed estimator. An estimator and theoretical properties in the scenario that incomplete trajectories observed with measurement error are introduced in Sect. 3.2. Section 4 illustrates the finite sample performance of our proposed estimators through simulation studies, followed by a real data analysis in Sect. 5. Discussion is presented in Sect. 6. Proofs of theorems are given in the Appendix.

2   Functional Linear Model

Consider a functional linear model, in which the scalar response Y_i is linearly related to the functional covariate X_i,

$$Y_i = \alpha + \int_{\mathcal{T}} \gamma(t) X_i(t) dt + \epsilon_i, \tag{1}$$

where α is the intercept, $\{X_i(t) : t \in \mathcal{T}, i = 1, \ldots, n\}$ are the functional predictors, sampled from the stochastic process $\{X(t) : t \in \mathcal{T}\}$ with mean function μ, domain $\mathcal{T}$ is bounded and closed, γ is the slope function to be estimated, ϵ_i are random errors satisfying $E[\epsilon_i] = 0$, $E[\epsilon_i^2] = \sigma^2 < \infty$. We can easily get an estimator of intercept once we get an estimator of γ. So we focus on estimating γ in the following (Hall and Horowitz 2007). Let $\langle \cdot, \cdot \rangle$, $\|\cdot\|$ be the inner product and norm on $L^2(\mathcal{T})$, the set of all square integrable functions on $\mathcal{T}$, with $\langle f, g \rangle = \int_{\mathcal{T}} f(t)g(t)\mathrm{d}t$, $\|f\| = \langle f, f \rangle^{1/2}$ for any $f, g \in L^2(\mathcal{T})$.

We first recall the method FPCA in estimating the slope function for model (1) with the functional predictor X_i observed on the entire domain $\mathcal{T}$. For the stochastic process $X \in L^2(\mathcal{T})$, denote its mean function as μ: $\mu = E(X)$, and its covariance function as $c_X(s, t)$: $c_X(s, t) = \mathrm{cov}(X(s), X(t))$. Assume c_X is continuous on $\mathcal{T} \times \mathcal{T}$. The expression $c_X(s, t) = \sum_{j=1}^{\infty} \lambda_j \phi_j(s)\phi_j(t)$ exists by the Mercer Lemma (Riesz and Nagy 1955), where $\lambda_1 > \lambda_2 > \cdots > 0$; $\phi_1, \phi_2, \cdots$ are the eigenvalue sequence and the continuous orthonormal eigenfunction sequence of the linear operator C_X: $(C_X\phi)(\cdot) = \int_{\mathcal{T}} c_X(\cdot, t)\phi(t)\mathrm{d}t$, $\phi \in L^2(\mathcal{T})$, with the kernel c_X. On the other hand, by the Karhunen–Loève (K-L) expansion, one has $X_i(t) = \sum_{j=1}^{\infty} U_{ij}\phi_j(t)$, where the random variables $U_{ij} = \langle X_i - \mu, \phi_j \rangle$ are uncorrelated with $E[U_{ij}] = 0$, $E[U_{ij}^2] = \lambda_j$, and $\gamma(t) = \sum_{j=1}^{\infty} \gamma_j\phi_j(t)$ with $\gamma_j = \langle \gamma, \phi_j \rangle$.

The full model (1) is then equivalent to $Y_i - EY_i = \sum_{j=1}^{\infty} \gamma_j U_{ij} + \epsilon_i$ based on K-L expansion, which can be approximated by $\sum_{j=1}^{m} \gamma_j U_{ij} + \epsilon_i$ by using the first m terms. To simplify notations, we assume that $\{Y_i, i = 1, \cdots, n\}$ are centered. Let $\mathbf{Y} = (Y_1, \cdots, Y_n)^T$, $\gamma = (\gamma_1, \cdots, \gamma_m)^T$, $\hat{\mu}$ be an estimator of μ, $\{\hat{\lambda}_j\}$ and $\{\hat{\phi}_j\}$ be estimators of the sequence $\{\lambda_j\}$ and $\{\phi_j\}$ with $\hat{\lambda}_1 > \hat{\lambda}_2 > \cdots > 0$. The least square estimator $\hat{\gamma}$ is then given as

$$\hat{\gamma} = \left(\hat{\mathbf{U}}_m^T \hat{\mathbf{U}}_m\right)^{-1} \hat{\mathbf{U}}_m \mathbf{Y}, \tag{2}$$

provided that $(\hat{\mathbf{U}}_m^T \hat{\mathbf{U}}_m)^{-1}$ exists with $\hat{U}_{ij} = \langle X_i - \hat{\mu}, \hat{\phi}_j \rangle$, $\hat{\mathbf{U}}_m = (\hat{U}_{ij})_{i=1,\cdots,n;\ j=1,\cdots,m}$. Moreover, for the estimator $\hat{\gamma}_j$, $j = 1, \cdots, m$, it has the equivalent form as

$$\hat{\gamma}_j = \hat{\lambda}_j^{-1} \left\langle n^{-1} \sum_{i=1}^{n} (Y_i - \bar{Y}_0)(X_i - \hat{\mu}), \hat{\phi}_j \right\rangle.$$

Consequently, an estimator of γ is given by

$$\hat{\gamma}(t) = \sum_{j=1}^{m} \hat{\gamma}_j \hat{\phi}_j(t). \tag{3}$$

The number m of included eigenfunctions is chosen by fraction of variance explained criterion in practice (James et al. 2000): $m = \min\{k :$

$\sum_{l=1}^{k} \hat{\lambda}_l / \sum_{l=1}^{n} \hat{\lambda}_i \geq R\}$, with a given threshold R. For the asymptotic analysis, we assume m depends on sample size n such that $m \to \infty$ as $n \to \infty$.

3 Estimation Methods

The above analysis is based on the assumption the functional predictor is observed on the entire domain. We now consider the scenario that the predictor $X_i, i = 1, \cdots, n$ may be available only on parts of $\mathcal{T}$. We first give some notations and then make further analysis. Let $X_1, \cdots, X_n$ be an independent and identically distributed samples from the random function X. We denote the observed and missing parts of X_i by O_i and M_i with $O_i \cup M_i = \mathcal{T}$. Let $O_i = [L_i, R_i] \subseteq \mathcal{T}$, and assume that it is a random subinterval independent of X_i with $R_i - L_i > 0$ almost surely. The observed data for ith functional predictor is then given as $X_i(t), t \in O_i, i = 1, \cdots, n$, denoted by X_{iO_i}. In this section, our objective interest is to develop an estimation method for model (1) with partially observed functional observations without and with measurement error, respectively. And in these scenarios, our objective is to get estimators of the functional principal component scores $\{U_{ij}\}$ and the eigenfunctions $\{\phi_j\}$ as indicated in formulas (2) and (3). Depending on whether measurement error is presented in partially observed functional curves, two methods are developed: one is established by applying linear functionals of the observed parts of that trajectory, while the other one is based on principal component analysis through conditional expectation.

3.1 Partially Observed Functional Data Without Measurement Error

In the scenario that functional curves are partially observed on the domain without measurement error, to get an estimator of γ in model (1), we need to get estimators of U_{ij} and ϕ_j pertaining to this case. An estimator of U_{ij} is obtained based on the linear functional of the observed part X_{iO_i}, and an estimator of ϕ_j is obtained by giving estimators of mean and covariance function of X. The steps are given here.

Step 1: Estimate the mean μ and the covariance function c_X by sample mean and sample covariance.

Step 2: Estimate eigenvalues $\{\lambda_j\}$ and eigenfunctions $\{\phi_j\}$ by $\int_{\mathcal{T}} \hat{c}_X(s, t) \hat{\phi}_j(s) \, ds = \hat{\lambda}_j \hat{\phi}_j(t)$.

Step 3: Estimate principal component scores $U_{ij} = U_{ijO_i} + U_{ijM_i}$ with $\hat{U}_{ijO_i} = \langle X_{iO_i} - \hat{\mu}_{O_i}, \hat{\phi}_{jO_i} \rangle$, and estimate U_{ijM_i} by modeling it as linear functionals of X_{iO_i} given as $\hat{U}_{ijM_i} = \langle \hat{\xi}_{ijM_i}, X_{iO_i} - \hat{\mu}_{O_i} \rangle$.

Step 4:   Estimate γ based on formulas (2) and (3) for X_{iO_i} observed without measurement error.

We first address the problem of getting estimators of μ and c_X, denoted as $\hat{\mu}^{\text{NME}}$ and $\hat{c}_X^{\text{NME}}$, respectively, followed by establishing estimators of U_{ij} and eigenfunctions ϕ_j which are denoted as $\hat{U}_{ij}^{\text{NME}}$ and $\hat{\phi}_j^{\text{NME}}$. For simplicity of presentation, we suppress the notation on "NME" in this subsection unless otherwise stated.

Let $O_i(t) = \text{I}_{O_i}(t)$ with indicator function $\text{I}_{O_i}(t)$ being 1 if $t \in O_i$, and 0 otherwise, and let $W_i(s, t) = O_i(s)O_i(t)$. The estimators of the mean function μ and the covariance function c_X of X obtained from the observed points s, t of X_i, are given by,

$$\hat{\mu}(t) = \frac{1}{\sum_{i=1}^n O_i(t)} \sum_{i=1}^n O_i(t)X_i(t), \tag{4}$$

$$\hat{c}_X(s, t) = \frac{1}{\sum_{i=1}^n W_i(s, t)} \sum_{i=1}^n W_i(s, t)(X_i(s) - \hat{\mu}(s))(X_i(t) - \hat{\mu}(t)). \tag{5}$$

Therefore, we get the estimators $\{\hat{\lambda}_j\}$, $\{\hat{\phi}_j\}$ related to $\{\lambda_j\}$ and $\{\phi_j\}$ from $\hat{c}_X$ associated with the covariance operator $\hat{C}_X$.

We could not get estimators $\hat{U}_{ij}$ of FPC scores $\{U_{ij}\}$ of X_i directly from its definition if $O_i \neq \mathcal{T}$. To bridge the gap, U_{ij} is decomposed into two parts:

$$U_{ij} = \langle X_{iO_i} - \mu_{O_i}, \phi_{jO_i} \rangle + \langle X_{iM_i} - \mu_{M_i}, \phi_{jM_i} \rangle = U_{ijO_i} + U_{ijM_i}, \tag{6}$$

where μ_{O_i} and ϕ_{jO_i} denote the restriction of μ and the eigenfunction ϕ_j on O_i, respectively, and the definitions of μ_{M_i}, ϕ_{jM_i} are similar. The estimator $\hat{U}_{ijO_i}$ of U_{ijO_i} can be estimated directly from the observed part X_{iO_i} and the estimator $\hat{\phi}_j$, given as $\hat{U}_{ijO_i} = \langle X_{iO_i} - \hat{\mu}_{iO_i}, \hat{\phi}_{jO_i} \rangle$. For the term U_{ijM_i}, we consider using the linear functional form $\langle \xi_{ijM_i}, X_{iO_i} - \mu_{O_i} \rangle$ of the observed part X_{iO_i} to estimate it which is also considered in Kraus (2015), that is,

$$\hat{\xi}_{ijM_i} = \underset{\xi_{ijM_i} \in L^2}{\text{argmin}} \; n^{-1} \sum_{i=1}^n (\hat{U}_{ijM_i} - \langle \xi_{ijM_i}, X_{iO_i} - \hat{\mu}_{iO_i} \rangle)^2$$

with $\hat{U}_{ijM_i} = \langle X_{iM_i} - \hat{\mu}_{M_i}, \hat{\phi}_{jM_i} \rangle$. The estimator $\hat{\xi}_{ijM_i}$ has the explicit form: $\hat{\xi}_{ijM_i} = \hat{C}_{O_iO_i}^{-1}\hat{C}_{O_iM_i}\hat{\phi}_{jM_i}$, where $\hat{C}_{O_iO_i}$, $\hat{C}_{O_iM_i}$ are the empirical covariance operator for $C_{O_iO_i}$, $C_{O_iM_i}$ with the kernel being the covariance function $\hat{c}_X$ of X_i restricted to $O_i \times O_i$ and $O_i \times M_i$, respectively. To obtain a stable solution, we adopt ridge regularization, given by

$$\hat{\xi}_{ijM_i}^{(\rho)} = (\hat{C}_{O_iO_i}^{(\rho)})^{-1}\hat{C}_{O_iM_i}\hat{\phi}_{jM_i},$$

$$\hat{U}_{ijM_i}^{(\rho)} = \langle\hat{\xi}_{ijM_i}^{(\rho)}, X_{iO_i} - \hat{\mu}_{iO_i}\rangle, \quad i = 1, \cdots, n, \quad j = 1, \cdots, m, \tag{7}$$

where $\hat{C}_{O_iO_i}^{(\rho)} = \hat{C}_{O_iO_i} + \rho\mathcal{F}_{O_i}$, $\mathcal{F}_{O_i}$ is an identity operator defined on $L^2(O_i)$, ρ is a ridge parameter; see Kraus (2015) for further details. Let $\hat{U}_{ij}^{\text{NME}} = \hat{U}_{ijO_i} + \hat{U}_{ijM_i}^{(\rho)}$. The estimator $\hat{\gamma}^{\text{NME}}$ of γ using all of the information of the dataset is then obtained through replacing $\hat{U}_{ij}$ in (2) with $\hat{U}_{ij}^{\text{NME}}$,

$$\hat{\gamma}^{\text{NME}}(t) = \sum_{j=1}^m \hat{\gamma}_j\hat{\phi}_j(t). \tag{8}$$

To facilitate our theoretical analysis, we first impose some assumptions on observation points for partially observed functional curves, indicating the observation points asymptotically provide enough information in individual or pairwise crossover.

(A1) There exists $\delta_1 > 0$ s.t. $\sup\limits_{t\in[0,1]} \text{P}\{n^{-1}\sum_{i=1}^n I_{O_i}(t) \le \delta_1\} = O(n^{-2})$.

(A2) There exists $\delta_2 > 0$ s.t. $\sup\limits_{s,t\in[0,1]^2} \text{P}\{n^{-1}\sum_{i=1}^n W_i(s,t) \le \delta_2\} = O(n^{-2})$.

Moreover, we also introduce some regularity conditions necessary to derive theoretical properties for the estimate $\hat{\gamma}^{\text{NME}}$.

(A3) $\text{E}\|X - \mu\|^4 < \infty$.

(A4) $nm^{-1} \to \infty, n/(\sum_{j=1}^m \delta_j^{-2}) \to \infty$ with $\delta_j = \min_{j\ge1}\{\lambda_j - \lambda_{j+1}, \lambda_{j-1} - \lambda_j\}$ and $n\lambda_m^2 \to \infty$ as $m \to \infty$.

(A5) The ridge parameter ρ satisfies $\rho \to 0, n\rho^3 \to 0, nm^{-1}\rho^2 \to \infty$.

(A6) $\sum_{k=1}^\infty [\text{E}[YU_k]]^2/\lambda_k^2 < \infty$.

(A7) $\sum_{j=1}^\infty \sum_{k=1}^\infty \dfrac{r_{M_iO_ijk}^2}{\lambda_{O_iO_ik}^2} < \infty$, with $r_{M_iO_ijk} = \text{cov}(\langle X_{M_i} - \mu_{M_i}, \phi_{M_iM_ij}\rangle, \langle X_{M_i} - \mu_{M_i}, \phi_{O_iO_ik}\rangle)$.

Assumption (A3) is a common condition in the analysis of functional model by using the method of FPCA to guarantee the random functions have finite fourth moment (see Cardot et al. 1999). Note that if the eigenvalues $\{\lambda_j\}$ are exponentially or geometrically decreasing, the assumption (A4) holds. The same kind of conditions are also introduced in Cardot et al. (1999). Assumption (A5) is used to control the size of ridge effect. To define the convergence of the right hand of the formula $\gamma(s) = \sum_{k=1}^\infty (\text{E}[YU_k]/\lambda_k)\phi_k(s)$, in the L^2 sense, assumption (A6) is required that is similar to the condition (A1) in Yao et al. (2005b). Assumption (A7) is used to make the solution $\hat{\xi}_{ijM_i}$ valid which is commonplace in the theory of inverse problems as Picard condition (see Hansen 1990).

Let $\theta_n = \sum_{k=m}^{\infty} [E[YU_k]]^2/\lambda_k^2$. Then assumption (A6) indicates that $\theta_n \to 0$. Denote $\upsilon = \sum_{j=1}^{m} V_{ij}$ with $V_{ij} = \langle \phi_{jM_i}, (C_{M_iM_i} - C_{M_iO_i}C_{O_iO_i}^{-1}C_{O_iM_i})\phi_{jM_i}\rangle$. Based on the above assumptions, Theorem 1 gives the converge rate for the estimator $\hat{\gamma}^{\mathrm{NME}}$ in the L^2 sense.

Theorem 1 *Suppose that (A1)–(A7) are satisfied. Then*

$$\|\hat{\gamma}^{NME} - \gamma\|^2 = O_p(n^{-1}m\rho^{-2} + \iota_n + \theta_n + \upsilon),$$

with $\iota_n = n^{-1}\sum_{j=1}^{m}\delta_j^{-2}$.

Theorem 1 indicates that the approximation error rate of $\hat{\gamma}^{\mathrm{NME}}$ for γ is controlled by four terms. The first term depends on sample size n, tuning parameter m, ridge parameter ρ, which is of the higher order than the one given in Hall and Horowitz (2007) that is mainly due to functional curves observed on the part of the domain. The second term is related to the spacings between adjacent eigenvalues, and its effect on convergence rate of γ is also emphasized in Hall and Horowitz (2007). The third term is related to the convergence of γ in L^2 sense, which is also shown in Yao et al. (2005b) to get approximation error rate for functional coefficient. The fourth term is introduced by approximating U_{ijM_i} with $\tilde{U}_{ijM_i}$.

Note that in practice, the ridge parameter ρ included in the regularized estimation of the jth score of the ith functional observation is chosen by generalized cross-validation based on the set of samples observed on the entire domain (see Kraus 2015).

3.2 Partially Observed Functional Data with Measurement Error

In this subsection, we construct an estimator for the slope function γ for partially observed trajectories with measurement error. We suppose the functional observations are:

$$Z_{il} = X_i(t_{il}) + \varepsilon_{il}, \quad t_{il} \in O_i, i = 1, \cdots, n, l = 1, \cdots N_i, \tag{9}$$

where ε_{il} is independent from all the other variables $X_j, j \neq i$, with $\mathrm{E}(\varepsilon_{il}) = 0$, $\mathrm{var}(\varepsilon_{il}) = \sigma_X^2$.

To get an estimator of γ in (1) in the scenario that trajectories may be observed on parts of the domain with measurement error (WME), we need give estimators of FPC scores and eigenstructure pertaining to this case. Estimator of eigenstructure is established after using local linear smoothers to get estimators of mean and covariance function of X. We obtain estimators of FPC scores by using approach of principal component analysis via conditional expectation. The steps are given here.

Step 1:   Estimate the mean and covariance functions by local linear smoothers.

Step 2:   Estimate eigenvalues $\{\lambda_j\}$ and eigenfunctions $\{\phi_j\}$ by $\int_{\mathcal{T}} \hat{c}_X^{\text{WME}}(s, t)$ $\hat{\phi}_j^{\text{WME}}(s)ds = \hat{\lambda}_j^{\text{WME}}\hat{\phi}_j^{\text{WME}}(t)$.

Step 3:   Estimate FPC scores $\{U_{ij}\}$ by principal component analysis via conditional expectation (PACE): $\tilde{U}_{ij} = \text{E}[U_{ij}|\mathbf{Z}_i]$.

Step 4:   Based on obtained estimators $\tilde{U}_{ij}$ and $\hat{\phi}_j^{\text{WME}}$, we get estimator γ^{WME} for X_{iO_i} observed with measurement error.

We first calculate estimators for the mean and the covariance function of X in the scenario (9), denoted as $\hat{\mu}^{\text{WME}}$ and $\hat{c}^{\text{WME}}$, that are required to derive estimators for the FPC scores $U_{ij} = \int(X_i(t) - \mu(t))\phi_j(t)dt$. For simplicity of presentation, we suppress notation on "WME" unless otherwise stated in this subsection.

Let $K(\cdot)$ be a nonnegative univariate kernel function that is assumed to be a symmetric probability density function (pdf) with compact support $\text{supp}(K) = [-1, 1]$, and h_μ, h_c be the bandwidths for obtaining estimators of μ, c_X. Assume that the second derivatives of μ, c_X on $\mathcal{T}$, $\mathcal{T}^2$, respectively, exist. We use local linear smoothers for the mean function μ (Yao et al. 2005a,b; Kneip and Liebl 2020) defined as $\hat{\mu}(t) = \hat{\beta}_0$, where

$$(\hat{\beta}_0, \hat{\beta}_1) = \underset{\beta_0, \beta_1}{\text{argmin}} \sum_{i=1}^{n} \sum_{l=1}^{N_i} K\left(\frac{t_{il} - t}{h_\mu}\right) [Z_{il} - \beta_0 - \beta_1(t - t_{il})]^2. \tag{10}$$

Let $\hat{G}_{ilk} = (Z_{il} - \hat{\mu}(t_{il}))(Z_{ik} - \hat{\mu}(t_{ik}))$ be the raw covariance points. The local linear smoother for the covariance function c_X is defined as $\hat{c}_X = \hat{\tilde{\beta}}_0$, where

$$(\hat{\tilde{\beta}}_0, \hat{\tilde{\beta}}_1, \hat{\tilde{\beta}}_2) = \underset{\tilde{\beta}_0, \tilde{\beta}_1, \tilde{\beta}_2}{\text{arg min}} \sum_{i=1}^{n} \sum_{1 \leq l, k \leq N_i} K\left(\frac{t_{il} - t}{h_c}\right) K\left(\frac{t_{ik} - s}{h_c}\right)$$
$$\times [\hat{G}_{ilk} - \tilde{\beta}_0 - \tilde{\beta}_1(t_{il} - t) - \tilde{\beta}_2(t_{ik} - s)]^2. \tag{11}$$

Similar to the technique introduced in Yao et al. (2005a), the points $\hat{G}_{ill}, l = 1 \cdots, N_i$ are not included in (11). Let $\mathcal{T}_1 = [\inf\{L_i \in \mathcal{T}, i = 1, \cdots, n\} + |\mathcal{T}|/4, \sup\{R_i \in \mathcal{T}, i = 1, \cdots, n\} - |\mathcal{T}|/4]$ with $|\mathcal{T}|$ being the length of $\mathcal{T}$. The estimator of σ_X^2 is defined as $\hat{\sigma}_X^2$ if $\hat{\sigma}_X^2 > 0$, otherwise $\hat{\sigma}_X^2 = 0$ with

$$\hat{\sigma}_X^2 = 2 \int_{\mathcal{T}_1} (\hat{V}_X(t) - \tilde{G}(t))\text{dt}/|\mathcal{T}|,$$

where $\hat{V}_X(t)$ is the local linear estimator using the points $\{\hat{G}_{ill}\}$, $\tilde{G}(t)$ is the estimate $\hat{c}_X(s, t)$ restricted to $s = t$ (Staniswalis and Lee 1998; Yao et al. 2005a). The estimators of $\{\lambda_j, \phi_j\}_{j \geq 1}$ are the corresponding solutions of the eigen-equations

$$\int_{\mathcal{T}} \hat{c}_X(s,t)\hat{\phi}_j(s)\mathrm{d}s = \hat{\lambda}_j\hat{\phi}_j(t).$$

Based on the K-L expansion of X_i, model (9) can be rewritten as

$$Z_{il} = \mu(t_{il}) + \sum_{j=1}^{\infty} U_{ij}\phi_j(t_{il}) + \varepsilon_{il}, \quad t_{il} \in O_i, i = 1 \cdots, n, l = 1 \cdots, N_i.$$

Let $\mathbf{X}_i = (X_i(t_{i1}), \cdots, X_i(t_{iN_i}))^T$, $\mathbf{Z}_i = (Z_{i1}, \cdots, Z_{iN_i})^T$, $\mu_i = (\mu(t_{i1}), \cdots, \mu(t_{iN_i}))^T$, $\phi_{ij} = (\phi_j(t_{i1}), \cdots, \phi_j(t_{iN_i}))^T$. Assume that U_{ij} and ε_{il} are jointly Gaussian. Following Yao et al. (2005a), the best prediction of U_{ij} of the ith subject given the observations $(Z_{il}, t_{il}), l = 1, \cdots, N_i$ is obtained as

$$\tilde{U}_{ij} = \lambda_j\phi_{ij}^T \Sigma_{\mathbf{Z}_i}^{-1}(\mathbf{Z}_i - \mu_i),$$

where $\Sigma_{\mathbf{Z}_i} = \mathrm{cov}(\mathbf{Z}_i, \mathbf{Z}_i) = \mathrm{cov}(\mathbf{X}_i, \mathbf{X}_i) + \sigma_X^2 \mathbf{I}_{N_i}$ with identity matrix $\mathbf{I}_{N_i}$. That is, the (u,v)th element of $\Sigma_{\mathbf{Z}_i}$ is $(\Sigma_{\mathbf{Z}_i})_{u,v} = c_X(t_{iu}, t_{iv}) + \sigma_X^2 I_{uv}$ with $I_{uv} = 1$ if $u = v$, and 0 otherwise. Then the estimator of U_{ij} is given through substituting μ, λ_j, ϕ_j with $\hat{\mu}, \hat{\lambda}_j, \hat{\phi}_j$ as

$$\hat{U}_{ij}^{\mathrm{WME}} = \hat{\lambda}_j\hat{\phi}_{ij}^T \hat{\Sigma}_{\mathbf{Z}_i}^{-1}(\mathbf{Z}_i - \hat{\mu}_i), \tag{12}$$

where the (u,v)th entry of $\hat{\Sigma}_{\mathbf{Z}_i}$ is $(\hat{\Sigma}_{\mathbf{Z}_i})_{u,v} = \hat{c}_X(t_{iu}, t_{iv}) + \hat{\sigma}_X^2 I_{uv}$. Replacing $\hat{U}_{ij}$ in (2) with $\hat{U}_{ij}^{\mathrm{WME}}$, we then get the estimator $\hat{\gamma}^{\mathrm{WME}}$ of γ from (3)

$$\hat{\gamma}^{\mathrm{WME}}(t) = \sum_{j=1}^{m} \hat{\gamma}_j\hat{\phi}_j,$$

where $\hat{\gamma}_j$ is the jth entry of $\hat{\gamma}$ with $\hat{U}_{ij}^{\mathrm{WME}}$ in (2).

Next, we give some theoretical results for $\hat{\gamma}^{\mathrm{WME}}(t)$. We assume the following regularity conditions which are similar to the assumptions in Kneip and Liebl (2020), Yao et al. (2005b).

(B1) The observational points $\{t_{il}, l = 1, \cdots, N_i\}$ given O_i for the ith subject are i.i.d. random variables with pdf $f_{t|O_i}(u) > 0$ for all $u \in O_i \subseteq \mathcal{T}$ and zero else. For the marginal pdf f_t of observation times t_{ij}, $f_t(u) > 0$ for all $u \in \mathcal{T}$.

(B2) Let $N = \min\{N_i, i = 1, \cdots, n\}$. $N \asymp n^r$ with $0 < r < \infty$, where $a_n \asymp b_n$ means that there exists a constant $0 < L < \infty$ such that $a_n/b_n \to L$ as $n \to \infty$.

(B3) $h_\mu \to 0$, $h_c \to 0$, $nNh_\mu \to \infty$, $nMh_c \to \infty$ as $n \to \infty$ with $M = N^2 - N$.

(B4) K is a second order kernel with compact support $[-1, 1]$.

(B5) Let $G_{ilk} = (Z_{il} - \mu(t_{il}))(Z_{ik} - \mu(t_{ik}))$. Define f_{Zt}, f_{tt}, f_{Gtt} as the joint pdf of (Z_{il}, t_{il}) on $\mathbb{R} \times \mathcal{T}$, (t_{il_1}, t_{il_2}) on $\mathcal{T}^2$, $(G_{ilk}, t_{il}, t_{ik})$ on $\mathbb{R} \times \mathcal{T}^2$, respectively. All of the second derivatives of f_{Zt}, f_{tt}, f_{Gtt} are uniformly continuous and bounded. Moreover, f_t is uniformly continuous and bounded on $\mathcal{T}$.

(B6) Let $\Lambda = \mathrm{diag}\{\lambda_1, \cdots, \lambda_m\}$, $\Xi = (\lambda_1 \phi_{i1}, \cdots, \lambda_m \phi_{im})^T$, $\Upsilon = \Lambda - \Xi \Sigma_{Z_i}^{-1} \Xi^T$ and $\varsigma_n \equiv \mathrm{trace}(\Upsilon)$. Denote $r_\mu = h_\mu^2 + 1/\sqrt{nNh_\mu} + 1/\sqrt{n}$, $r_c = h_c^2 + 1/\sqrt{nMh_c^2} + 1/\sqrt{n}$. $\upsilon_n \equiv m r_\mu \to 0$, $\tau_n \equiv r_c(\sum_{j=1}^m \delta_j^{-1}) \to 0$.

Theorem 2 *Under the regularity conditions (A3), (A6), (B1)–(B6), we have that*

$$\|\hat{\gamma}^{WME} - \gamma\|^2 = O_p(\upsilon_n + \tau_n + \varsigma_n + \theta_n).$$

Theorem 2 gives the rate of convergence of the estimator $\hat{\gamma}^{WME}$ in the L^2 sense. The rate of convergence of $\hat{\gamma}^{WME}$ depends on the sample size and bandwidths which is common for estimating curves or surface by local linear smoothers for functional data analysis (see Li and Hsing 2010). Related results of Theorem 2 can also be found in Yao et al. (2005b). The terms υ_n, τ_n are related to rates of convergence of estimators for the mean and covariance function by using local linear smoothers. The term ς_n is introduced by approximating U_{ij} with $\tilde{U}_{ij}$.

4   Simulation Studies

In this section, we use the simulated datasets to evaluate the finite sample properties of our proposed methods in Sect. 3. These studies are based on $n \in \{50, 100, 200\}$ i.i.d. samples $\{X_i, Y_i\}_{i=1}^n$ and equally spaced grid $\{t_1, \cdots, t_{30}\}$ on $[0, 1]$ with $t_1 = 0, t_{30} = 1$. For the ith functional observation $X_i(t)$, the missing interval M_i takes the form $[R_i - E_i, R_i + E_i]$, with $R_i = a_1 T_{i1}^{1/2}$, $E_i = a_2 T_{i2}$, where T_{i1}, T_{i2} are independent random variables uniformly distributed on $[0, 1]$, $a_1, a_2 \in \mathbb{R}$. We consider $(a_1, a_2) = (1.5, 0.2)$, $(a_1, a_2) = (1.5, 0.4)$ with the expected missing length over the domain being 0.4 and 0.8, respectively. We set the intercept $\alpha = 0$. To evaluate the performance of an estimator $\hat{\gamma}$ of γ, mean integrated square error (MISE) is used below as an evaluation criterion, given by,

$$\mathrm{MISE} = \frac{1}{N} \sum_{l=1}^N \int_0^1 (\hat{\gamma}_l(t) - \gamma(t))^2 dt,$$

where N is the number of Monte Carlo replications.

For functional predictors $\{X_i\}$ without measurement error, the trajectories are generated as follows. The simulated random function X_i has zero mean, the covariance function is generated from two eigenfunctions, $\phi_1(t) = \sqrt{2}\sin(\pi t/2)$, $\phi_2(t) = \sqrt{2}\sin(3\pi t/2)$. For the eigenvalues, we take $\lambda_1 = (\pi/2)^{-2}$, $\lambda_2 =$

Table 1 MISEs of the estimators of γ under different methods with 1000 Monte Carlo replications for functional predictors without measurement error

Method	(a_1, a_2)	$n = 50$	$n = 100$	$n = 200$
ORI[a]		2.0295	1.0767	0.3670
NME[b]	$(1.5, 0.2)$	2.8653	1.6650	0.7343
	$(1.5, 0.4)$	3.5650	2.4412	1.3497
SUB[c]	$(1.5, 0.2)$	3.5632	1.8844	0.8322
	$(1.5, 0.4)$	4.600	2.6664	1.4401

[a] The estimator is obtained with the original dataset $\{X_i, Y_i\}$ with functional predictors observed in entire domain $[0, 1]$ (ORI)
[b] The estimator $\hat{\gamma}^{NME}$ introduced in Sect. 3.1 (NME)
[c] The estimator is obtained by deleting the functional predictors with missing parts (SUB)

$(3\pi/2)^{-2}$, $\lambda_k = 0$, for $k \geq 3$. The error ϵ_i in (1) is assumed to be standard normal. For the slope function γ in (1), we take the form $\gamma(t) = \phi_1(t) + 3\phi_2(t)$. We compare the finite sample performance of our proposed method with the method that gives an estimator for γ through formula (2), (3) with deleting the incomplete functional observations in the datasets denoted as "SUB." Moreover, the estimator of γ based on the original complete dataset is also considered in this scenario and denotes it as "ORI." We conduct 1000 simulation runs in each setup. Table 1 reports the results.

As shown in Table 1, in the scenario where incomplete functional predictors are observed without measurement error, the estimation method in Sect. 3.1 performs better than "SUB" method. This is because some useful information the dataset has will be lost if we delete them directly, while the "NME" method can take advantage of the whole information about the dataset. Specially, in each setting for (a_1, a_2), MISEs from the "NME" method have smaller values relative to the "SUB" method. These simulation results also demonstrate that MISEs decrease with increasing sample size n for these three methods. And MISEs increase with longer missing length on $[0, 1]$ at fixed n indicating that a large error is introduced for the "NME" method in imputing missing scores of incomplete functional predictors through little available information from functional samples. In further, the difference of MISEs among these three methods are reduced with increasing sample size n, and the "NME" method still performs better than the "SUB" method, those imply the "NME" method is promising.

For functional predictors X_i with measurement error, they are generated according to $Z_i(t_{il}) = X_i(t_{il}) + \varepsilon_{il}$, $l = 1, \cdots, 30$, as follows. We take $X_i(t) = \sum_{j=1}^{50} U_{ij}\phi_j(t)$ with $U_{ij} = (-1)^{j+1}j^{-1.1/2}W_{ij}$, where W_{ij} is uniformly distributed on $[-\sqrt{3}, \sqrt{3}]$, $\phi_1(t) = 1$, $\phi_j(t) = \sqrt{2}\cos(j\pi t)$ for $j \geq 2$. The additional random error ε_{il}, $l = 1 \cdots, 30$ and the error ϵ_i in (1) are assumed to be normal with mean zero, variance 0.25. For the slope function γ, we take $\gamma = \sum_{j=1}^{50} \gamma_j\phi_j(t)$ with $\gamma_1 = 0.3$, $\gamma_j = 4(-1)^{j+1}j^{-2}$ for $j \geq 2$ (Hall and Horowitz 2007). We conduct 100 simulation runs in each setup. To demonstrate the superior performance of our proposed method in Sect. 3.2, we compare it with the other two methods after we

Table 2 MISEs of the estimators of γ under different methods with 100 Monte Carlo replications for functional predictors with measurement error

Method	(a_1, a_2)	$n = 50$	$n = 100$	$n = 200$
WME[a]	(1.5, 0.2)	0.1535	0.1176	0.0753
	(1.5, 0.4)	0.2033	0.1607	0.1057
IN[a]	(1.5, 0.2)	0.1702	0.1560	0.1024
	(1.5, 0.4)	0.2671	0.2374	0.1974
NME[c]	(1.5, 0.2)	0.6312	0.4517	0.3320
	(1.5, 0.4)	0.7249	0.5086	0.3808

[a] The estimator is obtained by using the method in Sect. 3.2 (WME)
[b] The estimator is obtained by using integration method to get estimators of the principal component scores U_{ij} (IN)
[c] The estimator is obtained by using the method in Sect. 3.1 (NME)

get estimators of $\mu(t)$ and $c_X(s, t)$ by solving the optimization problems (10), (11), respectively: one is that an estimator of γ is established by applying integration method to get the FPC scores $\hat{U}_{ij}$ in (2) instead of using formula (12), denoted as "IN"; the other one is that an estimator of γ is obtained by using the method in Sect. 3.1 with dataset $\{Z_i, Y_i\}$ with measurement error being ignored. The results are summarized in Table 2.

We find from Table 2 that the "WME" method has the best performance relative to the other two methods in each setup, and the gains are dramatic when switching from the "NME" method to the "WME" method with the "NME" method ignoring observation errors for functional predictors. Specifically, for the case of $n = 100$, comparing with the "NME" method, the MISEs are reduced by 74%, 68% using the "WME" method with $(a_1, a_2) = (1.5, 0.2)$ and $(a_1, a_2) = (1.5, 0.4)$, respectively. For the "IN" method, it provides a reasonable estimator for γ and has better performance than the "NME" method, but nevertheless the "WME" method still performs better than "IN" method with improvement of 25%, 32% with respect to $(a_1, a_2) = (1.5, 0.2)$ and $(a_1, a_2) = (1.5, 0.4)$. In addition, these simulation results show that the MISEs decrease with increasing sample size n that is consistent with the derived theoretical results.

To sum up, in the scenario that incomplete functional predictors observed without measurement error, the "NME" method taking advantage of the whole information of the dataset produces a better estimator compared with the "SUB" method; in the scenario that incomplete functional predictors observed with measurement error, the "WME" method is preferred for giving the smallest MISE relative to the "IN" and "NME" methods. Both MISEs of the estimators of γ decrease with increasing sample size n that is consistent with the derived theoretical properties.

5 Real Data Analysis

A real diffusion tensor imaging (DTI) dataset considered here is from NIH Alzheimer's Disease Neuroimaging Initiative (ADNI) study with 212 subjects, and is obtained through http://adni.loni.usc.edu/. The primary goal of ADNI study is to test whether serial magnetic resonance imaging (MRI), positron emission tomography (PET), biological markers, and neuropsychological assessment can be combined to measure the progression of mild cognitive impairment (MCI) and early Alzheimer's disease (AD). DTI obtained using mathematical method to represent the anisotropic diffusion of the water molecule in brain organization can be used to learn MCI and AD. The concrete measure of anisotropy includes fractional anisotropy (FA), relative anisotropy (RA), Volume ratio (VR), and FA is commonly adopted for its advantage in contrast ratio of grey-white matter. More details about preprocessing and methods of this study can be found in Zhu et al. (2012) and Yu et al. (2016).

Our main interest is characterizing the dynamic relationship between FA and mini-mental state examination (MMSE) score which is seen as a reliable and valid clinical measure in quantitatively assessing the severity of cognitive impairment. FA is measured at 83 equally spaced grid along the corpus callosum (CC) fiber tract that is the largest fiber tract in human brain, is responsible for much of the communication between two hemispheres, and connects homologous areas in two cerebral hemispheres.

To demonstrate the usefulness of the proposed method in Sect. 3.1, we artificially delete some observed points of FA, and then compare the estimator of γ obtained by using these incomplete functional observations with the estimator obtained by applying original complete dataset. For the ith FA curve, the missing domain has the same form with the interval given in Sect. 4 with $(a_1, a_2) = (1.5, 0.2)$ and $(a_1, a_2) = (1.5, 0.4)$. A part of complete and incomplete individual trajectories are displayed in Fig. 1.

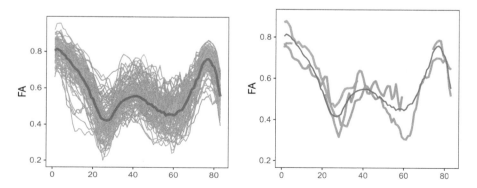

Fig. 1 A part of complete (left) and incomplete (right) FA curves with mean function (purple line)

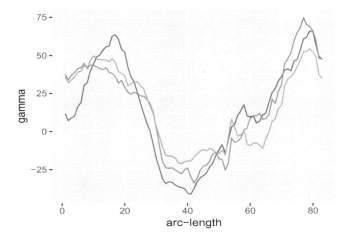

Fig. 2 Estimators of γ with different expected missing length on $[0, 1]$. Blue line: the estimator using original complete dataset; Red line: the estimator with $(a_1, a_2) = (1.5, 0.2)$; Green line: the estimator with $(a_1, a_2) = (1.5, 0.4)$

Estimators of functional coefficient obtained by both complete and incomplete FA dataset are illustrated in Fig. 2. It shows that estimators obtained by incomplete dataset with different missing domain (red line and green line) are similar to the estimator obtained from original complete dataset (blue line). This reveals that the proposed framework is useful in getting an estimator for the model with incomplete functional predictors.

Next, we focus on the problem of recovering the missing parts X_{iM_i} of X_i. Assume that the infinite-dimensional process X_i is well approximated by the projection onto the function space $L^2(\mathcal{T})$ via the first m eigenfunctions (Yao et al. 2005a). In practice, the prediction for the trajectory $X_i(t)$ of the ith subject using the first m eigenfunctions given in Sect. 3.1 can be approached by

$$\hat{X}_i(t) = \hat{\mu}^{\mathrm{NME}}(t) + \sum_{k=1}^{m} \hat{U}_{ij}^{(\rho)} \hat{\phi}_j^{\mathrm{NME}}(t).$$

We randomly select four FA curves with different missing parts. The predicted profiles for these four curves are presented in Fig. 3, showing that the predicted profiles are close to the real part. This demonstrates the "NME" method by recovering the missing parts of incomplete trajectories encourages a better estimator comparing with the "SUB" method with deleting them directly.

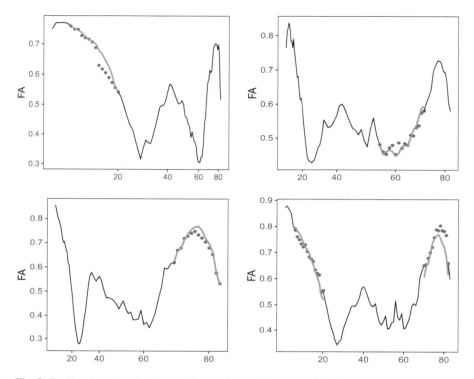

Fig. 3 Predicted profiles for four randomly chosen FA curves with different missing parts with $(a_1, a_2) = (1.5, 0.2)$. Missing parts of trajectories from left to right and top to down: missing in left side, middle side, right side, both left and right side. Blue point: real data point; Red line: predicted profile

6 Discussion

In this paper, we address the problem for getting estimators of γ in (1) with partially observed trajectories without and with measurement error. Basic elements of our approach are estimators of FPC scores for each partially observed trajectory. Specially, in the scenario that incomplete functional predictors observed without measurement error, we achieve it by modeling FPC scores of the missing part as linear functionals of the observed part of that trajectory. In the scenario where incomplete functional data is observed with measurement error, we obtain estimators of FPC scores via conditional expectation. Rates of convergence of the proposed estimators $\hat{\gamma}^{\mathrm{NME}}$, $\hat{\gamma}^{\mathrm{WME}}$ under different scenarios are established. We also compare the proposed methods with the "SUB" or "IN" method. We conclude from simulation studies that both the "NME" and "WME" methods borrowing strength from entire samples to get estimators of γ in model (1) perform well in practice.

The methods proposed here can be extended to other models in terms of functional regression with partially observed trajectories, such as partial functional linear regression (see Shin 2009). The framework established in this paper is based on the assumption that missing parts of trajectories are missing completely at random. In a number of applications, it is common to encounter that the underlying missing mechanism for dataset depends on systematic strategies (Liebl and Rameseder 2019) that clearly violate MCAR assumption. Extension to this scenario is also of interest and significance in practice.

Appendix

Lemma 1 (Kraus (2015), Proposition 1)

(a) Let $E\|X\|^2 < \infty$ and assumption (A1) be satisfied. Then $E(\|\hat{\mu}^{NME} - \mu\|^2) = O(n^{-1})$ for $n \to \infty$.

(b) Let $E\|X\|^4 < \infty$ and observation pattern (A2) holds. Then $E(\|\hat{C}_X^{NME} - C_X\|_S^2) = O(n^{-1})$ for $n \to \infty$ (here $\|\cdot\|_S$ denotes the Hilbert–Schmidt norm).

Lemma 2 (Kneip and Liebl (2020), Theorem 4.1) *Under the assumptions (B1)–(B5), we have that*

(a) $\sup_{t \in \mathcal{T}} |\hat{\mu}^{WME}(t) - \mu(t)| = O_p(r_\mu)$ with $r_\mu = h_\mu^2 + 1/\sqrt{nNh_\mu} + 1/\sqrt{n}$.

(b) $\sup_{(s,t) \in \mathcal{T}^2} |\hat{c}^{WME}(s,t) - c_X(s,t)| = O_p(r_\mu + r_c)$ with $r_c = h_c^2 + 1/\sqrt{nMh_c^2} + 1/\sqrt{n}$.

Proof of Theorem 1 The following results can be derived from the theory developed by Bhatia et al. (1983):

$$\sup_{j \geq 1} |\hat{\lambda}_j^{NME} - \lambda_j| \leq \|\hat{C}_X^{NME} - C_X\|,$$

$$\sup_{j \geq 1} \delta_j \|\hat{\phi}_j^{NME} - \phi_j\| \leq 8^{1/2} \|\hat{C}_X^{NME} - C_X\|. \tag{13}$$

Therefore, we obtain from Lemma 1,

$$\sup_{j \geq 1} |\hat{\lambda}_j^{NME} - \lambda_j| = O_p(n^{-1/2}),$$

$$\sup_{j \geq 1} \delta_j \|\hat{\phi}_j^{NME} - \phi_j\| = O_p(n^{-1/2}). \tag{14}$$

Note that,

$$\int_{\mathcal{T}} (\hat{\gamma}^{\mathrm{NME}}(s) - \gamma(s))^2 ds$$

$$= \int_{\mathcal{T}} \left\{ \sum_{j=1}^{m-1} \left[\frac{n^{-1}\sum_{i=1}^{n}[Y_i \hat{U}_{ij}^{\mathrm{NME}}]}{\hat{\lambda}_j^{\mathrm{NME}}} \hat{\phi}_j^{\mathrm{NME}}(s) - \frac{E[YU_j]}{\lambda_j}\phi_j(s) \right] \right\}^2 ds$$

$$+ \int_{\mathcal{T}} \left\{ \sum_{j=m}^{\infty} \frac{E[YU_j]}{\lambda_j}\phi_j(s) \right\}^2 ds$$

$$+ 2\int_{\mathcal{T}} \left\{ \sum_{j=1}^{m-1} \left[\frac{n^{-1}\sum_{i=1}^{n}[Y_i \hat{U}_{ij}^{\mathrm{NME}}]}{\hat{\lambda}_j^{\mathrm{NME}}} \hat{\phi}_j^{\mathrm{NME}}(s) - \frac{E[YU_j]}{\lambda_j}\phi_j(s) \right] \right\} \left\{ \sum_{j=m}^{\infty} \frac{E[YU_j]}{\lambda_j}\phi_j(s) \right\} ds$$

$$:= A_1(n) + A_2(n) + A_3(n). \tag{15}$$

For simplicity, we suppress the notation on "NME." Assumption (A6) implies that $A_2(n) \to 0$ as $m \to \infty$. For $A_3(n)$, Cauchy–Schwarz inequality implies that $A_3^2(n) \le A_1^2(n) \times A_2^2(n) \overset{p}{\to} 0$. Combing the result (14), and the formula (15), we see that the result of the theorem follows if we can get the convergence rate of $\hat{U}_{ij}$ of the trajectories per subject with $\hat{U}_{ij} = \hat{U}_{ijO_i} + \hat{U}_{ijM_i}^{(\alpha)}$.

Denote the estimates of U_{ijM_i}, $C_{O_iO_i}$, $C_{O_iM_i}$, ϕ_{jM_i} as $\hat{U}_{ijM_i(-i)}$, $\hat{C}_{O_iO_i(-i)}$, $\hat{C}_{O_iM_i(-i)}$, $\hat{\phi}_{jM_i(-i)}$ with deleting the ith curves $X_i(t)$. Let $\tilde{\xi}_{ijM_i}^{(\rho)} = (C_{O_iO_i}^{(\rho)})^{-1} C_{O_iM_i}\phi_{jM_i}$ with $C_{O_iO_i}^{(\rho)} = C_{O_iO_i} + \rho\mathcal{F}_{O_i}$, $\tilde{U}_{ijM_i}^{(\rho)} = \langle \tilde{\xi}_{ijM_i}^{(\rho)}, X_{iO_i} \rangle$, and the notation $\tilde{\xi}_{ijM_i}$ $\tilde{U}_{ijM_i}$ are corresponded to the symbols $\tilde{\xi}_{ijM_i}^{(\rho)}, \tilde{U}_{ijM_i}^{(\rho)}$ with $\rho = 0$. Since

$$E\left\| \hat{U}_{ijM_i}^{(\rho)} - \tilde{U}_{ijM_i} \right\|^2 = E\left\| \hat{U}_{ijM_i}^{(\rho)} - \tilde{U}_{ijM_i}^{(\rho)} + \tilde{U}_{ijM_i}^{(\rho)} - \tilde{U}_{ijM_i} \right\|^2$$

$$= 2E\left\| \hat{U}_{ijM_i}^{(\rho)} - \tilde{U}_{ijM_i}^{(\rho)} \right\|^2 + 2\left\| \tilde{U}_{ijM_i}^{(\rho)} - \tilde{U}_{ijM_i} \right\|^2$$

$$\le 4E\left\| \hat{U}_{ijM_i}^{(\rho)} - \hat{U}_{ijM_i(-i)}^{(\rho)} \right\|^2 + 4E\left\| \hat{U}_{ijM_i(-i)}^{(\rho)} - \tilde{U}_{ijM_i}^{(\rho)} \right\|^2$$

$$+ 2\left\| \tilde{U}_{ijM_i}^{(\rho)} - \tilde{U}_{ijM_i} \right\|^2, \tag{16}$$

we then analyze the terms $E\|\hat{U}_{ijM_i}^{(\rho)} - \hat{U}_{ijM_i(-i)}^{(\rho)}\|^2$, $E\|\hat{U}_{ijM_i(-i)}^{(\rho)} - \tilde{U}_{ijM_i}^{(\rho)}\|^2$, $\|\tilde{U}_{ijM_i}^{(\rho)} - \tilde{U}_{ijM_i}\|^2$ in turn. Let $\hat{\xi}_{ijM_i(-i)}^{(\rho)} = (\hat{C}_{O_iO_i(-i)}^{(\rho)})^{-1}\hat{C}_{O_iM_i(-i)}\hat{\phi}_{jM_i(-i)}$. Then

$$E\|\hat{U}_{ijM_i(-i)}^{(\rho)} - \tilde{U}_{ijM_i}^{(\rho)}\|^2$$

$$= E\langle \hat{\xi}_{ijM_i(-i)}^{(\rho)} - \tilde{\xi}_{ijM_i}^{(\rho)}, X_{iO_i} \rangle^2$$

$$= E\{E[\langle \hat{\xi}_{ijM_i(-i)}^{(\rho)} - \tilde{\xi}_{ijM_i}^{(\rho)}, X_{iO_i} \rangle^2 | \{X_{kO_i}, k \ne i\}]\}$$

$$= \mathrm{E}||C_{O_iO_i}^{1/2}((\hat{C}_{O_iO_i(-i)}^{(\rho)})^{-1}\hat{C}_{O_iM_i(-i)}\hat{\phi}_{jM_i(-i)} - (C_{O_iO_i}^{(\rho)})^{-1}C_{O_iM_i}\phi_{jM_i})||^2$$

$$\leq 4\left\{ \mathrm{E}||C_{O_iO_i}^{1/2}(\hat{C}_{O_iO_i(-i)}^{(\rho)})^{-1}(\hat{C}_{O_iM_i(-i)} - C_{O_iM_i})(\hat{\phi}_{jM_i(-i)} - \phi_{jM_i})||^2 \right.$$

$$+ \mathrm{E}||C_{O_iO_i}^{1/2}(\hat{C}_{O_iO_i(-i)}^{(\rho)})^{-1}C_{O_iM_i}(\hat{\phi}_{jM_i(-i)} - \phi_{jM_i})||^2$$

$$+ \mathrm{E}||C_{O_iO_i}^{1/2}(\hat{C}_{O_iO_i(-i)}^{(\rho)})^{-1}(\hat{C}_{O_iM_i(-i)} - C_{O_iM_i})\phi_{jM_i}||^2$$

$$\left. + \mathrm{E}||C_{O_iO_i}^{1/2}((\hat{C}_{O_iO_i(-i)}^{(\rho)})^{-1} - (C_{O_iO_i}^{(\rho)})^{-1})C_{O_iM_i}\phi_{jM_i}||^2 \right\}$$

$$:= B_1 + B_2 + B_3 + B_4. \tag{17}$$

Let $\mathcal{F}_m = \{\frac{\lambda_m}{2} < \hat{\lambda}_m < \frac{3}{2}\lambda_m\}$. Suppose the event $\mathcal{F}_m$ holds. Otherwise, we have $\mathrm{P}(|\hat{\lambda}_m - \lambda_m| \geq \frac{\lambda_m}{2}) \leq \mathrm{P}(||\hat{C}_X^{\mathrm{NME}} - C_X|| \geq \frac{\lambda_m}{2}) \to 0$ from assumption (A4). We have the following results for terms B_1 to B_4 with the equality

$$\left(\hat{C}_{O_iO_i(-i)}^{(\rho)}\right)^{-1} - \left(C_{O_iO_i}^{(\rho)}\right)^{-1} = (\hat{C}_{O_iO_i(-i)} - C_{O_iO_i})\left(C_{O_iO_i}^{(\rho)}\right)^{-1}\left(\hat{C}_{O_iO_i(-i)}^{(\rho)}\right)^{-1}.$$

For the term B_1,

$$B_1 \leq \mathrm{E}\left[\left\|C_{O_iO_i}^{1/2}\right\|_2^2 \cdot \left\|\left(\hat{C}_{O_iO_i(-i)}^{(\rho)}\right)^{-1}\right\|_\infty^2 \cdot \left\|\hat{C}_{O_iM_i(-i)} - C_{O_iM_i}\right\|_2^2 \cdot \left\|\hat{\phi}_{jM_i(-i)} - \phi_{jM_i}\right\|^2\right]$$

$$= O\left(n^{-2}\delta_j^{-2}\right) \cdot O(\rho^{-2}).$$

Denote $\|\cdot\|_\infty$ as the operator norm. For the term B_2, under the assumption (A7), $\mathrm{E}\|C_{O_iO_i}^{1/2}\|_\infty^2 < \infty$ and the result (14), it is clear that

$$B_2 \leq \mathrm{E}\left[\left\|C_{O_iO_i}^{1/2}\right\|_\infty^2 \cdot \left\|\left(\hat{C}_{O_iO_i(-i)}^{(\rho)}\right)^{-1}C_{O_iM_i}\right\|_2^2 \cdot \left\|\hat{\phi}_{jM_i(-i)} - \phi_{jM_i}\right\|^2\right]$$

$$\leq \sum_j \sum_k \frac{r_{M_iO_ijk}^2}{(\lambda_{O_iO_ik} + \rho)^2} \cdot O\left(n^{-1}\delta_j^{-2}\right) = O\left(n^{-1}\delta_j^{-2}\right).$$

For the term B_3,

$$B_3 \leq \mathrm{E}\left[\|C_{O_iO_i}^{1/2}\|_2^2 \cdot \|(\hat{C}_{O_iO_i(-i)}^{(\rho)})^{-1}\|_\infty^2 \cdot \|\hat{C}_{O_iM_i(-i)} - C_{O_iM_i}\|_2^2 \cdot \|\phi_{jM_i}\|^2\right]$$

$$= O(n^{-1}\rho^{-2}).$$

Note that $\frac{\rho\lambda_{O_iO_ik}}{(\lambda_{O_iO_ik} + \rho)^2} < 1$. Under the assumption (A7), we have that

$$B_4 \leq \mathrm{E}\left[\|C_{O_iO_i}^{1/2} \cdot (C_{O_iO_i}^{(\rho)})^{-1} \cdot (\hat{C}_{O_iO_i(-i)}^{(\rho)})^{-1} \cdot C_{O_iM_i}\|_2^2 \cdot \|\hat{C}_{O_iO_i(-i)} - C_{O_iO_i}\|_2^2 \cdot \|\phi_{jM_i}\|^2\right]$$

$$\leq \left\{\sum_j \sum_k \frac{\rho\lambda_{O_iO_ik}}{(\lambda_{O_iO_ik} + \rho)^2} \cdot \frac{r_{O_iM_ijk}^2}{(\lambda_{O_iO_ik} + \rho)^2} \cdot \rho^{-1}\right\} \cdot O(n^{-1})$$

$$= O(n^{-1}) \cdot O(\rho^{-1}).$$

These results combined with (17) indicate

$$\mathrm{E}\|\hat{U}_{ijM_i(-i)}^{(\rho)} - \tilde{U}_{ijM_i}^{(\rho)}\|^2 = O\left(n^{-1}\rho^{-2} + n^{-1}\delta_j^{-2}\right). \tag{18}$$

We then analyze $\mathrm{E}\|\hat{U}_{ijM_i}^{(\rho)} - \hat{U}_{ijM_i(-i)}^{(\rho)}\|^2$,

$$\mathrm{E}\|\hat{U}_{ijM_i}^{(\rho)} - \hat{U}_{ijM_i(-i)}^{(\rho)}\| = \mathrm{E}\langle\hat{\xi}_{ijM_i}^{(\rho)} - \hat{\xi}_{ijM_i(-i)}^{(\rho)}, X_{iO_i}\rangle$$

$$\leq \{\mathrm{E}\|\hat{\xi}_{ijM_i}^{(\rho)} - \hat{\xi}_{ijM_i(-i)}^{(\rho)}\|^2\}^{1/2}\{\mathrm{E}\|X_{iO_i}\|^2\}^{1/2}$$

$$\leq L\{\mathrm{E}\|\hat{\xi}_{ijM_i}^{(\rho)} - \hat{\xi}_{ijM_i(-i)}^{(\rho)}\|^2\}^{1/2}, \tag{19}$$

where the last inequality holds from the finite second moment of X that is bounded by constant L. We also have,

$$\mathrm{E}\|\hat{\xi}_{ijM_i}^{(\rho)} - \hat{\xi}_{ijM_i(-i)}^{(\rho)}\|^2 = \mathrm{E}\|\left((\hat{C}_{O_iO_i}^{(\rho)})^{-1}\hat{C}_{O_iM_i} - (\hat{C}_{O_iO_i(-i)}^{(\rho)})^{-1}\hat{C}_{O_iM_i(-i)}\right)\hat{\phi}_{jM_i(-i)}\|^2$$

$$= \mathrm{E}\|\left[\left((\hat{C}_{O_iO_i}^{(\rho)})^{-1} - (\hat{C}_{O_iO_i(-i)}^{(\rho)})^{-1}\right)\hat{C}_{O_iM_i}\right.$$

$$\left. + (\hat{C}_{O_iO_i(-i)}^{(\rho)})^{-1}(\hat{C}_{O_iM_i} - \hat{C}_{O_iM_i(-i)})\right]\hat{\phi}_{jM_i(-i)}\|^2$$

$$\leq 2\left\{\mathrm{E}\|\left((\hat{C}_{O_iO_i}^{(\rho)})^{-1} - (\hat{C}_{O_iO_i(-i)}^{(\rho)})^{-1}\right)\hat{C}_{O_iM_i}\|^2\right.$$

$$\left. + \mathrm{E}\|(\hat{C}_{O_iO_i(-i)}^{(\rho)})^{-1}(\hat{C}_{O_iM_i} - \hat{C}_{O_iM_i(-i)})\|^2\right\}. \tag{20}$$

Note that

$$\mathrm{E}\|\hat{C}_{O_iM_i} - \hat{C}_{O_iM_i(-i)}\|^2 = O(n^{-2}),$$

$$\mathrm{E}\|\left((\hat{C}_{O_iO_i}^{(\rho)})^{-1} - (\hat{C}_{O_iO_i(-i)}^{(\rho)})^{-1}\right)\hat{C}_{O_iM_i}\|^2 = O(n^{-2}),$$

$$\mathrm{E}\|(\hat{C}_{O_iO_i(-i)}^{(\rho)})^{-1}(\hat{C}_{O_iM_i} - \hat{C}_{O_iM_i(-i)})\|^2 = O(n^{-2}\rho^{-2}).$$

Combining formulas (19) and (20), we deduce that

$$E\|\hat{U}_{ijM_i}^{(\rho)} - \hat{U}_{ijM_i(-i)}^{(\rho)}\|^2 = O(n^{-2}\rho^{-2}). \tag{21}$$

On the other hand,

$$E \parallel \tilde{U}_{ijM_i}^{(\rho)} - \tilde{U}_{ijM_i} \parallel^2 = O(\rho), \tag{22}$$

$$\text{var}(\tilde{U}_{ijM_i} - U_{ijM_i}) = \langle \phi_{jM_i}, C_{M_iM_i}\phi_{jM_i} \rangle - \langle \phi_{jM_i}, C_{M_iO_i}C_{O_iO_i}^{-1}C_{O_iM_i}\phi_{jM_i} \rangle$$

$$:= V_{ij}. \tag{23}$$

Therefore, with $n\rho^3 \to 0$ and the formulas (16), (18), (21)–(23), we have that

$$E\|\hat{U}_{ijM_i}^{(\rho)} - U_{ijM_i}\|^2 = O\left(n^{-1}\rho^{-2} + n^{-1}\delta_j^{-2} + V_{ij}\right).$$

Then the results are proved with $n\rho^3 \to 0$.

Proof of Theorem 2 Let $\tilde{\mathbf{U}}_i = (\tilde{U}_{i1}, \cdots, \tilde{U}_{im})^T$, $\mathbf{U}_i = (U_{i1}, \cdots, U_{im})^T$. The covariance matrix of $\tilde{\mathbf{U}}_i$ is $\text{var}(\mathbf{U}_i) = \varXi \mathbf{\Sigma}_{\mathbf{Z}_i}^{-1}\varXi^T$ with $\varXi = \text{cov}(\tilde{\mathbf{U}}_i, \mathbf{Z}_i) = (\lambda_1\boldsymbol{\phi}_{i1}, \cdots, \lambda_m\boldsymbol{\phi}_{im})^T$. Moreover, $\text{var}(\tilde{\mathbf{U}}_i - \mathbf{U}_i) = \mathbf{\Lambda} - \varXi \mathbf{\Sigma}_{\mathbf{Z}_i}\varXi^T$. Combining these results with formulas (14), (12) and the results of Lemma 2, the result of Theorem 3 is obtained by replacing $\hat{U}_{ij}^{\text{NME}}$ with $\hat{U}_{ij}^{\text{WME}}$ in (15) with assumptions (B1)–(B6).

References

Besse, P., & Ramsay, J. O. (1986). Principal components analysis of sampled functions. *Psychometrika, 51*(2), 285–311.

Bhatia, R., Davis, C., & McIntosh, A. (1983). Perturbation of spectral subspaces and solution of linear operator equations. *Linear Algebra and its Applications, 52*, 45–67.

Cardot, H., Ferraty, F., & Sarda, P. (1999). Functional linear model. *Statistics & Probability Letters, 45*(1), 11–22.

Che, M., Kong, L., Bell, R. C., & Yuan, Y. (2017). Trajectory modeling of gestational weight: A functional principal component analysis approach. *PloS One, 12*(10), e0186761.

Crambes, C., Kneip, A., & Sarda, P. (2009). Smoothing splines estimators for functional linear regression. *The Annals of Statistics, 37*(1), 35–72.

Delaigle, A., & Hall, P. (2016). Approximating fragmented functional data by segments of Markov chains. *Biometrika, 103*(4), 779–799.

Goldberg, Y., Ritov, Y., & Mandelbaum, A. (2014). Predicting the continuation of a function with applications to call center data. *Journal of Statistical Planning and Inference, 147*, 53–65.

Hall, P., & Horowitz, J. L. (2007). Methodology and convergence rates for functional linear regression. *The Annals of Statistics, 35*(1), 70–91.

Hall, P., Müller, H.-G., & Wang, J.-L. (2006). Properties of principal component methods for functional and longitudinal data analysis. *The Annals of Statistics, 34*(3), 1493–1517.

Hansen, P. C. (1990). The discrete Picard condition for discrete ill-posed problems. *BIT Numerical Mathematics, 30*(4), 658–672.

Horváth, L., & Kokoszka, P. (2012). *Inference for functional data with applications*, vol. 200. Berlin: Springer.

James, G. M., Hastie, T. J., & Sugar, C. A. (2000). Principal component models for sparse functional data. *Biometrika, 87*(3), 587–602.

Kneip, A., & Liebl, D. (2020). On the optimal reconstruction of partially observed functional data. *Annals of Statistics, 48*(3), 1692–1717.

Kraus, D. (2015). Components and completion of partially observed functional data. *Journal of the Royal Statistical Society: Series B (Statistical Methodology), 77*(4), 777–801.

Li, Y., & Hsing, T. (2010). Uniform convergence rates for nonparametric regression and principal component analysis in functional/longitudinal data. *The Annals of Statistics, 38*(6), 3321–3351.

Liebl, D. (2013). Modeling and forecasting electricity spot prices: A functional data perspective. *The Annals of Applied Statistics, 7*(3), 1562–1592.

Liebl, D., & Rameseder, S. (2019). Partially observed functional data: The case of systematically missing parts. *Computational Statistics and Data Analysis, 131*, 104–115.

Marx, B. D. & Eilers, P. H. (1999). Generalized linear regression on sampled signals and curves: a p-spline approach. *Technometrics, 41*(1), 1–13.

Morris, J. S. (2015). Functional regression. *Annual Review of Statistics and Its Application, 2*, 321–359.

Ramsay, J. (2005). Functional data analysis. In B. S. Everitt & D. C. Howell (Eds.) *Encyclopedia of Statistics in Behavioral Science* (Vol. 2. pp. 675–678). Chichester: John Wiley & Sons Ltd.

Ramsay, J. O., & Dalzell, C. (1991). Some tools for functional data analysis. *Journal of the Royal Statistical Society: Series B (Methodological), 53*(3), 539–561.

Reiss, P. T., Goldsmith, J., Shang, H. L., & Ogden, R. T. (2017). Methods for scalar-on-function regression. *International Statistical Review, 85*(2), 228–249.

Rice, J. A., & Silverman, B. W. (1991). Estimating the mean and covariance structure non-parametrically when the data are curves. *Journal of the Royal Statistical Society: Series B (Methodological), 53*(1), 233–243.

Riesz, F., & Nagy, S. (1955). B.(1990). functional analysis. *Dover Publications, Inc., New York. First published in, 3*(6), 35.

Shang, H. L. (2014). A survey of functional principal component analysis. *AStA Advances in Statistical Analysis, 98*(2), 121–142.

Shin, H. (2009). Partial functional linear regression. *Journal of Statistical Planning and Inference, 139*(10), 3405–3418.

Staniswalis, J. G., & Lee, J. J. (1998). Nonparametric regression analysis of longitudinal data. *Journal of the American Statistical Association, 93*(444), 1403–1418.

Wang, Y., Kong, L., Jiang, B., Zhou, X., Yu, S., Zhang, L., & Heo, G. (2019). Wavelet-based lasso in functional linear quantile regression. *Journal of Statistical Computation and Simulation, 89*(6), 1111–1130.

Yao, F., Müller, H.-G., & Wang, J.-L. (2005a). Functional data analysis for sparse longitudinal data. *Journal of the American Statistical Association, 100*(470), 577–590.

Yao, F., Müller, H.-G., & Wang, J.-L. (2005b). Functional linear regression analysis for longitudinal data. *The Annals of Statistics, 33*(6), 2873–2903.

Yu, D., Kong, L., & Mizera, I. (2016). Partial functional linear quantile regression for neuroimaging data analysis. *Neurocomputing, 195*, 74–87.

Zhao, Y., Ogden, R. T., & Reiss, P. T. (2012). Wavelet-based lasso in functional linear regression. *Journal of computational and graphical statistics, 21*(3), 600–617.

Zhu, H., Li, R., & Kong, L. (2012). Multivariate varying coefficient model for functional responses. *Annals of Statistics, 40*(5), 2634–2666.

Profile Estimation of Generalized Semiparametric Varying-Coefficient Additive Models for Longitudinal Data with Within-Subject Correlations

Yanqing Sun and Fang Fang

Abstract In this paper, we study several profile estimation methods for the generalized semiparametric varying-coefficient additive model for longitudinal data by utilizing the within-subject correlations. The model is flexible in allowing time-varying effects for some covariates and constant effects for others, and in having the option to choose different link functions which can used to analyze both discrete and continuous longitudinal responses. We investigated the profile generalized estimating equation (GEE) approaches and the profile quadratic inference function (QIF) approach. The profile estimations are assisted with the local linear smoothing technique to estimate the time-varying effects. Several approaches that incorporate the within-subject correlations are investigated including the quasi-likelihood (QL), the minimum generalized variance (MGV), the quadratic inference function, and the weighted least squares (WLS). The proposed estimation procedures can accommodate flexible sampling schemes. These methods provide a unified approach that works well for discrete longitudinal responses as well as for continuous longitudinal responses. Finite sample performances of these methods are examined through Monto Carlo simulations under various correlation structures for both discrete and continuous longitudinal responses. The simulation results show efficiency improvement over the working independence approach by utilizing the within-subject correlations as well as comparative performances of different approaches.

Keywords Discrete and continuous longitudinal responses · Generalized estimating equations · Generalized semiparametric varying-coefficient additive model · Local linear smoothing · Quadratic inference function · Quasi-likelihood approach · Within-subject correlation

Y. Sun (✉)
Department of Mathematics and Statistics, University of North Carolina at Charlotte, Charlotte, NC, USA
e-mail: yasun@uncc.edu

F. Fang
Corporate Model Risk at Wells Fargo, Charlotte, NC, USA
e-mail: Fang.Fang2@wellsfargo.com

© The Author(s), under exclusive license to Springer Nature Switzerland AG 2022
W. He et al. (eds.), *Advances and Innovations in Statistics and Data Science*, ICSA
Book Series in Statistics, https://doi.org/10.1007/978-3-031-08329-7_8

159

1 Introduction

The repeated measurements on same individuals over time are common in medical and public health researches. In AIDS clinical trials, for example, the viral load and CD4 cell counts, which are considered as surrogate endpoints for HIV disease progression and HIV transmission to others, are measured repeatedly during the course of studies for trial participants. The repeated measurements in the longitudinal follow-up often display temporal effects and are correlated. We investigate several estimation methods for analyzing longitudinal data under the generalized semiparametric varying-coefficient additive models by incorporating the within-subject correlations.

Suppose that there is a random sample of n subjects. For the ith subject, let $Y_i(t)$ be the response at time t and let $X_i(t)$ and $Z_i(t)$ be the possibly time-dependent covariates of dimensions $p + 1$ and q, respectively, over the time interval $[0, \tau]$, where τ is the end of follow-up. Let $\mu_i(t) = E\{Y_i(t)|X_i(t), Z_i(t)\}$ be the conditional expectation of $Y_i(t)$ given $X_i(t)$ and $Z_i(t)$ at time t. The generalized semiparametric regression model speculates that

$$\mu_i(t) = g^{-1}\{\alpha^T(t)X_i(t) + \beta^T Z_i(t)\}, \qquad i = 1, \ldots, n, \qquad (1)$$

for $0 \leq t \leq \tau$, where $g(\cdot)$ is a known link function, $\alpha(t)$ is a $(p + 1)$-dimensional vector of unspecified functions and β is a q-dimensional vector of unknown parameters. The notation θ^T represents transpose of a vector or matrix θ. When the link function $g(\cdot)$ is the identity function, model (1) is known as the semiparametric additive model. When the link function is the natural logarithm function and $X_i(t) = 1$, model (1) is known as the proportional means model. Setting the first component of $X_i(t)$ as 1 gives a nonparametric baseline function. Under model (1), the effects of some covariates are constant while others are time-varying. Model (1) is more flexible than the parametric regression model where all the regression coefficients are time-independent and more desirable for model building than the nonparametric regression model where every covariate effect is an unspecified function of time. Different link functions can be selected to provide a rich family of models for longitudinal data. Both the categorical and continuous longitudinal responses can be modeled with appropriately chosen link functions. For example, the identity and logarithm link functions can be used for the continuous response variables while the logit link function can be used for the binary responses.

The semiparametric additive model for longitudinal data has been studied extensively for decades. These approaches include the nonparametric kernel smoothing by Hoover et al. (1998), the joint modeling of longitudinal responses and sampling times by Martinussen and Scheike (1999) and Lin and Ying (2001), the backfitting method by Zeger and Diggle (1994) and Wu and Liang (2004), and the profile kernel smoothing approach by Sun and Wu (2005). Fan and Li (2004) considered the profile local linear approach and the joint modeling for partially linear models. Hu et al. (2004) showed that for partially linear models, the backfitting is less efficient than the profile kernel method. Sun et al. (2013) investigated the generalized semiparametric additive model (1) using the local linear profile estimation method. The aforementioned estimation and inference procedures are derived without considering the correlations of longitudinal responses within subjects known as the working independence approach. The estimation methods under the working independence are valid and yield asymptotically unbiased estimators.

Correlation among repeated measurements on the same subject often exists for longitudinal data or clustered data. Incorporating such within-subject correlation into estimation procedure can lead to improved efficiency. Liang and Zeger (1986) introduced the idea of using a working correlation matrix with a small set of nuisance parameters to avoid specification of correlation between measurements within the cluster. Severini and Staniswalis (1994) and Lin and Carroll (2001a,b) estimated $\alpha(t)$ using the kernel method by ignoring the within-subject correlation while estimating β using weighted least squares by accounting for the within-subject correlation when $X_i(t) \equiv 1$. Chen and Jin (2006) studied the method of generalized estimating equations by modeling the within-cluster correlation. Using piecewise local polynomial approximation of $\alpha(t)$, Chen and Jin (2006) showed that the weighted least square estimator of β achieves the semiparametric efficiency. Fan et al. (2007) proposed a profile local linear approach by imposing certain correlation structure for the longitudinal data for improved efficiency. Fan et al. (2007) proposed two methods to estimate for the within-subject correlation by optimizing the quasi-likelihood (QL) and by minimizing the generalized variance of the estimator of β (MGV). Following the generalized method of moments of Hansen (1982) and Qu et al. (2000) proposed the quadratic inference function method (QIF) by representing the inverse of working correlation matrix by a linear combination of basis matrices. Song et al. (2009), Madsen et al. (2011), and Tang et al. (2019) studied a mean-correlation parametric regression method for a family of discrete longitudinal responses by assuming that the marginal distributions of longitudinal responses follow an exponential family distribution and the joint distributions of the discrete responses from the same subject are modeled by a copula model. These approaches have a limitation of not allowing for time-varying covariate effects.

Semiparametric statistical modeling of discrete longitudinal responses beyond the marginal approach has been understudied. We investigate several profile estimation methods for the generalized semiparametric varying-coefficient additive model (1) by incorporating the within-subject correlations including the profile generalized estimating equation (GEE) approaches and the quadratic inference function approach. These methods provide a unified approach that work well for discrete longitudinal responses as well as for continuous longitudinal responses. Different methods for estimating the within-subject correlations such as the QL and MGV methods as well as a newly proposed profile weighted least square (WLS) approach fall under the umbrella of profile GEE approaches. The performances of these different methods are examined through extensive simulation studies under a variety of models and the within-subject correlation structures. The proposed semiparametric methods utilizing the within-subject correlations work well for discrete longitudinal responses as well as for continuous longitudinal responses.

The rest of the paper is organized as follows. The profile GEE estimation using fixed working covariance matrices is presented in Sect. 2.1. The methods for estimating the correlations are described in Sect. 2.2. An alternative profile estimation of model (1) via quadratic inference function is proposed in Sect. 2.3. The computational algorithms of the proposed procedures are summarized in Sect. 2.4. Section 3 presents the results of simulation studies for evaluating the finite sample performances of different methods. The results of simulation studies for continuous longitudinal responses are presented in Sect. 3.1 and the results of simulation studies for discrete longitudinal responses are given in Sect. 3.2. Some concluding remarks are given in Sect. 4.

2   Profile GEE Estimation Procedures

This section presents several profile estimation methods for the generalized semi-parametric varying-coefficient additive model (1) by incorporating the within-subject correlations and the approaches for estimating the within-subject correlations. Choices of kernel function, bandwidth, and link function are also discussed.

2.1   Model Estimation Using Fixed Working Covariance Matrices

Suppose that the longitudinal response $Y_i(t)$ and the possibly time-dependent covariates $X_i(t)$ and $Z_i(t)$ are observed at the sampling times $T_{i1} < T_{i2} < \cdots < T_{iJ_i}$, where J_i is the total number of observations on the ith subject. Let $Y_{ij} = Y_i(T_{ij})$, $X_{ij} = X_i(T_{ij})$ and $Z_{ij} = Z_i(T_{ij})$. Let $Y_i = (Y_{i1}, \cdots, Y_{iJ_i})^T$ be the vector of responses for individual i. Similarly, define $X_i = (X_{i1}, \cdots, X_{iJ_i})^T$, $Z_i = (Z_{i1}, \cdots, Z_{iJ_i})^T$ and $T_i = (T_{i1}, \cdots, T_{iJ_i})$. The sampling times $\{T_{ij}, j = 1, \ldots, J_i\}$ varies among individuals under random designs, while they are not dependent on i under fixed designs. We propose the kernel assisted profile method to estimate the nonparametric functions $\alpha(t)$ and parametric coefficients β under model (1) by taking into consideration of the within-subject correlations.

For given β, let $\alpha(t) = \alpha(t_0) + \dot{\alpha}(t_0)(t - t_0) + O((t - t_0)^2)$ be the first-order Taylor expansion of $\alpha(\cdot)$ for $t \in \mathcal{N}_{t_0}$, a neighborhood of t_0, where $\dot{\alpha}(t_0)$ is the derivative of $\alpha(t)$ at $t = t_0$. Denote $\alpha^*(t_0) = (\alpha^T(t_0), \dot{\alpha}^T(t_0))^T$ and $X_i^*(t, t - t_0) = X_i(t) \otimes (1, t - t_0)^T$, where $\otimes$ is the Kronecker product. Then for $t \in \mathcal{N}_{t_0}$, model (1) can be approximated by

$$\tilde{\mu}(t, t_0, \alpha^*(t_0), \beta | X_i(t), Z_i(t)) = g^{-1}\{\alpha^{*T}(t_0)X_i^*(t, t - t_0) + \beta^T Z_i(t)\}. \quad (2)$$

Let $X_{ij}^*(t_0) = X_{ij} \otimes (1, T_{ij} - t_0)^T$, $j = 1, \ldots, J_i$. The approximated conditional expectation of Y_{ij} for $T_{ij} \in \mathcal{N}_{t_0}$ is given by $\mu_{ij}^*(t_0) = \mu\{\alpha^{*T}(t_0)X_{ij}^*(t_0) + \beta^T Z_{ij}\}$, where $\mu(\cdot) = g^{-1}(\cdot)$. Denote $\dot{\mu}_{ij}^*(t_0) = \dot{\mu}\{\alpha^{*T}(t_0)X_{ij}^*(t_0) + \beta^T Z_{ij}\}$ where $\dot{\mu}(\cdot)$ is the first derivative of $\mu(\cdot)$. Let $\mu_i^*(t_0) = (\mu_{i1}^*(t_0), \cdots, \mu_{iJ_i}^*(t_0))^T$. Let $X_i^*(t_0)$ denote a $2(p + 1) \times J_i$ matrix with the jth column vector being the $X_{ij}^*(t_0)$, $j = 1, \ldots, J_i$.

Let $K(\cdot)$ be a nonnegative kernel function and $h = h_n > 0$ a bandwidth parameter. Let $K_{ih}(t_0) = diag\{K_h(T_{ij} - t_0), j = 1, \ldots, J_i\}$ be the $J_i \times J_i$ diagonal matrix with $\{K_h(T_{ij} - t_0), j = 1, \ldots, J_i\}$, on the diagonal and zero elsewhere, where $K_h(\cdot) = K(\cdot/h)/h$. At each t_0 and for fixed β, we consider the following local linear estimating function for $\alpha^*(t_0)$:

$$U_\alpha(\alpha^*; \beta, t_0) = \sum_{i=1}^n X_i^*(t_0)\Delta_i^*(t_0)K_{ih}^{1/2}(t_0)V_{1i}^{-1}K_{ih}^{1/2}(t_0)\left[Y_i - \mu_i^*(t_0)\right], \quad (3)$$

where $\Delta_i^*(t_0) = diag\{\dot{\mu}_{ij}^*(t_0), j = 1, \ldots, J_i\}$ and V_{1i}^{-1} is the inverse of the working covariance matrix for estimating $\alpha^*(t_0)$. The solution to the equation $U_\alpha(\alpha^*; \beta, t_0) = 0$ is denoted by $\tilde{\alpha}^*(t_0, \beta)$. We denote the first $p + 1$ components of $\tilde{\alpha}^*(t_0, \beta)$ by $\tilde{\alpha}(t_0, \beta)$.

Let $\tilde{\mu}_{ij}(\beta) = \mu\{\tilde{\alpha}^T(T_{ij}, \beta)X_{ij} + \beta^T Z_{ij}\}$ and $\tilde{\mu}_i(\beta) = (\tilde{\mu}_{i1}(\beta), \ldots, \tilde{\mu}_{iJ_i}(\beta))^T$. The profile weighted least squares estimator $\hat{\beta}$ is obtained by minimizing the following profile least squares function:

$$\ell_\beta(\beta) = \frac{1}{n}\sum_{i=1}^n [Y_i - \tilde{\mu}_i(\beta)]^T V_{2i}^{-1}[Y_i - \tilde{\mu}_i(\beta)], \quad (4)$$

where V_{2i}^{-1} is the inverse of the working covariance matrix for estimating β.

Let $A_{ij} = \partial\tilde{\alpha}^T(T_{ij}, \beta)/\partial\beta$ be the derivative of $\tilde{\alpha}^T(T_{ij}, \beta)$ with respect to β, which is a $q \times (p + 1)$ matrix with the kth row having the partial derivative of $\tilde{\alpha}^T(T_{ij}, \beta)$ with respect to the kth component of β_k, $1 \leq k \leq q$. Let $\frac{\partial\tilde{\alpha}^T(T_i, \beta)}{\partial\beta} = \left(\frac{\partial\tilde{\alpha}^T(T_{i1}, \beta)}{\partial\beta}, \cdots, \frac{\partial\tilde{\alpha}^T(T_{iJ_i}, \beta)}{\partial\beta}\right)$ and $\tilde{X}_i = diag\{X_{ij}, j = 1, \ldots, J_i\}$. Then $\frac{\partial\tilde{\alpha}^T(T_i, \beta)}{\partial\beta}\tilde{X}_i = \left(\frac{\partial\tilde{\alpha}^T(T_{i1}, \beta)}{\partial\beta}X_{i1}, \cdots, \frac{\partial\tilde{\alpha}^T(T_{iJ_i}, \beta)}{\partial\beta}X_{iJ_i}\right)$ is a $q \times J_i$ matrix.

Taking the derivative of $\ell_\beta(\beta)$ with respect to β, we have the score function

$$U_\beta(\beta) = \sum_{i=1}^n \left\{\frac{\partial\tilde{\alpha}^T(T_i, \beta)}{\partial\beta}\tilde{X}_i + \tilde{Z}_i\right\}\tilde{\Delta}_i V_{2i}^{-1}\left[Y_i - \tilde{\mu}_i(\beta)\right], \quad (5)$$

where $\tilde{\Delta}_i = diag\{\dot{\tilde{\mu}}_{ij}, j = 1, \ldots, J_i\}$, $\dot{\tilde{\mu}}_{ij} = \dot{\mu}\{\tilde{\alpha}^T(T_{ij}, \beta)X_{ij} + \beta^T Z_{ij}\}$, and $\tilde{Z}_i = (Z_{i1}, \cdots, Z_{iJ_i})$ is a $q \times J_i$ matrix.

For given working covariance matrices V_{1i} and V_{2i}, the profile GEE estimator $\hat{\beta}$ of β is obtained by solving the estimating equation $U_\beta(\beta) = 0$. The profile GEE estimator for $\alpha(t)$ is given by $\hat{\alpha}(t) = \tilde{\alpha}(t, \hat{\beta})$.

Note that $\partial\tilde{\alpha}^T(t, \beta)/\partial\beta$ is the first $p + 1$ columns of $\partial\alpha^{*T}(t, \beta)/\partial\beta$. Next we show that $\partial\alpha^{*T}(t, \beta)/\partial\beta$ can be expressed in terms of the partial derivatives of $U_\alpha(\alpha^*; \beta, t)$ at $\alpha^* = \tilde{\alpha}^*(t, \beta)$. Specifically, since $U_\alpha(\tilde{\alpha}^*(t, \beta); \beta, t) \equiv \mathbf{0}_{2(p+1)}$ by (3), it follows that $\tilde{\alpha}^*(t, \beta)$ satisfies

$$\left\{\frac{\partial U_\alpha(\alpha^*; \beta, t)}{\partial\alpha^*}\frac{\partial\tilde{\alpha}^{*T}(t, \beta)}{\partial\beta} + \frac{\partial U_\alpha(\alpha^*; \beta, t)}{\partial\beta}\right\}\Bigg|_{\alpha^*=\tilde{\alpha}^*(t,\beta)} = \mathbf{0}_{2(p+1)}.$$

Therefore,

$$\frac{\partial\tilde{\alpha}^{*T}(t, \beta)}{\partial\beta} = -\left\{\frac{\partial U_\alpha(\alpha^*; \beta, t)}{\partial\alpha^*}\right\}^{-1}\frac{\partial U_\alpha(\alpha^*; \beta, t)}{\partial\beta}\Bigg|_{\alpha^*=\tilde{\alpha}^*(t,\beta)}, \tag{6}$$

where

$$\frac{\partial U_\alpha(\alpha^*; \beta, t)}{\partial\alpha^*} = -\sum_{i=1}^{n} X_i^*(t)\Delta_i^*(t)K_{ih}^{1/2}(t)V_{1i}^{-1}K_{ih}^{1/2}(t)\Delta_i^*(t)X_i^{*T}(t), \tag{7}$$

and

$$\frac{\partial U_\alpha(\alpha^*; \beta, t)}{\partial\beta} = -\sum_{i=1}^{n} X_i^*(t)\Delta_i^*(t)K_{ih}^{1/2}(t)V_{1i}^{-1}K_{ih}^{1/2}(t)\Delta_i^*(t)\tilde{Z}_i^T. \tag{8}$$

Under the identity link in model (1), $\tilde{\alpha}^*(t, \beta)$ and $\hat{\beta}$ can be solved explicitly as the roots of the score functions (3) and (5), respectively. When there are no explicit solutions, the Newton–Raphson iterative algorithm can be used to solve the equations. The estimation procedure iteratively updates estimates of the nonparametric component $\tilde{\alpha}^*(t, \beta)$ and the parametric component $\hat{\beta}$ until convergence. We denote the first $p + 1$ components of the convergent $\tilde{\alpha}^*(t, \beta)$ as $\hat{\alpha}(t)$.

Let $\dot{\hat{\mu}}_{ij} = \dot{\mu}\{\hat{\alpha}^T(T_{ij})X_{ij} + \beta^T Z_{ij}\}$ and $\hat{\Delta}_i = diag\{\dot{\hat{\mu}}_{ij}\}$. Define $\hat{E}_{11}(t) = n^{-1}\sum_{i=1}^{n} X_i\hat{\Delta}_i K_{ih}^{1/2}(t) V_{1i}^{-1}K_{ih}^{1/2}(t)\hat{\Delta}_i X_i^T$ and $\hat{E}_{12}(t) = n^{-1}\sum_{i=1}^{n} X_i$ $\hat{\Delta}_i K_{ih}^{1/2}(t)V_{1i}^{-1}K_{ih}^{1/2}(t)$ $\hat{\Delta}_i Z_i^T$. Let $\hat{B}_{ij} = -\hat{E}_{12}^T(T_{ij})$ $\hat{E}_{11}^{-1}(T_{ij})X_{ij} + Z_{ij}$ and $\hat{B}_i = (\hat{B}_{i1}, \cdots, \hat{B}_{iJ_i})^T$. Following the derivations in Fan et al. (2007), we estimate the variance of $\hat{\beta}$ by $\hat{P}^{-1}\hat{D}\hat{P}^{-1}$ for given covariance matrices V_{1i} and V_{2i}, where

$$\hat{P} = n^{-1} \sum_{i=1}^{n} \left[\hat{B}_i^T \hat{\Delta}_i V_{2i}^{-1} \hat{\Delta}_i \hat{B}_i \right],$$

and

$$\hat{D} = n^{-1} \sum_{i=1}^{n} \left[\hat{B}_i^T \hat{\Delta}_i V_{2i}^{-1} (Y_i - \hat{\mu}_i)(Y_i - \hat{\mu}_i)^T V_{2i}^{-1} \hat{\Delta}_i \hat{B}_i \right].$$

2.2 Estimation of the Within-Subject Covariance Matrix

The conditional within-subject correlation of longitudinal responses $Y_i(\cdot)$ at times $s, t \in [0, \tau]$ can be measured by the Pearson correlation coefficient $\rho_i(s, t) = Corr\big(Y_i(s), Y_i(t) | X_i(\cdot), Z_i(\cdot)\big) = Cov\big(Y_i(s), Y_i(t) | X_i(\cdot), Z_i(\cdot)\big)/(\sigma_i(s)\sigma_i(t))$, where $\sigma_i(t)$ be the conditional standard deviation of $Y_i(t)$ given $X_i(t)$ and $Z_i(t)$, $0 \le t \le \tau$. For simplicity, we assume that both $\sigma_i(t)$ and $\rho_i(s, t)$ do not depend on the covariates $X_i(\cdot)$ and $Z_i(\cdot)$. Thus we use the notations $\sigma(t)$ and $\rho(s, t)$ in place of $\sigma_i(t)$ and $\rho_i(s, t)$, respectively. In practice, the correlation structure $\rho(s, t)$ is often unknown or complex, and a working correlation is employed by assuming a correlation model for $\rho(s, t)$. The working independence corresponds to assuming $\rho(s, t) = 0$ for $s \ne t$. Other commonly used correlation models include the compound symmetry or exchangeable structure (Exchangeable) with $\rho(s, t) = \theta$, $|\theta| < 1$; a generalized the first-order autoregressive (AR(1)) with $\rho(s, t) = \theta^{|s-t|}$, $0 < \theta < 1$, which is a generalization of AR(1) model in time series to allow the possibility of unequally spaced times; and a generalization of the first-order autoregressive moving-average (ARMA(1,1)) with $\rho(s, t) = pq^{|s-t|}$, where $|p| < 1$ and $q > 0$. Fan et al. (2007) considered more complex correlation structure by embedding the working correlation into a collection of the correlation families $\rho_0(s, t, \theta_0), \ldots, \rho_m(s, t)$:

$$\rho(s, t, \theta) = b_0 \rho_0(s, t; \theta_0) + b_1 \rho_1(s, t, \theta_1) + \cdots + b_m \rho_m(s, t, \theta_m), \qquad (9)$$

where $\theta = (\theta_0, b_0, \theta_1, b_1, \ldots, b_m, \theta_m)$ and $b_0 + \cdots + b_m = 1$ with all $b_i \ge 0$.

Let $\rho_k(s, t, \theta)$, $\theta \in \Theta$, be the working correlation function for $Y_i(t)$, $0 \le t \le \tau$, for $k = 1, 2$. We consider decomposition of the working covariance V_{ki} of $(Y_{i1}, \cdots, Y_{iJ_i})$ into

$$V_{ki} = A_i R_{ki}(\theta) A_i, \qquad (10)$$

where $A_i = diag\{\sigma(T_{ij}), j = 1, \ldots, J_i\}$, and $R_{ki}(\theta)$ is the working correlation matrix of $(Y_{i1}, \cdots, Y_{iJ_i})$ under the working correlation model $\rho_k(s, t, \theta)$ for $k = 1, 2$.

The examples of correlation matrices $R_i(\theta)$ of $(Y_{i1}, \cdots, Y_{iJ_i})$ at the measurement times $t_1, \ldots, t_{J_i}$ for $J_i = 4$ for Exchangeable, AR(1) and ARMA(1,1) correlations are shown in the following:

$$
\begin{bmatrix}
1 & \theta & \theta & \theta \\
 & 1 & \theta & \theta \\
 & & 1 & \theta \\
 & & & 1
\end{bmatrix},
\quad
\begin{bmatrix}
1 & \theta^{|t_1-t_2|} & \theta^{|t_1-t_3|} & \theta^{|t_1-t_4|} \\
 & 1 & \theta^{|t_2-t_3|} & \theta^{|t_2-t_4|} \\
 & & 1 & \theta^{|t_3-t_4|} \\
 & & & 1
\end{bmatrix},
\quad
\begin{bmatrix}
1 & pq^{|t_1-t_2|} & pq^{|t_1-t_3|} & pq^{|t_1-t_4|} \\
 & 1 & pq^{|t_2-t_3|} & pq^{|t_2-t_4|} \\
 & & 1 & pq^{|t_3-t_4|} \\
 & & & 1
\end{bmatrix}.
$$

(a) Exchangeable   (b) AR(1)   (c) ARMA(1,1)

The GEE estimation of the regression coefficients is consistent even when the true correlation matrix is not an element of the class of working correlation matrices, and are efficient when the working correlation is correctly specified (Liang and Zeger 1986). Lin and Carroll (2000) showed that the most efficient estimation of the nonparametric component $\alpha(t)$ can be achieved by ignoring the within-subject correlation. However, more efficient estimation for the parametric component β is obtained by letting V_{2i} in (5) to be to the inverse of true covariance matrix of Y_i; see Lin and Carroll (2001a,b), Wang et al. (2005), and Fan et al. (2007). Thus we set $R_{1i}(\theta)$ to be the identity matrix and focus on discussing the approaches for estimating A_i and $R_{2i}(\theta)$. For convenience, we use the notation $\rho(s, t, \theta)$ for $\rho_2(s, t, \theta)$ and $R_i(\theta)$ for $R_{2i}(\theta)$.

2.2.1 Estimation of Marginal Variance

Let $\hat{\alpha}_0(t)$ and $\hat{\beta}_0$ be the marginal estimators of $\alpha(t)$ and β in Sect. 2 by setting V_{ki} to the identity matrix for $k = 1, 2$. Define the residual $\hat{r}_{ij} = Y_{ij} - \hat{\mu}_{ij}$, where $\hat{\mu}_{ij} = g^{-1}\{\hat{\alpha}_0^T(T_{ij})X_{ij} + \hat{\beta}_0^T Z_{ij}\}$. Following Fan et al. (2007), we estimate the marginal variance of response $Y_i(t)$ when it is continuous using kernel smoothing:

$$
\hat{\sigma}^2(t) = \frac{\sum_{i=1}^n \sum_{j=1}^{J_i} \hat{r}_{ij}^2 K_h^*(t - T_{ij})}{\sum_{i=1}^n \sum_{j=1}^{J_i} K_h^*(t - T_{ij})},
\tag{11}
$$

where $K_h^*(\cdot) = K^*(\cdot/h)/h$, $K^*(\cdot)$ is a nonnegative kernel function and $h = h_n > 0$ a bandwidth parameter.

When the response $Y_i(t)$ is a discrete random variable, the variance estimation can take different form to account for the model structure of the particular distribution family. For example, $\hat{r}_{ij}^2$ is replaced by $\hat{\mu}_{ij}(1 - \hat{\mu}_{ij})$ if the response $Y_i(t)$ is a Bernoulli random variable, and by $\hat{\mu}_{ij}$ if $Y_i(t)$ is a Poisson random variable. We refer to Liang and Zeger (1986) for the relationship between variance and the model parameters when marginal distribution of $Y_i(t)$ belongs to an exponential family.

2.2.2   Estimation of Correlation Coefficients

We study different approaches to estimate θ of the correlation matrix $R(\theta)$. Two of the methods, the quasi-likelihood approach and the minimum generalized variance approach, were adopted from Fan et al. (2007) for model (1) with the identity link function. We also propose the minimum weighted least squares approach to estimate θ.

The QL estimation of θ is obtained by maximizing the quasi-likelihood function:

$$\hat{\theta} = \arg\max_{\theta \in \Theta} \left(-\frac{1}{2} \sum_{i=1}^{n} \{\log |R_i(\theta)| + \hat{r}_i^T \hat{A}_i^{-1} R_i^{-1}(\theta) \hat{A}_i^{-1} \hat{r}_i\} \right), \tag{12}$$

where $R_i(\theta)$ and $\hat{A}_i = diag\{\hat{\sigma}(T_{ij}), j = 1, \ldots, J_i\}$ are defined the same as in Eq. (10), $\hat{r}_i = \{\hat{r}_{i1}, \ldots, \hat{r}_{iJ_i}\}$ is the estimator for vector ϵ_i and $\hat{r}_{ij}$ are defined above.

Let $\Sigma_{\hat{\beta}}(\hat{\sigma}^2, \theta)$ be the estimated covariance matrix of $\hat{\beta}$ under the working correlation model $\rho_k(s, t, \theta)$, which depends on the estimated marginal variance $\hat{\sigma}^2$ and the correlation parameter vector θ. Defining the generalized variance of $\hat{\beta}$ as the determinant $|\Sigma_{\hat{\beta}}(\hat{\sigma}^2, \theta)|$ of $\Sigma_{\hat{\beta}}(\hat{\sigma}^2, \theta)$. By Dempster (1969, Section 3.5), the volume of the ellipsoid of $(\hat{\beta} - \beta)^T \Sigma_{\hat{\beta}}^{-1}(\hat{\sigma}^2, \theta) (\hat{\beta} - \beta) < c$ for any positive constant c equals $\pi^{q/2} c^{1/2} |\Sigma_{\hat{\beta}}(\hat{\sigma}^2, \theta)|^{1/2} / \Gamma(\frac{q}{2} + 1)$, where $\Gamma(\cdot)$ is the gamma function. It follows that minimizing the volume of the confidence ellipsoid of $(\hat{\beta} - \beta)^T \Sigma_{\hat{\beta}}^{-1}(\hat{\sigma}^2, \theta) (\hat{\beta} - \beta) < c$ over $\theta \in \Theta$ is equivalent to minimizing $|\Sigma_{\hat{\beta}}(\hat{\sigma}^2, \theta)|$ for $\theta \in \Theta$ and that the minimizer of the volume of the confidence ellipsoid over $\theta \in \Theta$ is not affected by c. Here c can be viewed as a constant associated with a confidence level. The MGV estimation of θ by Fan et al. (2007) is obtained by minimizing the generalized variance of $\hat{\beta}$:

$$\hat{\theta} = \arg\min_{\theta \in \Theta} |\Sigma_{\hat{\beta}}(\hat{\sigma}^2, \theta)|. \tag{13}$$

Following the idea of the quasi-likelihood approach of Fan et al. (2007), we also study estimation of θ obtained by minimizing the weighted least squares:

$$\hat{\theta} = \arg\min_{\theta} \left(\hat{r}_i^T \hat{A}_i^{-1} R_i^{-1}(\theta) \hat{A}_i^{-1} \hat{r}_i \right). \tag{14}$$

2.3   Profile Estimation via Quadratic Inference Function

Qu et al. (2000) proposed the method of quadratic inference functions that does not involve direct estimation of the correlation parameter. The idea is to represent the inverse of the working correlation matrix by the linear combination of basis matrices:

$$R^{-1} \approx a_1 M_1 + a_2 M_2 + \cdots + a_K M_K, \tag{15}$$

where M_1 is the identity matrix, and $M_2, \cdots, M_K$ are symmetric matrices, and $a_1, \cdots, a_K$ are constant coefficients. The representation is applicable to many commonly used working correlations (Qu et al. 2000). For example, if the correlation structure exchangeable, then $R(\theta)$ has 1's on the diagonal, and θ's everywhere off the diagonal. The inversion R^{-1} can be written as $a_1 M_1 + a_2 M_2$, where M_1 is the identity matrix, and M_2 is a matrix with 0 on the diagonal and 1 off the diagonal. For the AR(1) correlation with $\rho(s, t) = \theta^{|s-t|}$, the inversion R^{-1} of a $J \times J$ correlation matrix can be written as a linear combination of three basis matrices, where M_1 is the identity matrix, and M_2 has 1 on the two main off-diagonals and 0 elsewhere, and M_2 has 1 on the corners $(1, 1)$ and (J, J), and 0 elsewhere.

Applying the QIF approach, we propose an alternative profile estimation of model (1). We replace the GEE estimator of β that solves $U_\beta(\beta) = 0$ in Sect. 2 by the estimator that minimizes the quadratic inference function while keep the estimation for $\tilde{\alpha}(t, \beta)$ as the root of (3) unchanged. Applying idea of the QIF, we define the "extended score" function:

$$
\begin{aligned}
g_n(\beta) &= \frac{1}{n} \sum_{i=1}^{n} g_i(\beta) \\
&= \frac{1}{n} \sum_{i=1}^{n} \begin{pmatrix} \left\{ \frac{\partial \tilde{\alpha}^T(T_i, \beta)}{\partial \beta} \tilde{X}_i + \tilde{Z}_i \right\} \Delta_i \hat{A}_i^{-1/2} M_1 \hat{A}_i^{-1/2} \left[Y_i - \tilde{\mu}_i(\beta) \right] \\ \vdots \\ \left\{ \frac{\partial \tilde{\alpha}^T(T_i, \beta)}{\partial \beta} \tilde{X}_i + \tilde{Z}_i \right\} \Delta_i \hat{A}_i^{-1/2} M_K \hat{A}_i^{-1/2} \left[Y_i - \tilde{\mu}_i(\beta) \right] \end{pmatrix}. \tag{16}
\end{aligned}
$$

The quadratic inference function is defined as $Q_n(\beta) = g_n^T(\beta) C_n^{-1}(\beta) g_n(\beta)$, where $C_n(\beta) = (1/n^2) \sum_{i=1}^{n} g_i(\beta) g_i^T(\beta)$. The profile QIF estimator is the minimizer of $Q_n(\beta)$:

$$\hat{\beta} = \arg \min_\beta Q_n(\beta). \tag{17}$$

Following the derivations of the asymptotic properties shown in Qu et al. (2000), we estimate the variance of the QIF estimator $\hat{\beta}$ by $\{\dot{g}_n(\hat{\beta}) C_n^{-1}(\hat{\beta}) \dot{g}_n^T(\hat{\beta})\}^{-1}$, where

$$
\dot{g}_n(\beta) = \frac{1}{n} \sum_{i=1}^{n} \begin{pmatrix} \left\{ \frac{\partial \tilde{\alpha}^T(T_i, \beta)}{\partial \beta} \tilde{X}_i + \tilde{Z}_i \right\} \hat{\Delta}_i \hat{A}_i^{-1/2} M_1 \hat{A}_i^{-1/2} \hat{\Delta}_i \left\{ \frac{\partial \tilde{\alpha}(T_i, \beta)}{\partial \beta} \tilde{X}_i + \tilde{Z}_i \right\}^T \\ \vdots \\ \left\{ \frac{\partial \tilde{\alpha}^T(T_i, \beta)}{\partial \beta} \tilde{X}_i + \tilde{Z}_i \right\} \hat{\Delta}_i \hat{A}_i^{-1/2} M_K \hat{A}_i^{-1/2} \hat{\Delta}_i \left\{ \frac{\partial \tilde{\alpha}(T_i, \beta)}{\partial \beta} \tilde{X}_i + \tilde{Z}_i \right\}^T \end{pmatrix}. \tag{18}
$$

2.4 Computational Algorithms

The iterative algorithms of the procedures using the QL, MGV, WLS, and QIF approaches for estimating $\alpha(t)$ and β under model (1) are outlined in the following.

1. Calculate the estimates of $\alpha(t)$ and β using the working independence approach and use them as the initial estimates $\hat{\alpha}^{\{0\}}(t)$ and $\hat{\beta}^{\{0\}}$;
2. Given the m-step estimates $\hat{\alpha}^{\{m\}}(t)$ and $\hat{\beta}^{\{m\}}$, calculate $\hat{r}_{ij} = Y_{ij} - g^{-1}\{(\hat{\alpha}^{\{m\}}(T_{ij}))^T X_{ij} + (\hat{\beta}^{\{m\}})^T Z_{ij}\}$ and obtain the matrix $\hat{A}_i^{\{m\}}$ whose diagonal elements are estimated by (11);
3. For the QL, MGV, and WLS approaches for estimating the correlation matrix, obtain the estimate $\hat{\theta}^{\{m\}}$ using one of the QL, MGV, and WLS methods described in Sect. 2.2.2; Set $\hat{V}_{2i}^{\{m\}} = \hat{A}_i^{\{m\}} R_i(\hat{\theta}^{\{m\}}) \hat{A}_i^{\{m\}}$ as in (10); Then update the estimate of β to $\hat{\beta}^{\{m+1\}}$ by solving (5) and the estimate of $\alpha(t)$ to $\hat{\alpha}^{\{m+1\}}(t) = \tilde{\alpha}(t, \hat{\beta}^{\{m+1\}})$;
4. For the QIF approach, update the estimate of β to $\hat{\beta}^{\{m+1\}}$ obtained by minimizing $Q_n(\beta) = g_n^T(\beta) C_n^{-1}(\beta) g_n(\beta)$ where and $\hat{A}_i$ in $g_n(\beta)$ is replaced by $\hat{A}_i^{\{m\}}$, and then update the estimate of $\alpha(t)$ to $\hat{\alpha}^{\{m+1\}}(t) = \tilde{\alpha}(t, \hat{\beta}^{\{m+1\}})$;
5. Repeating steps 2 to 4 until convergence, which is usually achieved within a few iterations.

2.5 Choices of Kernel Function, Bandwidth, and Link Function

We employ local linear techniques to estimate the nonparametric time-varying effects $\alpha(t)$. The kernel function is designed to give greater weight to observations with sampling time near t than those further away. In kernel density estimation, the Epanechnikov kernel function $K(x) = \frac{3}{4}(1 - x^2)_+$ is asymptotically optimal with the smallest mean integrated squared error among probability density functions. Silverman (1986, p.43) showed that there is not much variation in the efficiency in the choice of kernel function: the asymptotic relative efficiency of the Tukey kernel function $K(x) = \frac{15}{16}(1 - x^2)_+^2$ compared to the optimal Epanechnikov kernel is 99%, the Gaussian kernel has a relative efficiency of 95% and the rectangular kernel has a relative efficiency about 93%. We expect that the choice of kernel function has little effect on the performance of the proposed estimators for model (1) as well. It is common to assume compact support for technical simplicity. This assumption can be relaxed to include the Gaussian kernel (Silverman 1986, p.38).

The bandwidth, on the other hand, is much more of a concern. The cross-validation bandwidth selection is widely used to choose the bandwidth. Rice and Silverman (1991) suggested a leave-one-subject-out cross-validation approach. We recommend the K-fold cross-validation bandwidth selection considered by Sun et al. (2013) in the marginal estimation approach for the generalized semiparametric regression model (1). Specifically, subjects are divided into K approximately equal-sized groups. Let D_k denote the kth subgroup of data, then the kth prediction error is given by

$$PE_k(h) = \sum_{i \in D_k} \sum_{t_1 \leq T_{ij} \leq t_2} \left[Y_{ij} - g^{-1} \{ (\hat{\alpha}_{(-k)}(T_{ij}))^T X_{ij} + \hat{\beta}_{(-k)}^T Z_{ij} \} \right]^2, \quad (19)$$

for $k = 1, \ldots, K$, where $\hat{\alpha}_{(-k)}(t)$ and $\hat{\beta}_{(-k)}$ are the estimators of $\alpha(t)$ and β based on the data without the subgroup D_k, and $[t_1, t_2] \subset (0, \tau)$. The subset $[t_1, t_2]$ is considered to avoid possible instability in estimating $\alpha(t)$ near the boundary. In practice, this interval can be taken to be close to $[0, \tau]$. The data-driven bandwidth selection based on the K-fold cross-validation is to choose the bandwidth h that minimizes the total prediction error $PE(h) = \sum_{k=1}^{K} PE_k(h)$. The K-fold cross-validation bandwidth selection provides a working tool for locating an appropriate bandwidth.

The proposed estimation procedure holds for a wide class of link functions under model (1). A link function needs to be selected for a particular data application. The choice may be clear for some applications based on prior knowledge, but more often one needs to choose a link function that gives the "best fit" of the data. One criterion proposed by Sun et al. (2013) is to access the model fit by the regression deviation defined as

$$RD(g(\cdot), h_{cv}) = \sum_{i=1}^{n} \sum_{t_1 \leq T_{ij} \leq t_2} \left[Y_{ij} - g^{-1} \{ (\hat{\alpha}_g(T_{ij}))^T X_{ij} + \hat{\beta}_g^T Z_{ij} \} \right]^2, \quad (20)$$

where h_{cv} is the bandwidth selected based on the K-fold cross-validation method for the given link function $g(\cdot)$ described above, and $\hat{\alpha}_g(t)$ and $\hat{\beta}_g$ are the estimators of $\alpha(t)$ and β under model (1) with the bandwidth h_{cv}. In practice, the link function $g(\cdot)$ can be selected to minimize the regression deviation. Further examination of model fitness should be accompanied by model assessment tools such as the residual plots and formal goodness-of-fit tests.

3 Simulation Studies

In this section, we conduct a simulation study to assess the performances of the profile estimation methods using the QL, MGV, WLS, and QIF approaches presented in Sect. 2 under various models for longitudinal responses, different types of the within-subject correlation structures and different models for the measurement times. For convenience, we refer to the profile estimators resulted from these approaches as the QL, MGV, WLS, and QIF estimators. Section 3.1

presents a study of model (1) for continuous longitudinal responses and Sect. 3.2 shows the performances of these approaches for discrete longitudinal responses.

3.1 Continuous Longitudinal Responses

We study the performances of the proposed methods for continuous longitudinal responses under model (1) with the identity link function: $Y_i(t) = \alpha^T(t)X_i(t) + \beta^T Z_i(t) + \epsilon_i(t)$. We consider two simulation settings. In the first simulation setting (C1), the true correlation structure of the longitudinal responses is ARMA(1,1) and the measurement times are independent of covariates. In the second simulation setting (C2), the true correlation structure of the longitudinal responses is Exchangeable and the measurement times are dependent of covariates.

Simulation Setting (C1) Similar to Fan et al. (2007), for each subject i, we consider time-independent covariates $X_i(t) = (X_{1i}(t), X_{2i}(t))^T$ and $Z_i(t) = (Z_{1i}(t), Z_{2i})^T$, where $X_{1i} = 1$, $(X_{2i}(t), Z_{1i}(t))$ are time-varying covariates having a bivariate normal distribution with mean 0, variance 1 and correlation coefficient of 0.5 at each time t, and Z_{2i} is a time-independent covariate from Bernoulli distribution with success probability 0.5. We take $\alpha(t) = (\sqrt{t/12}, \sin(2\pi t/12))^T$ and $\beta = (1, 2)^T$. The error $\epsilon_i(t)$ is a Gaussian process with mean 0, variance varying with time $\sigma^2(t) = 0.5\exp(t/12)$ and of the ARMA(1,1) correlation structure, i.e., $Corr(Y_i(s), Y_i(t)) = \gamma\rho^{|t-s|}$ for $s \neq t$. We take $(\gamma, \rho) = (0.85, 0.9)$ and $(0.85, 0.6)$ for strong and moderate, respectively. All subjects have the same scheduled measurement time points, $\{0,1,2,\ldots,12\}$, but each of the scheduled time points has a 20% probability of being skipped except for the time 0. A random perturbation generated from the uniform distribution on $[0, 1]$ is added to the non-skipped scheduled time points. Every subject has approximately 7 to 13 observations with an average of 11.

Simulation Setting (C2) Similar to Sun et al. (2013), for each subject i, we let $Z_{1i}(t)$ be a time-varying covariate from a uniform distribution on $[0, 1]$, Z_{2i} a time-independent Bernoulli random variable with the success probability of 0.5, $X_{1i} = 1$, and $X_{2i}(t)$ a time-varying Bernoulli random variable with the success probability of 0.5 at each time t. Let $\alpha(t) = (0.5\sqrt{t}, 0.5\sin(2t))^T$ and $\beta = (0.5, 1)^T$. The error $\epsilon_i(t)$ has a normal distribution with mean ϕ_i and variance ν^2, where ϕ_i is a random variable from $N(0, 1)$. Thus $\epsilon_i(t)$ has an Exchangeable correlation structure with the correlation coefficients equal to $\theta = 0.8$ and $\theta = 0.5$ for $\nu = 0.5$ and $\nu = 1$, respectively. The measurement times T_{ij} for each subject i follow a Poisson process with the intensity $h_i(t) = 0.6\exp(0.7Z_{2i})$, for $0 \leq t \leq \tau$ with $\tau = 3.5$. The censoring times C_i are generated from a uniform distribution on $[1.5, 8]$. There are approximately three observations per subject on $[0, \tau]$ and about 30% of subjects are censored before $\tau = 3.5$.

The performances of the profile GEE estimators using the QL, MGV, and WLS approaches for estimating the correlation parameter θ as well as the profile estimators via the QIF approach are examined under the settings (C1) and (C2). We let V_{1i} to be the identity matrix for all the estimators while using different correlation structures are assumed for V_{2i}. The working independence estimator (WI) is obtained by letting V_{2i}^{-1} be the identity matrix. The Epanechnikov kernel function $K(x) = \frac{3}{4}(1 - x^2)_+$ is used in the study.

The simulation results for estimating β under the setting (C1) and ARMA(1,1) correlation with strong and moderate correlations are shown in Tables 1 and 2, respectively. The simulation results for estimating β under the setting (C2) and Exchangeable correlation with strong and moderate correlations are shown in Tables 3 and 4, respectively. The tables summarize the estimation bias (Bias), the sample standard error of estimates (SEE), the sample mean of the estimated standard errors (ESE), and the 95% empirical coverage probability (CP) for $n = 200$. Each entry of the table is calculated based on 1000 repetitions. The bandwidth used for each table is selected based on the 10-fold cross-validation of a single simulation that minimizes the total prediction error $PE(h)$ for h in [0.7, 1.3] and carried it over for all 1000 repetitions.

The results for WI is obtained by assuming working independence case. The performances of the estimators QL, MGV, WLS and QIF are examined under

Table 1 Summary of Bias, SEE, ESE and CP under different estimation methods for β_1 and β_2 with $n = 200$, $h = 0.8$ based on 1000 simulations under the model setting (C1) and the strong ARMA(1,1) correlation with $(\gamma, \rho) = (0.85, 0.9)$

	$\beta_1 = 1$				$\beta_2 = 2$			
Method	Bias	SEE	ESE	CP	Bias	SEE	ESE	CP
Working independence								
WI	0.0013	0.0244	0.0235	0.938	0.0059	0.1016	0.1011	0.944
Assuming exchangeable correlation (Misspecification)								
QL	0.0001	0.0166	0.0160	0.937	0.0041	0.1096	0.1020	0.938
MGV	0.0001	0.0166	0.0160	0.936	0.0041	0.1061	0.0992	0.940
QIF	0.0003	0.0168	0.0160	0.930	0.0053	0.0954	0.0915	0.940
WLS	0.0004	0.0171	0.0164	0.934	0.0052	0.0946	0.0912	0.941
Assuming ARMA(1,1) Correlation (True)								
QL	0.0005	0.0130	0.0127	0.936	0.0030	0.0955	0.0848	0.914
MGV	0.0008	0.0147	0.0140	0.929	0.0052	0.0936	0.0918	0.943
QIF	0.0005	0.0143	0.0136	0.931	0.0051	0.0926	0.0877	0.939
WLS	0.0006	0.0142	0.0136	0.935	0.0050	0.0926	0.0897	0.942
Assuming mixed correlation								
QL	0.0005	0.0131	0.0127	0.937	0.0030	0.0956	0.0847	0.916
MGV	0.0005	0.0145	0.0138	0.930	0.0047	0.0934	0.0895	0.942
QIF	0.0004	0.0142	0.0133	0.928	0.0053	0.0925	0.0864	0.932
WLS	0.0006	0.0142	0.0136	0.934	0.0051	0.0927	0.0897	0.942

Table 2 Summary of Bias, SEE, ESE and CP under different estimation methods for β_1 and β_2 with $n = 200$, $h = 0.8$ based on 1000 simulations under the model setting (C1) and the moderate ARMA(1,1) correlation with $(\gamma, \rho) = (0.85, 0.6)$

| Method | $\beta_1 = 1$ | | | | $\beta_2 = 2$ | | | |
	Bias	SEE	ESE	CP	Bias	SEE	ESE	CP
Working independence								
WI	0.0009	0.0242	0.0236	0.942	0.004	0.0672	0.0666	0.946
Assuming exchangeable correlation (Misspecification)								
QL	0.0003	0.0220	0.0210	0.937	0.0033	0.0665	0.0634	0.941
MGV	0.0001	0.0221	0.0212	0.939	0.0024	0.0937	0.0895	0.949
QIF	0.0004	0.0221	0.0209	0.931	0.0035	0.0647	0.0618	0.943
WLS	0.0005	0.0222	0.0212	0.937	0.0035	0.0645	0.0623	0.943
Assuming ARMA(1,1) Correlation (True)								
QL	0.0008	0.0182	0.0174	0.935	0.0028	0.0618	0.0601	0.938
MGV	0.0007	0.0187	0.0179	0.933	0.0031	0.0618	0.0604	0.942
QIF	0.0007	0.0195	0.0182	0.928	0.0036	0.0629	0.0606	0.941
WLS	0.0008	0.0194	0.0184	0.933	0.0033	0.0622	0.0609	0.941
Assuming Mixed Correlation								
QL	0.0008	0.0182	0.0174	0.935	0.0028	0.0619	0.0601	0.937
MGV	0.0005	0.0192	0.0183	0.942	0.0027	0.0659	0.0630	0.945
QIF	0.0007	0.0196	0.0181	0.924	0.0036	0.0633	0.0600	0.944
WLS	0.0008	0.0193	0.0184	0.933	0.0033	0.0622	0.0609	0.941

Table 3 Summary of Bias, SEE, ESE and CP under different estimation methods for β_1 and β_2 with $n = 200$, $h = 1.2$ based on 1000 simulations under the model setting (C2) and the strong Exchangeable correlation with $\theta = 0.8$

| Method | $\beta_1 = 1$ | | | | $\beta_2 = 2$ | | | |
	Bias	SEE	ESE	CP	Bias	SEE	ESE	CP
Working Independence								
WI	0.0023	0.1535	0.1544	0.949	0.0048	0.1691	0.1629	0.934
Assuming ARMA(1,1) Correlation								
QL	0.0064	0.0884	0.0878	0.949	−0.0084	0.1605	0.1427	0.915
MGV	0.0047	0.0974	0.0973	0.948	0.0008	0.1574	0.1466	0.933
QIF	0.0048	0.1064	0.1019	0.935	−0.0001	0.1576	0.1434	0.917
WLS	0.0051	0.0945	0.0948	0.953	−0.0004	0.1564	0.1451	0.929
Assuming Exchangeable Correlation (True)								
QL	0.0069	0.0853	0.0855	0.956	−0.0145	0.1625	0.1423	0.910
MGV	0.0044	0.1113	0.1119	0.950	0.0022	0.1588	0.1493	0.928
QIF	0.0066	0.1069	0.1037	0.950	0.0021	0.1584	0.1473	0.922
WLS	0.0053	0.0942	0.0945	0.956	−0.0009	0.1563	0.1449	0.926
Assuming Mixed Correlation								
QL	0.0068	0.0855	0.0853	0.953	−0.0134	0.1622	0.1422	0.911
MGV	0.0031	0.1246	0.1249	0.949	0.0033	0.1616	0.1532	0.929
QIF	0.0060	0.1044	0.0976	0.930	−0.0003	0.1573	0.1421	0.914
WLS	0.0052	0.0942	0.0944	0.954	−0.0008	0.1563	0.1448	0.927

Table 4 Summary of Bias, SEE, ESE and CP under different estimation methods for β_1 and β_2 with $n = 200$, $h = 1.2$ based on 1000 simulations under the model setting (C2) and the moderate Exchangeable correlation with $\theta = 0.5$

Method	$\beta_1 = 1$				$\beta_2 = 2$			
	Bias	SEE	ESE	CP	Bias	SEE	ESE	CP
Working Independence								
WI	0.006	0.1952	0.196	0.949	0.0062	0.1863	0.1787	0.94
Assuming ARMA(1,1) Correlation								
QL	0.0112	0.1611	0.1597	0.953	0.0006	0.1774	0.1647	0.932
MGV	0.0113	0.1723	0.1667	0.946	0.0020	0.1785	0.1665	0.929
QIF	0.0091	0.1740	0.1684	0.939	0.0033	0.1815	0.1658	0.917
WLS	0.0090	0.1661	0.1655	0.952	0.0039	0.1778	0.1667	0.927
Assuming exchangeable correlation (True)								
QL	0.0118	0.1602	0.1591	0.954	−0.0001	0.1773	0.1646	0.935
MGV	0.0083	0.1723	0.1731	0.952	0.0048	0.1795	0.1695	0.933
QIF	0.0114	0.1676	0.1637	0.951	0.0045	0.1787	0.1659	0.928
WLS	0.0092	0.1659	0.1654	0.956	0.0037	0.1777	0.1666	0.927
Assuming mixed correlation								
QL	0.0116	0.1602	0.1588	0.951	0.0001	0.1773	0.1646	0.933
MGV	0.0042	0.1837	0.1777	0.949	0.0055	0.1806	0.1710	0.936
QIF	0.0106	0.1692	0.1611	0.946	0.0039	0.1793	0.1632	0.921
WLS	0.0092	0.1658	0.1652	0.954	0.0037	0.1777	0.1665	0.927

both the correctly specified correlation model and the misspecified correlation models. The results under "Assuming Exchangeable Correlation" are obtained by assuming exchangeable correlation in the estimation, the results under "Assuming ARMA(1,1) Correlation" are obtained by assuming ARMA(1,1) correlation in the estimation, while the results under "Assuming Mixed Correlation" are obtained by assuming the correlation to be the mix of the exchangeable and AR(1) correlation in the estimation. The basis matrices for the QIF estimator are taken as a combination the basis matrices for Exchangeable and AR(1) when ARMA(1,1) and Mixed Correlation Structures are assumed.

The simulation study shows that all estimators are consistent with small estimation bias. The WLS, QL, MGV and QIF estimators all perform well and improve the estimation efficiency compared with the working independence (WI) method. The methods utilizing the within-subject correlations show reduced estimation standard errors in SEE and ESE. More efficiency is gained by assuming the true or mixed correlation structures than the scenarios where correlation structures are misspecified. More efficiency gain is also observed in the settings with stronger within-subject correlations than with moderate within-subject correlations. For example, compared with the WI estimator, the sample standard errors of the QL, MGV, WLS, and QIF estimators for β_1 reduced between 30% to 46% in Table 1 for strong within-subject correlation and the sample standard errors reduced between 8% to 25% in Table 2 for moderate within-subject correlations under the true

ARMA(1,1) correlation. Similarly, compared with the WI estimator, the sample standard errors of the QL, MGV, WLS, and QIF estimators for β_1 reduced between 18% to 44% in Table 3 for strong within-subject correlation and the sample standard errors reduced between 6% to 18% in Table 4 for moderate within-subject correlations under the true Exchangeable correlation. The efficiency improved is more evident in estimating the effect of time-varying covariate than for the time-invariant covariate. This phenomenon also appeared in the simulation studies in Lin and Carroll (2001b) and Wang et al. (2005).

The performances of the estimators by assuming ARMA(1,1) working correlation and those under the mixed working correlation are close. The QL estimator appeared to achieve most efficiency gain out of these estimators in most scenarios. The above observations hold for both covariate-independent and covariate-dependent measurement times.

3.2   Discrete Longitudinal Responses

In this section we examine the performance of the proposed methods for model (1) for discrete longitudinal responses. We consider binary longitudinal responses in the simulation setting (D1), and Poisson count responses in the simulation setting (D2). Both settings have an Exchangeable correlation structure.

Simulation Setting (D1): The Bernoulli Model   For binary longitudinal responses, we let $g(\mu) = \log\{\mu/(1 - \mu)\}$ be the logistic link function. The observation times are generated similarly to the simulation setting (C1). All subjects have the same scheduled observation time points, $\{0,1,2,\ldots,8\}$, but each of the scheduled time points has a 20% probability of being skipped except for the time 0. A random perturbation generated from the uniform distribution on $[0, 1]$ is added to the non-skipped scheduled time points. The number of observations, J_i, ranges from 4 to 9. At each observation time T_{ij}, $j = 1, \ldots, J_i$, $X_{ij} = 1$, Z_{1ij} and Z_{2ij} are independent standard normal random variables that do not vary with time. Let $\alpha(t) = \sin(\pi t/30) - 0.5$ and $\beta = (0.01, 0.01)^T$ and $\mu_{ij} = P(Y_{ij} = 1|X_{ij}, Z_{ij})$. The binary longitudinal responses $Y_{ij} = Y_i(T_{ij})$, $j = 1, \ldots, J_i$, are generated with the marginal means following the logit model $\text{logit}(\mu_{ij}) = \alpha(T_{ij})X_{ij} + \beta^T Z_{ij}$ and with constant correlation coefficient $Corr(Y_i(s), Y_i(t)) = 0.5$ for $s \neq t$. We refer to Macke et al. (2009) for the techniques for simulating correlated binary responses. Our simulation used the Matlab code provided in the paper to generate the correlated binary variables with the specified mean and covariance.

Simulation Setting (D2): The Poisson Model   Suppose that T_{ij}, X_{ij} and Z_{ij} are the same as in the simulation setting (D1). We also use $\alpha(t) = \sin(\pi t/30) - 0.5$ and $\beta = (0.01, 0.01)^T$. Let $\mu_{ij} = E(Y_{ij}|X_{ij}, Z_{ij})$. Using the method of Macke et al. (2009), we generate Poisson longitudinal process $Y_{ij} = Y_i(T_{ij})$, $j = 1, \ldots, J_i$,

Table 5 Summary of Bias, SEE, ESE, and CP under different estimation methods for β_1 and β_2 with $n = 200, h = 1.2$ based on 1000 simulations under the Bernoulli model (D1) and the moderate Exchangeable correlation with $\theta = 0.5$

Method	$\beta_1 = 1$				$\beta_2 = 2$			
	Bias	SEE	ESE	CP	Bias	SEE	ESE	CP
Working Independence								
WI	0.0002	0.0524	0.0525	0.954	0.0014	0.0516	0.0525	0.962
Assuming ARMA(1,1) Correlation								
QL	−0.0002	0.0406	0.0404	0.945	−0.0012	0.0407	0.0405	0.948
MGV	−0.0004	0.0429	0.0428	0.937	−0.0005	0.0429	0.0429	0.950
QIF	−0.0002	0.0445	0.0434	0.932	−0.0008	0.0440	0.0435	0.942
WLS	0.0000	0.0411	0.0410	0.944	−0.0005	0.0410	0.0410	0.955
Assuming exchangeable correlation (True)								
QL	0.0000	0.0396	0.0395	0.947	−0.0013	0.0396	0.0395	0.949
MGV	0.0000	0.0396	0.0395	0.947	−0.0013	0.0396	0.0395	0.948
QIF	0.0003	0.0404	0.0397	0.944	−0.0012	0.0404	0.0397	0.943
WLS	0.0001	0.0408	0.0407	0.950	−0.0005	0.0406	0.0407	0.956
Assuming Mixed Correlation								
QL	0.0000	0.0396	0.0394	0.947	−0.0012	0.0396	0.0394	0.949
MGV	0.0003	0.0434	0.0432	0.946	0.0000	0.0428	0.0432	0.951
QIF	0.0001	0.0406	0.0393	0.941	−0.0014	0.0406	0.0393	0.936
WLS	0.0001	0.0408	0.0406	0.948	−0.0005	0.0406	0.0406	0.956

with the conditional marginal mean model $\log(\mu_{ij}) = \alpha(T_{ij})X_{ij} + \beta^T Z_{ij}$ and with constant correlation coefficient $Corr(Y_i(s), Y_i(t)) = 0.5$ for $s \neq t$.

The estimation results under the simulation settings (D1) and (D2) are summarized in Tables 5 and 6, respectively. The simulation shows that estimation bias is small for all estimators. The QL, MGV, WLS, and QIF estimators that utilize the within-subject correlations show improved efficiency compared with using the working independence (WI) method with the sample standard errors reduced between 17% to 24% in Table 5 and between 10% to 30% in Table 6. The QL estimator achieved most efficiency gain out of these estimators. Efficiency gains are slightly higher when the true or mixed correlation structures are assumed compared to assuming the ARMA(1,1) correlation structures.

4 Concluding Remarks

The generalized semiparametric varying-coefficient additive model (1) specifies a model for the conditional mean of longitudinal responses. The model allows time-varying effects for some covariates and constant effects for others and is an umbrella for many different models with selections of the link function. The intensively studied semiparametric additive model obtained by using the identity link function is

Table 6 Summary of Bias, SEE, ESE and CP under different estimation methods for β_1 and β_2 with $n = 200$, $h = 1.2$ based on 1000 simulations under the Poisson model (D2) and the moderate Exchangeable correlation with $\theta = 0.5$

	$\beta_1 = 1$				$\beta_2 = 2$			
Method	Bias	SEE	ESE	CP	Bias	SEE	ESE	CP
Working independence								
WI	−0.0008	0.0271	0.0268	0.944	−0.0005	0.0271	0.0269	0.943
Assuming ARMA(1,1) Correlation								
QL	−0.0005	0.0206	0.0202	0.954	−0.0008	0.0199	0.0203	0.955
MGV	−0.0008	0.0243	0.0241	0.943	−0.0011	0.0245	0.0240	0.949
QIF	−0.0005	0.0220	0.0216	0.952	−0.0010	0.0224	0.0217	0.940
WLS	−0.0006	0.0208	0.0205	0.954	−0.0007	0.0202	0.0205	0.954
Assuming exchangeable correlation (True)								
QL	−0.0006	0.0199	0.0197	0.951	−0.0007	0.0191	0.0197	0.955
MGV	−0.0007	0.0219	0.0216	0.947	−0.0006	0.0215	0.0217	0.950
QIF	−0.0005	0.0201	0.0197	0.950	−0.0006	0.0193	0.0197	0.953
WLS	−0.0006	0.0206	0.0203	0.952	−0.0007	0.0199	0.0203	0.954
Assuming mixed correlation								
QL	−0.0006	0.0199	0.0197	0.948	−0.0007	0.0192	0.0197	0.956
MGV	−0.0006	0.0222	0.0218	0.956	−0.0008	0.0219	0.0219	0.945
QIF	−0.0006	0.0202	0.0195	0.949	−0.0007	0.0194	0.0195	0.954
WLS	−0.0006	0.0206	0.0202	0.954	−0.0007	0.0200	0.0203	0.955

popular for modeling continuous longitudinal responses. Semiparametric statistical modeling of discrete longitudinal responses has been understudied. With selection of link functions, model (1) can be used to model both continuous and discrete responses. Sun et al. (2013) investigated the local linear profile marginal estimation method for model (1) under the working independence. The estimation methods under working independence that ignore the within-subject correlation are valid and yield asymptotically unbiased estimators.

In this paper, we studied several profile estimation methods for model (1) that utilize the within-subject correlations to improve estimation efficiency. Several profile estimation methods that utilize the within-subject correlations including the profile GEE approaches and the profile QIF approach were investigated. The profile estimations are assisted with the local linear smoothing technique by approximating the time-varying effects with linear functions in the neighborhood of each time. The profile GEE approaches include the quasi-likelihood, the minimum generalized variance, and the weighted least squares. These methods differ by different procedures used in estimating the within-subject correlations. The proposed profile estimation methods for the generalized semiparametric varying-coefficient additive model (1) provide a unified approach that work well for discrete longitudinal responses as well as for continuous longitudinal responses.

Finite sample performances of these different methods are examined through Monto Carlo simulations under various correlation structures for both discrete and continuous longitudinal responses. Our study showed significant efficiency improvement of all the estimators, the QL, WLS, WLS, and QIF estimators, over the working independence approach. The QL estimator appeared to achieve most efficiency gain out of all estimators in most scenarios. The efficiency improved is more evident in estimating the effects of time-varying covariates than for the time-invariant covariates. Efficiency gains are higher when the true or mixed correlation structures are assumed compared to the misspecified correlation structures. The above observations hold for both covariate-independent and covariate-dependent measurement times.

Acknowledgments We thank the editors for their handling of our manuscript. We also thank the reviewer's valuable comments and suggestions that have improved the paper. This research was partially supported by the NIAID NIH award number R37AI054165 and the National Science Foundation grant DMS1915829. The authors would like to thank professor Runzi Li for providing the program code for Fan, Huang and Li (2007).

References

Chen, K., & Jin, Z. (2006). Partial linear regression models for clustered data. *Journal of the American Statistical Association, 101*(473), 195–204.

Dempster, A. P. (1969). *Elements of continuous multivariate analysis*. Reading, MA: Addison-Wesley.

Fan, J., & Li, R. (2004). New estimation and model selection procedures for semiparametric modeling in longitudinal data analysis. *Journal of the American Statistical Association, 99*(467), 710–723.

Fan, J., Huang, T., & Li, R. (2007). Analysis of longitudinal data with semiparametric estimation of covariance function. *Journal of the American Statistical Association, 102*(478), 632–641.

Hansen, L. P. (1982). Large sample properties of generalized method of moments estimators. *Econometrica: Journal of the Econometric Society, 50*(4), 1029–1054.

Hoover, D. R., Rice, J. A., Wu, C. O., & Yang, L.-P. (1998). Nonparametric smoothing estimates of time-varying coefficient models with longitudinal data. *Biometrika, 85*(4), 809–822.

Hu, Z., Wang, N., & Carroll, R. J. (2004). Profile-kernel versus backfitting in the partially linear models for longitudinal/clustered data. *Biometrika, 91*(2), 251–262.

Liang, K.-Y. & Zeger, S. L. (1986). Longitudinal data analysis using generalized linear models. *Biometrika, 73*(1), 13–22.

Lin, X., & Carroll, R. J. (2000). Nonparametric function estimation for clustered data when the predictor is measured without/with error. *Journal of the American Statistical Association, 95*(450), 520–534.

Lin, X., & Carroll, R. J. (2001a). Semiparametric regression for clustered data. *Biometrika 88*(4), 1179–1185.

Lin, X., & Carroll, R. J. (2001b). Semiparametric regression for clustered data using generalized estimating equations. *Journal of the American Statistical Association, 96*(455), 1045–1056.

Lin, D., & Ying, Z. (2001). Semiparametric and nonparametric regression analysis of longitudinal data. *Journal of the American Statistical Association, 96*(453), 103–126.

Macke, J. H., Berens, P., Ecker, A. S., Tolias, A. S., & Bethge, M. (2009). Generating spike trains with specified correlation coefficients. *Neural Computation, 21*(2), 397–423.

Madsen, L., Fang, Y., Song, P. X.-K., Li, M., & Yuan, Y. (2011). Joint regression analysis for discrete longitudinal data. *Biometrics, 67*(3), 1171–1176.

Martinussen, T., & Scheike, T. H. (1999). A semiparametric additive regression model for longitudinal data. *Biometrika, 86*, 691–702.

Qu, A., Lindsay, B. G., & Li, B. (2000). Improving generalised estimating equations using quadratic inference functions. *Biometrika, 87*(4), 823–836.

Rice, J. A., & Silverman, B. W. (1991). Estimating the mean and covariance structure nonparametrically when the data are curves. *Journal of the Royal Statistical Society. Series B (Methodological), 53*(1), 233–243.

Severini, T. A., & Staniswalis, J. G. (1994). Quasi-likelihood estimation in semiparametric models. *Journal of the American statistical Association, 89*(426), 501–511.

Silverman, B. (1986). *Density estimation for statistics and data analysis*. London: Chapman and Hall.

Song, P. X.-K., Li, M., & Yuan, Y. (2009). Joint regression analysis of correlated data using gaussian copulas. *Biometrics, 65*(1), 60–68.

Sun, Y., & Wu, H. (2005). Semiparametric time-varying coefficients regression model for longitudinal data. *Scandinavian Journal of Statistics, 32*(1), 21–47.

Sun, Y., Sun, L., & Zhou, J. (2013). Profile local linear estimation of generalized semiparametric regression model for longitudinal data. *Lifetime Data Analysis, 19*(3), 317–349. PMCID: PMC3710313.

Tang, C. Y., Zhang, W., & Leng, C. (2019). Discrete longitudinal data modeling with a mean-correlation regression approach. *Statistica Sinica, 29*(2), 853–876.

Wang, N., Carroll, R. J., & Lin, X. (2005). Efficient semiparametric marginal estimation for longitudinal/clustered data. *Journal of the American Statistical Association, 100*(469), 147–157.

Wu, H., & Liang, H. (2004). Backfitting random varying-coefficient models with time-dependent smoothing covariates. *Scandinavian Journal of Statistics, 31*(1), 3–19.

Zeger, S. L., & Diggle, P. J. (1994). Semiparametric models for longitudinal data with application to cd4 cell numbers in HIV seroconverters. *Biometrics, 50*(3), 689–699.

Sieve Estimation of Semiparametric Linear Transformation Model with Left-Truncated and Current Status Data

Riyadh Rustam Al-Mosawi and Xuewen Lu

Abstract In this paper, we analyze the semiparametric linear transformation model with left-truncated and current status data. Sieve maximum likelihood estimation method based on techniques of constrained Bernstein polynomials is exploited to obtain estimators for both the regression coefficients and the baseline survival function. Under some regularity conditions, we have proved that the proposed parameter estimators are semiparametrically efficient and asymptotically normal base on the conditional likelihood given the truncation time, and the estimator for the nonparametric function achieves the optimal rate of convergence. Simulation studies are conducted to assure the theoretical results, and a real data set is analyzed using the proposed method.

Keywords Bernstein polynomials · Current status data · Efficient estimation · Left-truncated data · Linear transformation model

1 Introduction

Let T be a nonnegative random variable denoting the failure time of interest and Z be a d-dimensional vector of covariates. The linear transformation model (LTM) assumes that

$$H_0(T) = -\beta_0^\mathsf{T} Z + \epsilon, \tag{1}$$

R. R. Al-Mosawi (✉)
Department of Mathematics, College of Computer Science and Mathematics, University of Thi-Qar, Thi-Qar, Iraq
e-mail: riyadh1965@utq.edu.iq

X. Lu
Department of Mathematics and Statistics, University of Calgary, Calgary, AB, Canada
e-mail: xlu@ucalgary.ca

© The Author(s), under exclusive license to Springer Nature Switzerland AG 2022
W. He et al. (eds.), *Advances and Innovations in Statistics and Data Science*, ICSA Book Series in Statistics, https://doi.org/10.1007/978-3-031-08329-7_9

181

where H_0 is an unknown monotone increasing function with $H_0(0) = -\infty$, β_0 is d-vector of regression parameters and ϵ is an error term assumed to follow a known survival function S_ϵ, free of the covariate Z, for example, see Cheng et al. (1995). Here and throughout the paper, B^T denotes the transpose of a vector or matrix B. The importance of LTM in the survival analysis is its flexibility to include some well-known regression models. The model (1) with ϵ following the extreme value distribution and the logistic distribution correspond to the proportional hazards model and the proportional odds model, respectively Cheng et al. (1995); while the model (1) with ϵ following a standard normal distribution represents a generalization of the usual Box-Cox model (see Bickel et al. 1993). The conditional survival function of T given Z can be written as

$$S(t|Z) = P(T > t|Z) = S_\epsilon(H_0(t) + \beta_0^\mathsf{T} Z). \tag{2}$$

It is common in survival analysis to collect data with incomplete observations or missing information rather than complete observations due to some reasons, for example, the limitation of time or shortage in the budget. One form of incomplete data is left censoring and right censoring. An observation is left-censored if we know that the event has already happened at a time before the monitoring time while it is right-censored if the event has not happened at or before the observation time. The scheme of censoring in which each observation is either left-censored or right-censored is called interval censoring of case I or current status, see, for example, Sun (2006); Keiding (1991). In specific, assume for each subject there is an monitoring time C. In current status data, the lifetime of each subject, T, is only known to occur before the monitoring time (i.e., $T \leq C$) or after the monitoring time (i.e., $T > C$). Current status observations are often occur in cross-sectional studies and tumorigenicity experiments (Sun and Kalbfleisch 1996). It should be noted that, unlike to the usual right-censored data, here we do not have exact observations. Analyzing the semiparametric linear transformation model with censored data was investigated by many authors. For example, Cheng et al. (1995); Chen et al. (2002); McLain and Ghosh (2013) for right-censored data, Zhang et al. (2013) and Lu et al. (2019) for current status data and (Hu and Xiang 2016) interval-censored data with cure fraction. Another form of missing information can be represented by truncation. Truncation occurs when the incomplete nature of the observations is due to the design of the experiment rather than the limitations of resources. If we observe those individuals whose event time are greater than some truncation threshold, then the individuals are subject to left censoring. Assume for each subject, there is a left-truncation time L such that $L < C$. The lifetime of each subject can be observed whenever $T > L$. For example, suppose that we are interested in the incubation time of AIDS for patients who have already recorded positive HIV. Patients who have already onset of AIDS before the study starts represent left-truncated observations and they cannot be observed. Furthermore, patients in which the onset of AIDS is already recorded at the observation time represent left-censored otherwise they are considered as right-censored. Statistical models with left-truncation and interval-censored data were considered by several authors. Kim (2003), Pan and Chappell

(2002), Shen (2014) for the Cox model, (Wang et al. 2015) for additive hazard model and Shen et al. (2019) for transformation model without or with a cure fraction. The goal of this paper is to estimate the regression parameter β_0 in model (2) in the presence of the nuisance infinite dimensional parameter H_0 with left-truncated and current status data.

The rest of the paper is organized as follows. In Sect. 2, sieve maximum likelihood estimators of the unknown parameters using Bernstein polynomials technique are computed and the variances are estimated. Section 3 is devoted to derive the efficient score and efficient information bound for estimation of β. In Sect. 4, we investigate the asymptotic properties of the proposed estimators. In Sect. 5, we conduct a Monte-Carlo simulation method to assess the proposed method. In Sect. 6, we analyze a real data set for illustration of our method. In Sect. 7, we provide some concluding remarks and discussions about future work. Proofs of the lemmas and theorems are included in Appendix.

2 Sieve Maximum Likelihood Estimation

In this section, we compute the sieve maximum likelihood estimators of β and H using Bernstein polynomials. Let $V = (L, C, \Delta, Z)$ be a single observation, where L is the left-truncation random variable, C is the monitoring time random variable, $\Delta = I(T \geq C)$ is the censored indicator random variable, and Z is a d-dimensional vector of covariates. Let $V_i = (L_i, C_i, \Delta_i, Z_i), i = 1, \cdots, n$, be n independent copies of V and let $\mathbf{V} = (V_1, \cdots, V_n)$. Then the log-conditional likelihood (hereinafter abbreviated as log-likelihood) of β and H based on the observations, $\mathbf{V}$, given L, can be written (up to terms do not involve (β, H)) as

$$l_n(\beta, H | \mathbf{V}) = \sum_{i=1}^{n} \left[\delta_i \log \left(\frac{S_\epsilon(H(c_i) + \beta^\mathsf{T} z_i)}{S_\epsilon(H(l_i) + \beta^\mathsf{T} z_i)} \right) \right.$$
$$\left. + (1 - \delta_i) \log \left(1 - \frac{S_\epsilon(H(c_i) + \beta^\mathsf{T} z_i)}{S_\epsilon(H(l_i) + \beta^\mathsf{T} z_i)} \right) \right], \tag{3}$$

where l_i, c_i, δ_i, and z_i denote the observed values of L_i, C_i, Δ_i, and Z_i, respectively. From the Assumptions **C1** and **C2** in the appendix, we define the parameter space of (β, H) as $\Theta = \mathbb{B} \times \mathbb{H}$, where $\mathbb{B}$ is defined in **C1** and

$$\mathbb{H} = \{H(.) : B^- < H(t) < B^+, dH(t)/dt > 0, t \in (\tau_0, \tau_1)\},$$

B^- and B^+ are defined in **C2**. The sieve estimation of the nonparametric component is performed by approximating the function H (or the space $\mathbb{H}$) over the finite interval by a parametric function with finite number of parameters (or finite dimensional space). Using Bernstein polynomial of degree $q = O(n^v), 0 < v < 1$,

Lorentz (2013), $H(t)$ can be approximated by $H_n(t; \gamma)$, where

$$H_n(t; \gamma) = \sum_{i=0}^{q} \gamma_i \frac{q!}{i!(q-i)!} \left(\frac{t - \tau_0}{\tau_1 - \tau_0} \right)^i \left(1 - \frac{t - \tau_0}{\tau_1 - \tau_0} \right)^{q-i} := \gamma^\mathsf{T} \mathcal{A}(t),$$

$\gamma^\mathsf{T} = (\gamma_0, \cdots, \gamma_q)$ and $\mathcal{A}^\mathsf{T}(t) = (A_0(t), \cdots, A_q(t))$ with

$$A_i(t) = \frac{q!}{i!(q-i)!} \left(\frac{t - \tau_0}{\tau_1 - \tau_0} \right)^i \left(1 - \frac{t - \tau_0}{\tau_1 - \tau_0} \right)^{q-i}, \ i = 0, 1 \cdots, q. \tag{4}$$

The optimal value of v is given in Theorem 3. Here, β_0 and H_0 denote the true values of β and H, respectively. Due to the monotonicity of H, we define the sieve space $\mathbb{H}_n$ by Lorentz (2013)

$$\mathbb{H}_n = \left\{ \gamma^\mathsf{T} \mathcal{A}(t) : B^- < \gamma_0 \leq \cdots \leq \gamma_q < B^+, \sum_{j=0}^{q} |\gamma_j| \leq M_\gamma \right\}.$$

The quantity $M_\gamma = O(n^a)$ is a positive constant that controls the size of the sieve space (Shen 1997). Substituting the approximated expression, H_n, in the log-likelihood function gives us

$$l_n(\beta, \gamma | \mathbf{V}) = \sum_{i=1}^{n} \left\{ \delta_i \log \left(\frac{S_\epsilon(\gamma^\mathsf{T} \mathcal{A}(c_i) + \beta^\mathsf{T} z_i)}{S_\epsilon(\gamma^\mathsf{T} \mathcal{A}(l_i) + \beta^\mathsf{T} z_i)} \right) \right.$$

$$\left. + (1 - \delta_i) \log \left(1 - \frac{S_\epsilon(\gamma^\mathsf{T} \mathcal{A}(c_i) + \beta^\mathsf{T} z_i)}{S_\epsilon(\gamma^\mathsf{T} \mathcal{A}(l_i) + \beta^\mathsf{T} z_i)} \right) \right\}. \tag{5}$$

In the sieve estimation problem, the major issue is how to select the degree of smoothness of approximation, q, in the parameter space $\mathbb{H}_n$. Here, the selection procedure of q and the transformation distribution parameter r is to find the value that minimizes the BIC criterion given by (19) in the simulation study and real data analysis. To find sieve maximum likelihood estimator $(\hat{\beta}, \hat{H}_n)$, we need to find $(\hat{\beta}, \hat{\gamma})$ that maximizes the log-likelihood over the space $\Theta_n = \mathbb{B} \times \mathbb{H}_n$, i.e.,

$$(\hat{\beta}, \hat{\gamma}) = argmax_{(\beta, \gamma) \in \Theta_n} l_n(\beta, \gamma | \mathbf{V}).$$

The algorithm we utilize here to maximize the log-likelihood consists of the following steps. Suppose the values of β and γ at the k-th iteration are $\beta^{(k)}$ and $\gamma^{(k)}$, respectively.

Step 1:   Find $\gamma^{(k+1)}$ by maximizing the log-likelihood $l_n(\beta^{(k)}, \gamma^{(k)} | \mathbf{V})$ subject to monotone constraint on γ to update $\gamma^{(k)}$.

Step 2:   Find $\beta^{(k+1)}$ by maximizing the log-likelihood $l_n(\beta^{(k)}, \gamma^{(k+1)} | \mathbf{V})$ to update $\beta^{(k)}$.

Step 3:   Repeat **Step 1** and **Step 2** if $\|\gamma^{(k+1)} - \gamma^{(k)}\| + \|\beta^{(k+1)} - \beta^{(k)}\| > \eta$, for
a small pre-specified quantity $\eta > 0$, otherwise, set $\hat{\beta} = \beta^{(k+1)}$ and $\hat{\gamma} = \gamma^{(k+1)}$
and terminate the algorithm.

Clearly, **Step 1**, is a constraint optimization of the log-likelihood function under monotone constraints while **Step 2** is an unconstraint optimization of log-likelihood function. In the simulation section, the method that we used in **Step 1** is known as the adaptive barrier algorithm (Lange 1994) which is incorporated in **constrOptim.nl**() function in the R package **alabama** and **Step 2** is performed by Nelder-Mead simplex algorithm incorporated in the R function **optim**().

Estimation of the variance-covariance matrix of the sieve maximum likelihood estimators can be obtained by the observed information matrix evaluated at $(\hat{\beta}, \hat{\gamma})$. Specifically, the variance-covariance matrix of $\hat{\beta}$ can be estimated by

$$\Sigma^{11} = \left(\hat{\Sigma}_{11} - \hat{\Sigma}_{12}\hat{\Sigma}_{22}^{-1}\hat{\Sigma}_{12}^{\mathsf{T}}\right)^{-1}, \tag{6}$$

where

$$\hat{\Sigma}_{11} = -\frac{\partial^2 l_n(\beta, \gamma|\mathbf{V})}{\partial\beta\partial\beta^{\mathsf{T}}}\bigg|_{\beta=\hat{\beta},\gamma=\hat{\gamma}}, \quad \hat{\Sigma}_{12} = -\frac{\partial^2 l_n(\beta, \gamma|\mathbf{V})}{\partial\beta\partial\gamma^{\mathsf{T}}}\bigg|_{\beta=\hat{\beta},\gamma=\hat{\gamma}},$$

$$\hat{\Sigma}_{22} = -\frac{\partial^2 l_n(\beta, \gamma|\mathbf{V})}{\partial\gamma\partial\gamma^{\mathsf{T}}}\bigg|_{\beta=\hat{\beta},\gamma}.$$

However, as we have seen in the simulation study (the results are not reported here), this procedure gives unstable estimates and many times it experiences singular observed information matrix. Instead, we propose instead to use the observed profile information technique suggested by Murphy and Van der Vaart (2000). Let $\hat{\gamma}_\beta$ be the maximizer of log-likelihood $l_n(\beta, \hat{\gamma}_\beta|\mathbf{V})$ for any β in the neighborhood of $\hat{\beta}$. The profile log-likelihood for β is defined as $pl_n(\beta) = l_n(\beta, \hat{\gamma}_\beta|\mathbf{V})$. Let e_s be a vector in $\mathbb{R}^d$ with 1 in the sth position and 0 elsewhere and let h_n is a constant such that $h_n = O(n^{-1/2})$. The (s, t)th element of the information matrix of $\hat{\beta}$ can be approximated by

$$\hat{I}_{\beta_{s,t}} = -\frac{pl_n(\hat{\beta} + h_n e_s + h_n e_t|\mathbf{V}) - pl_n(\hat{\beta} + h_n e_s|\mathbf{V}) - pl_n(\hat{\beta} + h_n e_t|\mathbf{V}) + pl_n(\hat{\beta}|\mathbf{V})}{nh_n^2}.$$

Then we propose to estimate the covariance matrix of $\hat{\beta}$ by the inverse of the matrix whose (s, t)th element is $n\hat{I}_{\beta_{s,t}}, s, t = 1, \ldots, d$.

3 Efficient Estimation

In this section, we investigate the efficient estimation of the regression parameters, β, by computing the efficient score function and the efficient information. Assume $T > L$ a.s. and $C > T$ a.s. Let f_C and f_L denote the marginal densities of L and C, respectively, and let $f_{L,C}$ denote the joint density of (L, C). Without loss of generality, we assume $d = 1$ and consider a single observation $V = (L, C, \Delta, Z)$. Let

$$Q_\theta \equiv Q_{\beta,H}(l, c, z) = Pr(T \geq c | T > l, L = l, C = c, Z = z) = \frac{S_\epsilon(H(c) + \beta^\mathsf{T} z)}{S_\epsilon(H(l) + \beta^\mathsf{T} z)},$$

$$\dot{Q}_\beta = Q_\theta \left(\frac{\dot{S}_\epsilon^\beta(H(c) + \beta^\mathsf{T} z)}{S_\epsilon(H(c) + \beta^\mathsf{T} z)} - \frac{\dot{S}_\epsilon^\beta(H(l) + \beta^\mathsf{T} z)}{S_\epsilon(H(l) + \beta^\mathsf{T} z)} \right),$$

where

$$\dot{S}_\epsilon^\beta(H(t) + \beta^\mathsf{T} z) = \frac{\partial S_\epsilon(H(t) + \beta^\mathsf{T} z)}{z \partial \beta}.$$

The score function of β can be simply computed by differentiating the log-likelihood function with respect to β as

$$\dot{\ell}_\beta = \frac{z \dot{Q}_\beta (\delta - Q_\theta)}{Q_\theta (1 - Q_\theta)}. \tag{7}$$

Now, we construct the score function of H. Suppose that $\mathcal{H}_0 = \{H_s, |s| < 1\}$ is a regular parametric submodel of $\mathbb{H}$. Note that $\mathcal{H}_0$ passes through the true function H_0 at $s = 0$. Let $h(.) = \frac{dH_s(.)}{ds}\big|_{s=0}$. Let

$$\dot{S}_\epsilon^H(H(t) + \beta^\mathsf{T} z) = \frac{\partial S_\epsilon(H_s(t) + \beta^\mathsf{T} z)}{h(t) \partial s}\bigg|_{s=0}$$

and

$$\dot{Q}_t = Q_\theta \frac{\dot{S}_\epsilon^H(H(t) + \beta^\mathsf{T} z)}{S_\epsilon(H(t) + \beta^\mathsf{T} z)}.$$

Then the score operator for H in the direction h is

$$\dot{\ell}_H[h] = \frac{\partial l_n(\beta, H_s)}{\partial s}\bigg|_{s=0} = \frac{(\dot{Q}_c h(c) - \dot{Q}_l h(l))(\delta - Q_\theta)}{Q_\theta(1 - Q_\theta)}. \tag{8}$$

To find the efficient score vector and information bound, we need to find h^* in L_2 so that $\dot{\ell}_\beta - \dot{\ell}_H[h^*] \perp \dot{\ell}_H[h]$ for any function h in L_2 that is,

$$E((\dot{\ell}_\beta - \dot{\ell}_H[h^*])\dot{\ell}_H[h]) = 0, \tag{9}$$

where

$$L_2 = \left\{ a : \int_{\tau_0}^{\tau_1} a^2(t)dt < \infty \right\}.$$

Now, we present the main theorem of this section, the detailed proofs of Theorems 1 are deferred in the Appendix.

Theorem 1

(i) *The efficient score for* β *is* $\bar{\ell}_\beta = \dot{\ell}_\beta - \dot{\ell}_H[h^*(C)]$, *where* $h^*(t)$ *is the unique solution of the second-kind of Fredholm integral equation* $(I + A)[h^*(t)] = o(t)/g(t)$, *where*

$$A[h] = -\int h(s)r(t,s)ds/g(t), \tag{10}$$

$$g(t) = f_C(t)E\left(\frac{\dot{Q}_c^2}{Q_\theta(1-Q_\theta)} \Big| C = t\right) + f_L(t)E\left(\frac{\dot{Q}_l^2}{Q_\theta(1-Q_\theta)} \Big| L = t\right), \tag{11}$$

$$o(t) = f_C(t)E\left(\frac{\dot{Q}_c\dot{Q}_\beta Z}{Q_\theta(1-Q_\theta)} \Big| C = t\right) - f_L(t)E\left(\frac{\dot{Q}_l\dot{Q}_\beta Z}{Q_\theta(1-Q_\theta)} \Big| L = t\right), \tag{12}$$

$$r(t,s) = f_{L,C}(s,t)E\left(\frac{\dot{Q}_c\dot{Q}_l}{Q_\theta(1-Q_\theta)} \Big| C = t, L = s\right) +$$

$$f_{L,C}(t,s)E\left(\frac{\dot{Q}_c\dot{Q}_l}{Q_\theta(1-Q_\theta)} \Big| C = s, L = t\right), \tag{13}$$

   and I *is the identity operator.*
(ii) *The Efficient information for estimation of* β *is* $\bar{I} = E[\bar{\ell}_\beta \bar{\ell}_\beta^\top]$.

Remark 1 As a special case of Theorem 1, for the case of currents status data without truncation, we have $\dot{Q}_l = 0$, $Q_\beta = S_\epsilon(H(c) + \beta^\top z)$, $\dot{Q}_c = Q_\beta \dot{S}_\epsilon^H(H(t) + \beta^\top z)$,

$$g(t) = f_C(t)E\left(\frac{\dot{Q}_c^2}{Q_\beta(1-Q_\beta)} \Big| C = t\right),$$

$$o(t) = f_C(t)E\left(\frac{\dot{Q}_c^2 Z}{Q(1-Q)} \Big| C = t\right)$$

and $r(t,s) = 0$. Hence

$$h^*(t) = \frac{E\left(\frac{\dot{Q}_c^2 Z}{Q_\beta(1-Q_\beta)} \Big| C = t\right)}{E\left(\frac{\dot{Q}_c^2}{Q_\beta(1-Q_\beta)} \Big| C = t\right)},$$

the efficient score function and efficient information are

$$\tilde{\ell}_\beta = \frac{\dot{Q}_c(\Delta - Q_\beta)}{Q_\beta(1 - Q_\beta)}\left(Z - E\left(\frac{\dot{Q}_c^2 Z}{Q_\beta(1 - Q_\beta)}\Big|C\right)\left(E\left(\frac{\dot{Q}_c^2}{Q_\beta(1 - Q_\beta)}\Big|C\right)\right)^{-1}\right),$$

$$I = E\left[\left(\frac{\dot{Q}_c(\Delta - Q_\beta)}{Q_\beta(1 - Q_\beta)}\right)^2\left(Z - E\left(\frac{\dot{Q}_c^2 Z}{Q_\beta(1 - Q_\beta)}\Big|C\right)\left(E\left(\frac{\dot{Q}_c^2}{Q_\beta(1 - Q_\beta)}\Big|C\right)\right)^{-1}\right)^{\otimes 2}\right],$$

respectively, where $a^{\otimes 2} = aa^\mathsf{T}$. By replacing Δ with $1 - \Delta$ and after some simplifications, the above expressions reduce to the expressions (5) and (6) of Zhang et al. (2013).

Remark 2 As a second special case of Theorem 1, for the proportional hazards model with left-truncated and current-status data investigated by Kim (2003), let $S_\epsilon(t) = e^{-\Lambda(t)e^{\beta^\mathsf{T} z}}$, then we have $Q = e^{-(\Lambda(C) - \Lambda(L))e^{\beta^\mathsf{T} z}}$, $\dot{Q}_\beta = -Q(\Lambda(C) - \Lambda(L))e^{\beta^\mathsf{T} z}$ and $\dot{Q}_l = \dot{Q}_c = -Q_\beta e^{\beta^\mathsf{T} z}$. Therefore the expressions (11)–(13) reduce to

$$g(t) = -f_C(t)E\left(\frac{\dot{Q}_c^2}{Q_\beta(1 - Q_\beta)}\Big|C = t\right),$$

$$o(t) = -f_L(t)E\left(\frac{\dot{Q}_c \dot{Q}_\beta Z}{Q_\beta(1 - Q_\beta)}\Big|L = t\right),$$

$$r(t, s) = f_{L,C}(s, t)E\left(\frac{\dot{Q}_c^2}{Q_\beta(1 - Q_\beta)}\Big|C = t, L = s\right).$$

By multiplying both sides of the above expressions by $g(t)$, integrating with respect to t and after some algebraic simplifications, we get

$$h^*(C) - h^*(L) = (\Lambda(C) - \Lambda(L))\frac{E\left(\frac{Q_\beta}{1 - Q_\beta} Z \exp(2\beta^\mathsf{T} Z)\Big|L, C\right)}{E\left(\frac{Q_\beta}{1 - Q_\beta} \exp(2\beta^\mathsf{T} Z)\Big|L, C\right)}.$$

Now, by the above expression, the efficient score function and efficient information can be written as

$$\tilde{\ell}_\beta = \frac{-(\Delta - Q_\beta)(\Lambda(C) - \Lambda(L))\exp(\beta^\mathsf{T} Z)}{1 - Q_\beta}\left(Z - \frac{E\left(\frac{Q_\beta}{1 - Q_\beta} Z \exp(2\beta^\mathsf{T} Z)\Big|L, C\right)}{E\left(\frac{Q_\beta}{1 - Q_\beta} \exp(2\beta^\mathsf{T} Z)\Big|L, C\right)}\right),$$

$$I = E\left[\frac{(\Delta - Q_\beta)^2(\Lambda(C) - \Lambda(L))^2 \exp(2\beta^\mathsf{T} Z)}{(1 - Q_\beta)^2}\left(Z - \frac{E\left(\frac{Q_\beta}{1 - Q_\beta} Z \exp(2\beta^\mathsf{T} Z)\Big|L, C\right)}{E\left(\frac{Q_\beta}{1 - Q_\beta} \exp(2\beta^\mathsf{T} Z)\Big|L, C\right)}\right)^{\otimes 2}\right],$$

respectively. The above expressions are the same as given in Theorem 3.1. of Kim (2003) after replacing Δ with $1 - \Delta$.

4 Asymptotic Properties

In this section, we investigate the asymptotic properties of the sieve maximum likelihood estimator $(\hat{\beta}_n, \hat{H}_n)$. Let $\theta = (\beta, H) \in \Phi$. Similarly, let $\theta_0 = (\beta_0, H_0)$ and $\hat{\theta} = (\hat{\beta}, \hat{H})$ denote the true and the sieve maximum likelihood estimator, respectively. For $\theta_1, \theta_2 \in \Phi$, define the metric

$$d(\theta_1, \theta_2) = \|\beta_1 - \beta_2\| + \|H_1 - H_2\|_2,$$

where

$$\|H_1 - H_2\|_2 = \sqrt{E(H_1(C) - H_2(C))^2 + E(H_1(L) - H_2(L))^2}.$$

Here $\|\cdot\|$ denotes the Euclidean norm. To study the asymptotic properties of the maximum likelihood estimator in the semiparametric model, we need to impose several assumptions and they are included in the Appendix.

Theorem 2 (Consistency) *Suppose the assumptions C1–C7 hold. Then* $d(\hat{\theta}_n, \theta_0)$ $\to_p 0$ *and* $n \to \infty$.

Theorem 3 *(Rate of Convergence) the assumptions (C1), (C4), and (C5) hold. Let* $q = O(n^v)$, *where* $0 < v < 0.5$. *Then*

$$d(\hat{\theta}_n, \theta_0) = O_p(n^{-\min(rv, (1-v)/2)}).$$

By Theorem 3, the MLE of the nonparametric component of the model, H, achieves the optimal rate of convergence, $n^{r/(2r+1)}$, where r is the degree of smoothness of H. Consequently, the rate of convergence will be $n^{1/3}$ for $r = 1$ and $n^{2/5}$ for $r = 2$.

Now, we investigate the asymptotic distribution and efficiency of the sieve maximum likelihood estimators. Let $\delta_n = n^{-1/4}$. For any $\theta \in \Theta$ such that $d(\theta, \theta_0) = O(\delta_n)$, define the first directional derivative at the direction $w \in \mathbb{W}$, and the second directional derivative at the direction $w, \tilde{w} \in \mathbb{W}$, of the log-likelihood function, $l_n(\theta|\mathbf{V})$, as

$$\dot{l}_n(\theta|\mathbf{V})[w] = \frac{dl_n(\theta + sw|\mathbf{V})}{ds}\bigg|_{s=0}$$

and

$$\ddot{l}_n(\theta|\mathbf{V})[w, \tilde{w}] = \frac{d\dot{l}_n(\theta + s\tilde{w}|\mathbf{V})[w]}{ds}\bigg|_{s=0},$$

respectively, where $\mathbb{W}$ represents a vector space $\Theta - \theta_0 = \{\theta - \theta_0 : \theta \in \Theta\}$. For every $w, \tilde{w} \in \mathbb{W}$, define the Fisher inner product $\langle w, \tilde{w} \rangle = P\{\dot{l}_n(\theta_0|\mathbf{V})[w]\dot{l}_n(\theta_0|\mathbf{V})[\tilde{w}]\}$. Define $(\overline{\mathbb{W}}, \|\cdot\|)$ as a Hilbert space, where $\overline{\mathbb{W}}$ is the closed vector space of $\mathbb{W}$ and $\|\cdot\|$ is the Fisher norm defined by $\|w\| = \sqrt{\langle w, w \rangle}$, for $w \in \overline{\mathbb{W}}$.

Similar to Hu and Xiang (2016), define $\mathcal{Q}(\theta) = \alpha^{\mathsf{T}}\beta + \int_{\tau_0}^{\tau_1} \lambda(x)H(x)dx$ as a smooth functional of θ, where $\alpha \in \mathbb{R}^d$, $\|\alpha\| \leq 1$ and $\lambda \in \mathbb{H}$. Then, directional derivative of $\mathcal{Q}$ along the path $w = (w_\beta, w_H)$, where $w_\beta \in \mathbb{R}^d$ and $w_H \in \mathbb{H}$, can be computed as

$$\dot{\mathcal{Q}}(\theta)[w] = \frac{d\mathcal{Q}(\theta + sw)}{ds}\bigg|_{s=0} = \frac{d(\alpha^{\mathsf{T}}(\beta + sw_\beta) + \int_{\tau_0}^{\tau_1} \lambda(x)(H(x) + sw_H(x))dx)}{ds}\bigg|_{s=0}$$

$$= \alpha^{\mathsf{T}}w_\beta + \int_{\tau_0}^{\tau_1} \lambda(x)w_H(x)dx.$$

It can be seen that

$$\mathcal{Q}(\theta) - \mathcal{Q}(\theta_0) = \dot{\mathcal{Q}}(\theta_0)[\theta - \theta_0]. \tag{14}$$

By Riesz representation theorem and Assumption **C8**, there exists $w^* \in \overline{\mathbb{W}}$ such that

$$\dot{\mathcal{Q}}(\theta_0)[w] = \langle w^*, w \rangle \, for \, all \, w \in \overline{\mathbb{W}} \tag{15}$$

and $\|w^*\| = \|\dot{\mathcal{Q}}(\theta_0)\|$.

Theorem 4 *(Asymptotic Normality) Suppose the conditions (C1)–(C6),(C8) hold. For $0.25/r < v < 0.5$, we have*

$$\sqrt{n}(\mathcal{Q}(\hat{\theta}) - \mathcal{Q}(\theta_0)) \rightarrow_d N(0, \|\dot{\mathcal{Q}}(\theta_0)\|^2)$$

and $\mathcal{Q}(\hat{\theta})$ is semiparametrically efficient, where $\rightarrow_d$ denotes the convergence in distribution. Furthermore, the asymptotic variance $\|\dot{\mathcal{Q}}(\theta_0)\|^2$ can be consistently estimated by

$$(\alpha^{\mathsf{T}}, \Gamma^{\mathsf{T}})\Sigma^{-1}(\alpha^{\mathsf{T}}, \Gamma^{\mathsf{T}})^{\mathsf{T}},$$

where $\Gamma^{\mathsf{T}} = (\int_{\tau_0}^{\tau_1} \lambda(x)A_0(x)dx, \cdots, \int_{\tau_0}^{\tau_1} \lambda(x)A_q(x)dx)$, A_i is given in (4) and Σ is the observed information matrix of β and γ.

The detailed proofs of Theorems 2–4 are deferred in the Appendix.

Remark 3 Consider $\lambda \equiv 0$. Then $\mathcal{Q}(\theta) = \alpha^{\mathsf{T}}\beta$ and $\dot{\mathcal{Q}}(\theta_0)[w] = \alpha^{\mathsf{T}}w_\beta$. Then

$$\|\dot{\mathcal{Q}}(\theta_0)\|^2 = \sup_{w \in \overline{W}: \|w\| > 0} \frac{|\dot{\mathcal{Q}}(\theta_0)[w]|^2}{\|w\|^2}$$

$$= \sup_{w \in \overline{W}: \|w\| > 0} \frac{(\alpha^\mathsf{T} w_\beta)^2}{\|w\|^2}$$

$$= \sup_{w \in \overline{W}: \|w\| > 0} \frac{(\alpha^\mathsf{T} w_\beta)^2}{P(\dot{l}_n(\theta_0; W)[w])^2}$$

$$= \sup_{w \in \overline{W}: \|w\| > 0} \frac{(\alpha^\mathsf{T} w_\beta)^2}{P(\ell_\beta w_\beta + \ell_H[w_H])^2},$$

where ℓ_β and ℓ_H are the score functions of β and H given in (7) and (8). Let $w_H^* = -h^* w_\beta$, where h^* is the least-favorable direction given in Theorem 1. Then

$$\|\dot{\mathcal{Q}}(\theta_0)\|^2 = \frac{w_\beta^\mathsf{T} \alpha \alpha^\mathsf{T} w_\beta}{w_\beta^\mathsf{T} P(\ell_\beta - \ell_H[h^*])^2 w_\beta} = \alpha I^{-1} \alpha^\mathsf{T},$$

where I is the efficient information of β. This leads to

$$\sqrt{n}(\hat{\beta} - \beta_0) \to_d N(0, I^{-1}),$$

where I^{-1} can be consistently estimated by $\hat{\Sigma}^{11}$, where $\hat{\Sigma}^{11}$ is given in (6).

Remark 4 Consider $\alpha = 0$. Then $\mathcal{Q}(\theta) = \int_{\tau_0}^{\tau_1} \lambda(x) H(x) dx$ and $\dot{\mathcal{Q}}(\theta_0)[w] = \int_{\tau_0}^{\tau_1} \lambda(x) w_H(x) dx$. Then

$$\sqrt{n} \int_{\tau_0}^{\tau_1} \lambda(x)(\hat{H}_n(x) - H_0(x)) dx \to_d N(0, \|\dot{\mathcal{Q}}(\theta_0)\|^2).$$

The asymptotic variance can be consistently estimated by $\Gamma^\mathsf{T} \hat{\Sigma}^{22} \Gamma$, where $\hat{\Sigma}^{22} = (\hat{\Sigma}_{22} - \hat{\Sigma}_{21} \hat{\Sigma}_{11}^{-1} \hat{\Sigma}_{12})^{-1}$, where $\hat{\Sigma}_{22}$, $\hat{\Sigma}_{21}$, and $\hat{\Sigma}_{11}$ are defined in Sect. 1. We may use the above result in nonparametric test hypotheses as follows. Assume, for example, we are interested in testing the hypotheses $H_0(x) = \zeta_0 + \zeta_1 x$. Then we can adopt the test statistic

$$T_n = \frac{n \left(\int_{\tau_0}^{\tau_1} \lambda(x)(\hat{H}(x) - \zeta_0 - \zeta_1 x) dx \right)^2}{(\Gamma^\mathsf{T} \hat{\Sigma}^{22} \Gamma)^2} \sim \chi_1^2.$$

5 Simulation Study

In this section, we investigate the finite-sample performances of the proposed estimators using a Monte-Carlo simulation study. The linear transformation model is assumed to be

$$H(T) = -\beta_1 Z_1 - \beta_2 Z_2 + \epsilon, \tag{16}$$

where $H(\cdot)$ is the unknown transformation function. The performance of the proposed estimators is investigated across three different configurations of regression parameters β and the transformation function $H(\cdot)$. In specific, in configuration I, $\beta = (0.5, -0.5)^\mathsf{T}$ and $H(t) = \log(t/4)$, in configuration II, $\beta = (0.9, 0.5)$ and $H(t) = \log((t^2 + t)/5)$ and configuration III, $\beta = (-1, 1)$ and $H(t) = \log(\log(1 + t/2))$. The monitoring time C is uniformly distributed in $[0.5, 2]$ and the truncation variable L is uniformly distributed in $[0.01, 0.5]$. Under this setting, the left-truncation rate is of 0.19%. Moreover, the covariates Z_1 and Z_3 are assumed to fellow standard normal and Bernoulli with probability 0.5 distributions, respectively. The baseline survival function of the error, ϵ, is assumed to have the form $S(t) = (1 + r \exp(t))^{-1/r}$, where $0 \le r \le 1$ is a distribution parameter. Hence model (16) can be written as

$$S(T|Z) = [1 + r \exp\{H(T) + \beta_1 Z_1 + \beta_2 Z_2\}]^{-1/r}. \tag{17}$$

To approximate the function H, we use Bernstein polynomial with degree q. Following Huang and Rossini (1997) and Wang et al. (2016), in the simulation study, the value of q is set at $[n^{1/3}]$, which is the lower of the asymptotic convergence rates, where $[x]$ denotes the least integer greater than or equal to x. However, in practice, one can use a data-driven method such as BIC to select q and r, as we did in the data analysis. Table 1 reports the simulation results with sample sizes $n = 200, 500$ and $r = 0, 0.5, 1$, respectively, based on 1000 replications. For estimating the variances of $\hat{\beta}_1$ and $\hat{\beta}_2$ by the observed profile information method, we used the tuning constant $h_n = 0.56n^{-1/2}$. However, other values of h_n are also considered and the obtained results are similar to those given in Table 1. To assess the performance of the estimators of the nonparametric part, H, we calculate the Integrated Mean Square Error (IMSE) of each of these estimators. The IMSE is defined by

$$IMSE(H_n, H) = E \int (H_n(x) - H(x))^2 dx,$$

where $H_n(x)$ is the Bernstein estimator of $H(x)$. We approximate IMSE by

$$\widehat{IMSE} = \frac{1}{M} \sum_{i=1}^{M} \int (H_{n,i}(x) - H(x))^2 dx,$$

Table 1 Simulation results for estimation of (β_1, β_2) using the Bernstein MLE

Configuration	r	n		Bias	SSE	ESE	RMSE	CP
I	0	200	β_1	0.002	0.174	0.163	0.174	93.5
			β_2	−0.030	0.291	0.267	0.293	94.4
		500	β_1	0.001	0.107	0.103	0.107	95.1
			β_2	−0.007	0.185	0.168	0.185	95.3
	0.5	200	β_1	0.011	0.213	0.200	0.213	93.9
			β_2	−0.037	0.344	0.300	0.346	93.3
		500	β_1	0.007	0.126	0.124	0.126	95.4
			β_2	−0.010	0.208	0.187	0.209	94.5
	1	200	β_1	0.019	0.240	0.233	0.241	94.8
			β_2	−0.040	0.365	0.330	0.368	94.8
		500	β_1	0.012	0.144	0.143	0.144	95.2
			β_2	−0.010	0.223	0.205	0.223	95.2
II	0	200	β_1	0.028	0.150	0.151	0.152	94.0
			β_2	−0.005	0.191	0.165	0.191	94.1
		500	β_1	0.012	0.093	0.094	0.093	95.1
			β_2	0.007	0.112	0.103	0.113	95.1
	0.5	200	β_1	0.025	0.196	0.188	0.198	93.3
			β_2	−0.003	0.238	0.216	0.238	93.2
		500	β_1	0.012	0.113	0.117	0.114	95.3
			β_2	0.007	0.144	0.135	0.144	94.8
	1	200	β_1	0.031	0.253	0.227	0.255	93.8
			β_2	−0.003	0.299	0.267	0.298	93.8
		500	β_1	0.008	0.148	0.142	0.148	95.3
			β_2	0.006	0.184	0.178	0.184	95.1
III	0	200	β_1	−0.034	0.172	0.157	0.175	93.7
			β_2	−0.021	0.190	0.167	0.191	94.3
		500	β_1	−0.012	0.102	0.098	0.103	95.1
			β_2	−0.004	0.114	0.105	0.114	94.5
	0.5	200	β_1	−0.042	0.223	0.210	0.227	94.7
			β_2	−0.024	0.269	0.244	0.270	95.2
		500	β_1	−0.019	0.142	0.132	0.143	95.6
			β_2	−0.004	0.168	0.152	0.168	94.2
	1	200	β_1	−0.058	0.303	0.287	0.308	94.2
			β_2	−0.028	0.363	0.347	0.363	93.5
		500	β_1	−0.018	0.180	0.174	0.180	95.2
			β_2	−0.009	0.213	0.210	0.213	95.7

where M is the total number of simulation runs. The results of IMSE are presented in Table 2.

From Table 1, it can be seen that the biases (Bias) for the estimated values of $\beta = (\beta_1, \beta_2)^\top$ are reasonably small. The sampled standard errors (SSE) of the

Table 2 Integrated Mean Square Error (IMSE) of $\hat{H}$.

	Configuration I		Configuration II		Configuration III	
n	200	500	200	500	200	500
$r = 0$	0.379	0.170	0.702	0.281	0.321	0.137
$r = 0.5$	0.395	0.170	0.689	0.297	0.367	0.157
$r = 1$	0.426	0.164	0.678	0.285	0.354	0.148

estimator are close to the average estimated standard errors (ESE) and the root mean squared error (RMSE) of the estimator that are computed using the observed profile information matrix. The empirical coverage probabilities of 95% confidence intervals (CP), are very close to the nominal level especially when the sample size n is large (e.g., $n \geq 500$). Moreover, Table 2 shows that the values of IMSE of the Bernstein estimator for the unknown function, H. Clearly the IMSE values are reasonably small and these values significantly decrease as n increases. Figures 1, 2, 3, 4, 5, and 6 demonstrate the histograms for the estimated values of β_1, β_2 and the curve estimation of the function H in the three configurations: I, II, and III. The histograms show approximately normal distribution of the estimates of β_1 and β_2 and the figures show that the median estimated curves are close to the true curve. Moreover, Figs. 7, 8, and 9 show the effect of the degree of Bernstein binomial, q, on the estimation of the nonparametric part H in the three configurations. It is clear, from these figures, that for all the cases the estimated median curves of H are close to the true curves when the degree q of the Bernstein polynomials is close to $[n^{1/3}]$, the estimated curves become biased when q becomes smaller. From the above results, we conclude that the proposed estimation method performs very well.

6 Real Data Analysis

For further illustration, we apply the proposed method to an AIDS cohort study of hemophiliacs dataset proposed by De Gruttola and Lagakos (1989). The dataset was analyzed by many authors, for example, Sun (1995, 1997); Fang and Sun (2001); Kim (2003) and Wang et al. (2015), among others. The dataset consists of 257 patients with Type A or Type B hemophilia who had been treated at Hˆopital Kremlin Bicetre and Hôpital Coeur des Yvelines in France since 1978. These hemophiliacs were at risk for HIV-1 infection through the contaminated blood factor they received for their treatment. By the time of analysis, 188 were found to be infected with the virus, 41 of whom subsequently progressed to AIDS-related symptoms. The primary goal of this example is to apply the procedures described in the previous sections to assess the effects of level of treatment received for hemophilia on the risk of developing AIDS-related symptoms. The subjects are classified into two groups, lightly and heavily treated groups, according to the amount of blood they received. Patients in the heavily treated group (105) received

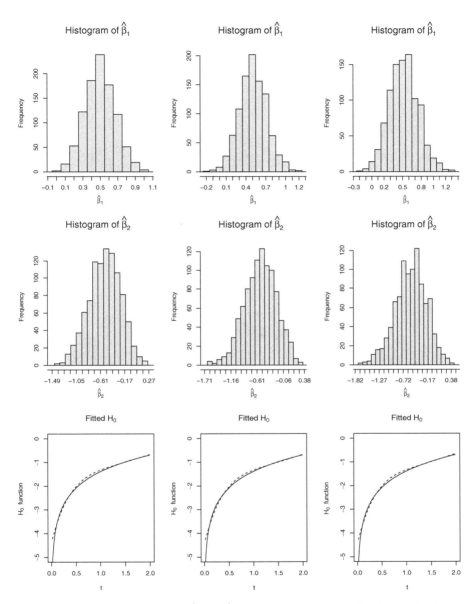

Fig. 1 Histograms of the estimators $\hat{\beta}_1$ and $\hat{\beta}_2$ and the estimated curves for the function H for $r = 0, 0.5, 1$, respectively, in the configuration I. Solid lines in the estimated curve of H: the true curves and dashed lines in the estimated curve of H: the median estimated curves. The results are based on Monte Carlo simulation with sample size $n = 200$ and 1000 simulation runs

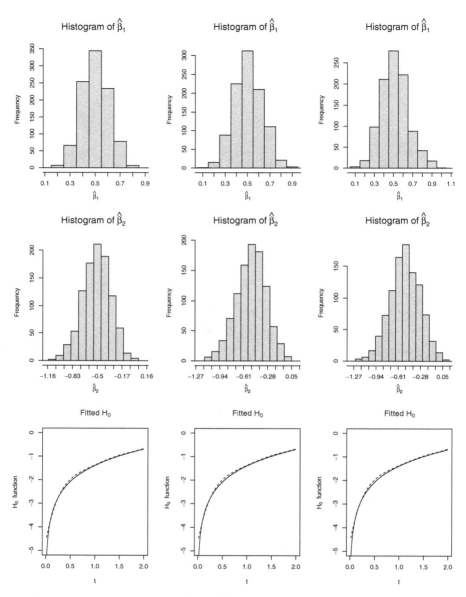

Fig. 2 Histograms of the estimators $\hat{\beta}_1$ and $\hat{\beta}_2$ and the estimated curves for the function H for $r = 0, 0.5, 1$, respectively, in the configuration I. Solid lines in the estimated curve of H: the true curves and dashed lines in the estimated curve of H: the median estimated curves. The results are based on Monte Carlo simulation with sample size $n = 500$ and 1000 simulation runs

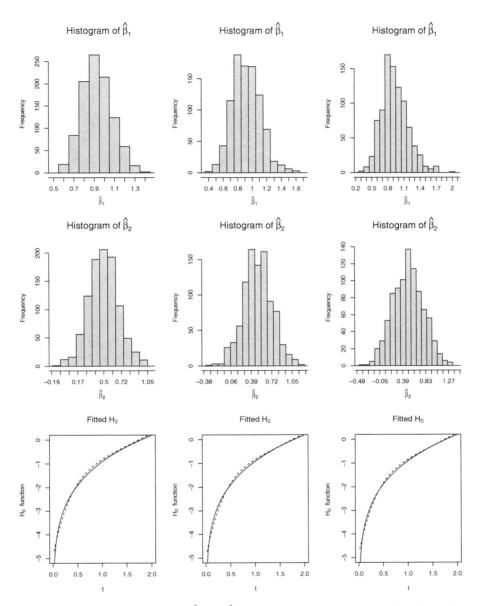

Fig. 3 Histograms of the estimators $\hat{\beta}_1$ and $\hat{\beta}_2$ and the estimated curves for the function H for $r = 0, 0.5, 1$, respectively, in the configuration II. Solid lines in the estimated curve of H: the true curves and dashed lines in the estimated curve of H: the median estimated curves. The results are based on Monte Carlo simulation with sample size $n = 200$ and 1000 simulation runs

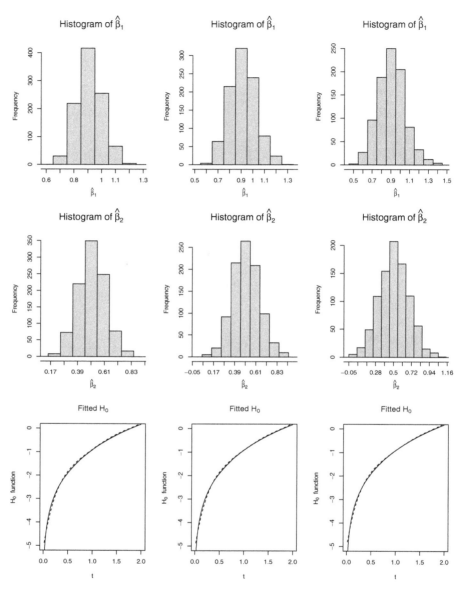

Fig. 4 Histograms of the estimators $\hat{\beta}_1$ and $\hat{\beta}_2$ and the estimated curves for the function H for $r = 0, 0.5, 1$, respectively, in the configuration II. Solid lines in the estimated curve of H: the true curves and dashed lines in the estimated curve of H: the median estimated curves. The results are based on Monte Carlo simulation with sample size $n = 500$ and 1000 simulation runs

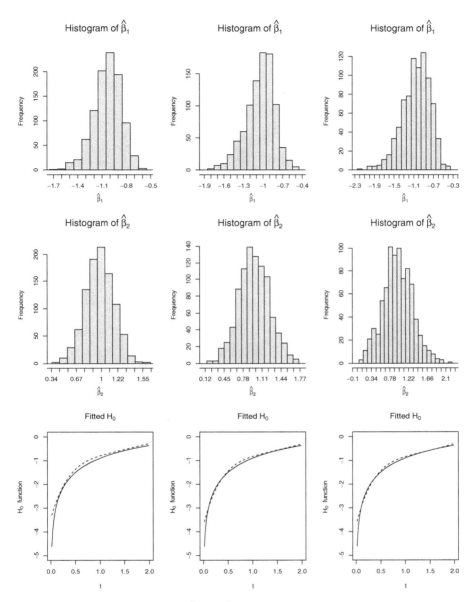

Fig. 5 Histograms of the estimators $\hat{\beta}_1$ and $\hat{\beta}_2$ and the estimated curves for the function H for $r = 0, 0.5, 1$, respectively, in the configuration III. Solid lines in the estimated curve of H: the true curves and dashed lines in the estimated curve of H: the median estimated curves. The results are based on Monte Carlo simulation with sample size $n = 200$ and 1000 simulation runs

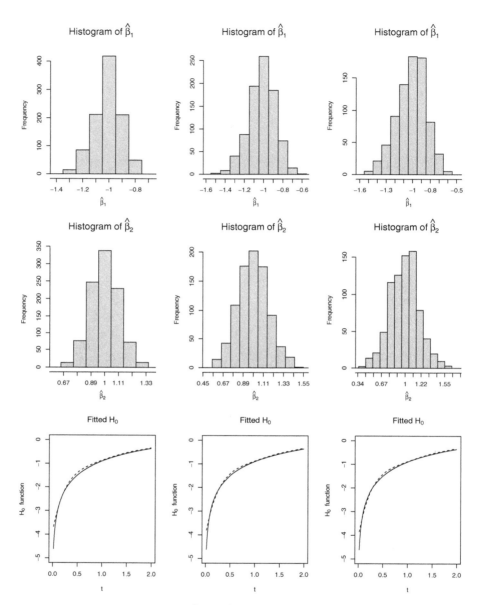

Fig. 6 Histograms of the estimators $\hat{\beta}_1$ and $\hat{\beta}_2$ and the estimated curves for the function H for $r = 0, 0.5, 1$, respectively, in the configuration III. Solid lines in the estimated curve of H: the true curves and dashed lines in the estimated curve of H: the median estimated curves. The results are based on Monte Carlo simulation with sample size $n = 500$ and 1000 simulation runs

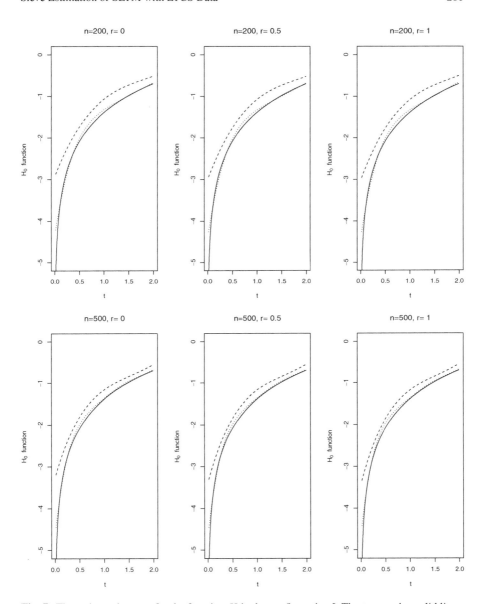

Fig. 7 The estimated curves for the function H in the configuration I. The top graphs; solid lines: the true curves, dashed lines: the median estimated curves for $q = 3$ and the dotted lines: the median estimated curves for $q = 6$. The bottom graphs; solid lines: the true curves, dashed lines: the median estimated curves for $q = 4$ and the dotted lines: the median estimated curves for $q = 8$

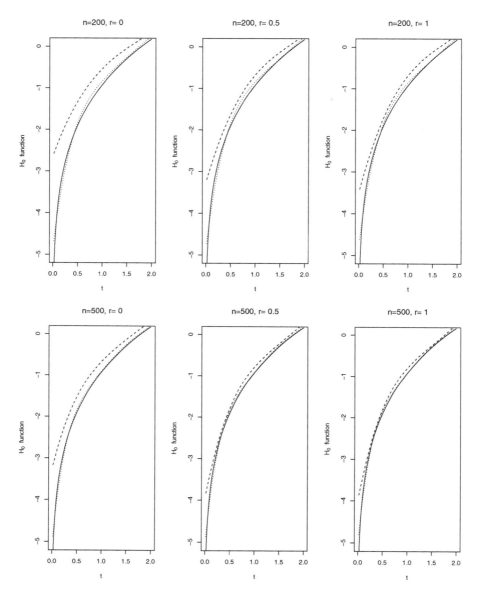

Fig. 8 The estimated curves for the function H in the configuration II. The top graphs; solid lines: the true curves, dashed lines: the median estimated curves for $q = 3$ and the dotted lines: the median estimated curves for $q = 6$. The bottom graphs; solid lines: the true curves, dashed lines: the median estimated curves for $q = 4$ and the dotted lines: the median estimated curves for $q = 8$

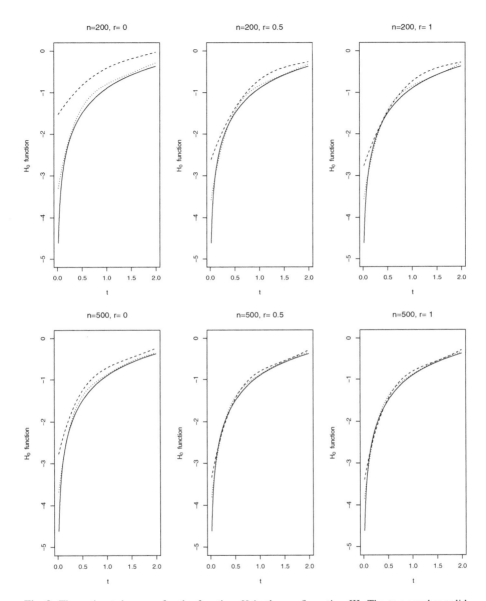

Fig. 9 The estimated curves for the function H in the configuration III. The top graphs; solid lines: the true curves, dashed lines: the median estimated curves for $q = 3$ and the dotted lines: the median estimated curves for $q = 6$. The bottom graphs; solid lines: the true curves, dashed lines: the median estimated curves for $q = 4$ and the dotted lines: the median estimated curves for $q = 8$

at least 1000, µg/kg of the blood factor while Patients in the lightly treated group (157) received less than 1000 µug/kg for at least 1 year between 1982 and 1985. By the time the study was terminated, it had been confirmed that 97 of these patients were infected with HIV-1, which is believed to have been due to the contaminated blood factor they received for their hemophilia. In the original data set, there are HIV-1 infection time intervals and AIDS-related-symptom diagnosis time intervals. The time unit is 6-months. Following Kim (2003) and Wang et al. (2015), we modify this data set into left-truncated and current status data by replacing HIV infection time interval and AIDS-related-symptom diagnosis time interval by the midpoint and the right end point of the interval, respectively. Define Z as binary covariate coded as $Z = 0$ for lightly treated group and $Z = 1$ for heavily treated group. In our analysis, we focus on the 188 patients (left-truncated data) who were found to be infected by HIV-1 at the time of analysis. among theme, 41 were found to have AIDS (left-censored) and the remaining 147 patients were found not developing AIDS (right-censored). It can be seen that the left-truncation rate is $69/257 = 0.27$. We apply the proposed transformation model given as follows to fit the data:

$$S(t|Z) = (1 + r \exp(H(t) + \beta Z))^{-1/r}. \tag{18}$$

In Table 3, we report the results of our analysis of HIV data set for different combinations of r and q and the values of BIC computed from the following defined Bayesian information criterion (BIC):

$$BIC = -2l_n(\hat{\beta}, r) + \log(n)(d + q + 1), \tag{19}$$

where $\hat{\beta} = (\hat{\beta}_1, \hat{\beta}_2)^\top$ denotes the MLE of $\beta = (\beta_1, \beta_2)^\top$, and to emphasize the dependence on β and r, the log-likelihood l_n has been expressed as $l_n(\hat{\beta}, r)$. The BIC selects $r = 0.1$ and $q = 3$ as an optimal model, this is a new result different from the proportional hazards model ($r = 0$) and the proportional odds model ($r = 1$). For the proportional hazards model with left-truncated and currents status data, (Kim 2003) computed the MLE of β as $\hat{\beta} = 0.765$ with the estimated standard error of 0.367 and p-value of 0.038 for testing $\beta = 0$. Kim et al. (1993) estimated β by 0.69 with the standard error of 0.34, using a discrete analogue of the proportional hazards model. Our sieve method yielded an estimate $\hat{\beta} = 0.737$ with the estimated

Table 3 Analysis of HIV dataset of De Gruttola and Lagakos (1989)

r	q	MLE	ESE	BIC	p-value
0	5	0.721	0.326	239.9	0.027
0.1	5	0.732	0.339	239.1	0.031
1	5	0.944	0.497	239.7	0.057
0	3	0.723	0.326	229.6	0.026
0.1	3	0.737	0.343	229.5	0.031
1	3	0.918	0.486	230.0	0.059

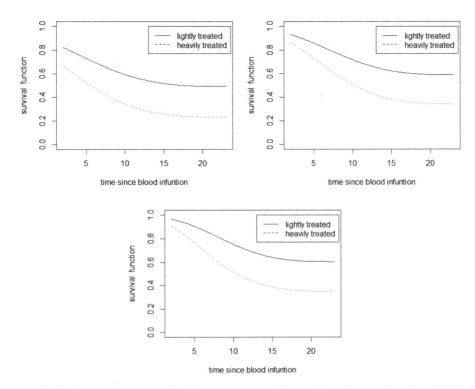

Fig. 10 Estimated survival function for the total AIDS diagnosis time for $q = 3$ and $r = 0, 0.1$ and 1, respectively

standard error of 0.343 and p-value of 0.031. Figure 10 shows the estimated survival functions for the two treatment groups with $q = 3$ and $r = 0, 0.1, 1$, respectively, where $r = 0.1$ and $q = 3$ correspond the proposed model. Similar to Kim et al. (1993) under the proportional hazards model and Wang et al. (2015) under the additive hazards model, the results show that the patients in the heavily treatment group had significantly greater risk of developing AIDS or being diagnosed to have AIDS than in the lightly treatment group.

7   Concluding Remarks and Future Work

In this paper, we develop an efficient estimation procedure to analyze left-truncated and current status data under a semiparametric linear transformation model. The importance of this model focuses on its form which includes two commonly used models: the linear proportional hazards and proportional odds models as special cases. In the theoretical part, by approximating the non-parametric parts using

Bernstein polynomial with suitable choice of Bernstein parameter q, we have shown that the estimators for the finite-dimensional parameters are consistent and asymptotically normal, and the estimators for the infinite-dimensional parameters achieve the optimal rate of convergence. A consistent estimation of the variance-covariance matrix is constructed using the observed information matrix to provide a reliable inference procedure for the regression parameters. By implementing Monte Carlo simulation experiments, we have shown that the proposed method performs well and the results assure the theory. A real dataset concerning HIV of De Gruttola and Lagakos (1989) is reanalyzed and the new results reveal a different model from the existing models. Our approach is a conditional approach, meaning that the analysis is conditional on truncation times. In consequence, these approaches may not be fully efficient. To improve the efficiency, in our future research, we can apply a pairwise pseudo-likelihood approach as Wang et al. (2020) did for the left-truncated and interval-censored data under the Cox model. For further studies, there exist several directions to extend the results of this paper. One is that, we may consider case II interval-censored data by imposing multiple observation times for each subject instead of one as in the case of currents status data.

Appendix

This Appendix devotes to sketch the proofs of Theorems 1–4. To study the asymptotic properties of the maximum likelihood estimator in the semiparametric model, we assume the following assumptions.

C1 The space of β, $\mathbb{B}$, is a compact subset of $\mathbb{R}^d$ and the true value β_0 is an interior point of $\mathbb{B}$.

C2 (i) The union of the supports of L and C is bounded by an interval $[\tau_0, \tau_1]$ where $0 < \tau_0 < \tau_1 < \infty$. (ii) There exist two finite values B^- and B^+ such that $B^- < H(t) < B^+$ for every $t \in [\tau_0, \tau_1]$.

C3 There exists a positive number η such that $C - L > \eta$ with probability one.

C4 The variable Z is bounded, that is, there exists k such that $||Z|| \le k$ with probability 1.

C5 The first derivative of H_0 is strictly positive and continuous on $[\tau_0, \tau_1]$ and its r-th ($r \ge 1$) derivative is bounded in $[\tau_0, \tau_1]$.

C6 The joint distribution function L and C has bounded second-order partial derivatives.

C7 (i) There exists $\varpi_1 \in (0, 1)$ such that

$$a^\mathsf{T} \mathrm{Var}(Z|L, C)a \ge \varpi a^\mathsf{T} E(ZZ^\mathsf{T}|L, C)a \ a.s. \ for \ all \ a \in \mathbb{R}^d.$$

(ii) There exists $\varpi_2 \in (0, 1)$ and $\mathrm{Var}(H(C) - H_0(C)|L) \ge \varpi_2 E((H(C) - H_0(C))^2|L)$.

C8 For any $w \in \overline{\mathbb{W}}$, $\mathcal{Q}(\theta_0 + tw)$ is continuously differentiable in $t \in [0, 1]$ near $t = 0$, and

$$\|\dot{\mathcal{Q}}(\theta_0)\| = \sup_{w \in \overline{\mathbb{W}}: \|w\| > 0} \frac{|\dot{\mathcal{Q}}(\theta_0)[w]|}{\|w\|} < \infty.$$

The above conditions are mild conditions and are commonly used in the literature of semiparametric models under interval censored data, see, for example, Huang and Rossini (1997), Huang and Wellner (1997) and Zhang et al. (2010). Assumptions **C1–C6** ensure that the survival function S_ϵ and its partial derivatives are bounded from 0 and finite which is necessary in proving the asymptotic properties of the MLE's. Assumption **C7** will be used in proving the consistency.

Remark 5 The assumption **C7** implies that $E(ZZ^\mathsf{T}|L, C)$ is a positive definite matrix and $E((H(C) - H_0(C))^2|L)$ is positive. By Wellner et al. (2007), the possible choice of ϖ_1 is $\varpi_1 = \lambda_d/\lambda_1$ where λ_d is the minimum eigen value of $\mathrm{Var}(Z|L, C)$ and λ_1 is the maximum eigen value of $E(ZZ^\mathsf{T}|L, C)$. Similarly, the choice of ϖ_2 is as follows. Let $k_1 < \mathrm{Var}(H(C) - H_0(C)|L)$ and $E((H(C) - H_0(C))^2|L) < k_2$. Clearly $0 < k_1 < k_2$. Then

$$\mathrm{Var}(H(C) - H_0(C)|L) > k_1 = \frac{k_1}{k_2}k_2 > \frac{k_1}{k_2}E((H(C) - H_0(C))^2|L).$$

Hence the possible choice of ϖ_2 is $\varpi_2 = k_1/k_2$.

Throughout this section we adopt the following notations. From Assumption **C1**, define $\mathbb{B} = \{\beta \in \mathbb{R}^d : \|\beta\| \leq K_\beta\}$, for some constant K_β. Define the class $\mathcal{L}_1 = \{l_n(\theta|\mathbf{V}); \theta \in \Theta_n\}$. Define P as the probability measure and P_n as the empirical measure of $V_i = 1, \cdots, n$. Define the expectations of a function f with respect to P and P_n by $Pf = \int f \, dP$ and $P_n f = \int f \, dP_n$, respectively. Let $\mathbb{M}(\theta) = Pl_n(\theta|\mathbf{V})$ and $\mathbb{M}_n(\theta) = P_n l_n(\theta|\mathbf{V})$. Define the space $L_1(P_n)$ as $\{g : P_n|g| < \infty\}$. Also let $\|g\|_F = \sup_{f \in F} |g(f)|$ and $\|g\|_\infty = \sup_x |g(x)|$. For $\varepsilon > 0$, define the ε-covering number $N(\varepsilon, \mathcal{L}_1, L_1(P_n))$ as the smallest value of k for which there exists $\{\theta^{(1)}, \cdots, \theta^{(k)}\}$ such that

$$\min_{j \in \{1,2,\cdots,k\}} P_n|l_n(\theta|\mathbf{V}) - l_n(\theta^{(j)}|\mathbf{V})| < \varepsilon, \ \ for \ all \theta \in \Theta_n.$$

Similarly, we can define the ε-covering number $N(\varepsilon, \mathcal{L}_1, \|\|)$. An ε-bracket, $[f_1, f_2]$, is the set of all functions f such that $f_1 \leq f \leq f_2$ and $\|f_1 - f_2\|_2 := \sqrt{P((f_1 - f_2)^2)} \leq \varepsilon$. The ε-bracketing number $N(\varepsilon, \mathcal{L}_1, L_2(P))$ as the minimum number of ε-brackets needed to cover $\mathcal{L}_1$. Throughout this section, we use $Q_\theta \equiv Q_{\beta,H}$ to refer to $S_\epsilon(H(c) + \beta^\mathsf{T}Z)/S_\epsilon(H(l) + \beta^\mathsf{T}Z)$ for $\theta \in \Theta_n$. Assume $K, K_1,$ and K_2 are universal constants.

Proof of Theorem 1 (*Efficient Score and Efficient Information*) We have

$$E(g(L, C, T, Z)) = E(g(L, C, T, Z)|T > L)P(T > L)$$
$$+ E(g(L, C, T, Z)|T < L)P(T < L)$$
$$= E(g(L, C, T, Z)|T > L),$$

since $P(L > L) = 1$. First, note that

$$E((\Delta - Q_\beta)^2|T > L, L = l, C = c, Z = z)$$
$$= E(\Delta^2|T > l, L = l, C = c, Z = z) - 2Q_\beta E(\Delta|T > l, L = l, C = c, Z = z) + Q_\beta^2$$
$$= E(\Delta|T > l, L = l, C = c, Z = z) - 2Q_\beta E(\Delta|T > l, L = l, C = c, Z = z) + Q_\beta^2$$
$$= P(T \geq c|T > l, L = l, C = c, Z = z)$$
$$- 2Q_\beta Pr(T \geq c|T > l, L = l, C = c, Z = z) + Q_\beta^2$$
$$= Q_\beta(1 - Q_\beta).$$

Then

$$E(\ell_\beta \ell_H[h]) = E\left(\frac{Z\dot{Q}_\beta(h(C)\dot{Q}_c - h(L)\dot{Q}_l)}{Q_\beta^2(1 - Q_\beta)^2}(\Delta - Q_\beta)^2\right)$$
$$= E\left(\frac{Z\dot{Q}_\beta(h(C)\dot{Q}_c - h(L)\dot{Q}_l)}{Q_\beta^2(1 - Q_\beta)^2}E((\Delta - Q_\beta)^2|T > l, L = l, C = c, Z = z)\right)$$
$$= E\left(\frac{Z\dot{Q}_\beta(h(C)\dot{Q}_c - h(L)\dot{Q}_l)}{Q_\beta(1 - Q_\beta)}\right), \tag{20}$$

and

$$E(\ell_H[h^*]\ell_H[h]) = E\left(\frac{(\dot{Q}_c h^*(C) - \dot{Q}_l h^*(L))(\dot{Q}_c h(C) - \dot{Q}_l h(L))}{Q_\beta^2(1 - Q_\beta)^2}(\Delta - Q_\beta)^2\right)$$
$$= E\left(\frac{(\dot{Q}_c h^*(C) - \dot{Q}_l h^*(L))(\dot{Q}_c h(C) - \dot{Q}_l h(L))}{Q_\beta(1 - Q_\beta)}\right)$$
$$= E\left(\frac{h(C)(\dot{Q}_c^2 h^*(C) - \dot{Q}_c \dot{Q}_l h^*(L))}{Q_\beta(1 - Q_\beta)}\right)$$
$$- E\left(\frac{h(L)(\dot{Q}_c \dot{Q}_l h^*(C) - \dot{Q}_l^2 h^*(L))}{Q_\beta(1 - Q_\beta)}\right). \tag{21}$$

Now, substituting (20) and (21) in (9) gives us

$$E\left(h(C)\frac{\dot{Q}_c \dot{Q}_\beta Z - \dot{Q}_c^2 h^*(C) + \dot{Q}_c \dot{Q}_l h^*(L)}{Q_\beta(1 - Q_\beta)} - h(L)\frac{\dot{Q}_l \dot{Q}_\beta Z - \dot{Q}_c \dot{Q}_l h^*(C) + \dot{Q}_l^2 h^*(L)}{Q_\beta(1 - Q_\beta)}\right) = 0$$

$$\Leftrightarrow E\Big(h(C)E\Big(\frac{\dot{Q}_c\dot{Q}_\beta Z - \dot{Q}_c^2 h^*(C) + \dot{Q}_c\dot{Q}_l h^*(L)}{Q_\beta(1-Q_\beta)}\Big|L,C\Big)$$

$$-h(L)E\Big(\frac{\dot{Q}_l\dot{Q}_\beta Z - \dot{Q}_c\dot{Q}_l h^*(C) + \dot{Q}_l^2 h^*(L)}{Q_\beta(1-Q_\beta)}\Big|L,C\Big)\Big) = 0$$

$$\Leftrightarrow E\Big(h(C)A_1(L,C) - h(L)A_2(L,C)\Big) = 0$$

$$\Leftrightarrow E\Big(h(C)A_1(L,C)\Big) - E\Big(h(L)A_2(L,C)\Big) = 0$$

$$\Leftrightarrow E(E(h(C)A_1(L,C)|C=t)) - E(E(h(L)A_2(L,C)|L=t)) = 0$$

$$\Leftrightarrow E(h(t)E(A_1(L,C)|C=t)) - E(h(t)E(A_2(L,C)|L=t)) = 0$$

$$\Leftrightarrow \int h(t)E(A_1(L,C)|C=t)f_C(t)dt - \int h(t)E(A_2(L,C)|L=t)f_L(t)dt = 0$$

$$\Leftrightarrow \int h(t)(E(A_1(L,C)|C=t)f_C(t) - E(A_2(L,C)|L=t)f_L(t))dt = 0,$$

where

$$A_1(L,C) = E\Big(\frac{\dot{Q}_c\dot{Q}_\beta Z}{Q_\beta(1-Q_\beta)}\Big|L,C\Big) - h^*(C)E\Big(\frac{\dot{Q}_c^2}{Q_\beta(1-Q_\beta)}\Big|L,C\Big)$$

$$+ h^*(L)E\Big(\frac{\dot{Q}_c\dot{Q}_l}{Q_\beta(1-Q_\beta)}\Big|L,C\Big)$$

and

$$A_2(L,C) = E\Big(\frac{\dot{Q}_l\dot{Q}_\beta Z}{Q_\beta(1-Q_\beta)}\Big|L,C\Big) - h^*(C)E\Big(\frac{\dot{Q}_c\dot{Q}_l}{Q_\beta(1-Q_\beta)}\Big|L,C\Big)$$

$$+ h^*(L)E\Big(\frac{\dot{Q}_l^2}{Q_\beta(1-Q_\beta)}\Big|L,C\Big).$$

Since the last equation holds for any function h in L_2, then we have

$$f_C(t)E(A_1(L,C)|C=t) - f_L(t)E(A_2(L,C)|L=t) = 0. \tag{22}$$

First, considering the first term on the left-hand side of (22), we have

$$f_C(t)E(A_1(L,C)|C=t)$$

$$= f_C(t)E\Big(E\Big(\frac{\dot{Q}_c\dot{Q}_\beta Z}{Q_\beta(1-Q_\beta)}\Big|L,C\Big) - h^*(C)E\Big(\frac{\dot{Q}_c^2}{Q_\beta(1-Q_\beta)}\Big|L,C\Big)$$

$$+ h^*(L)E\Big(\frac{\dot{Q}_c\dot{Q}_l}{Q_\beta(1-Q_\beta)}\Big|L,C\Big)\Big|C=t\Big)$$

$$
= f_C(t) E\left(\frac{\dot{Q}_c \dot{Q}_\beta Z}{Q_\beta(1 - Q_\beta)}\Big| C = t\right) - f_C(t) h^*(t) E\left(\frac{\dot{Q}_c^2}{Q_\beta(1 - Q_\beta)}\Big| C = t\right)
$$

$$
+ f_C(t) E\left(h^*(L) E\left(\frac{\dot{Q}_c \dot{Q}_l}{Q_\beta(1 - Q_\beta)}\Big| L, C\right)\Big| C = t\right). \tag{23}
$$

Similarly, the second term on the left-hand side of (22) is

$$
f_L(t) E(A_2(L, C)| L = t)
$$

$$
= f_L(t) E\left(E\left(\frac{\dot{Q}_l \dot{Q}_\beta Z}{Q_\beta(1 - Q_\beta)} | L, C\right) - h^*(C) E\left(\frac{\dot{Q}_c \dot{Q}_l}{Q_\beta(1 - Q_\beta)}\Big| L, C\right)\right.
$$

$$
\left. + h^*(L) E\left(\frac{\dot{Q}_l^2}{Q_\beta(1 - Q_\beta)} | L, C\right)\Big| L = t\right)
$$

$$
= f_L(t) E\left(\frac{\dot{Q}_l \dot{Q}_\beta Z}{Q_\beta(1 - Q_\beta)}\Big| L = t\right) - f_L(t) E\left(h^*(C) E\left(\frac{\dot{Q}_c \dot{Q}_l}{Q_\beta(1 - Q_\beta)}\Big| L, C\right)\Big| L = t\right)
$$

$$
+ f_L(t) h^*(t) E\left(\frac{\dot{Q}_l^2}{Q_\beta(1 - Q_\beta)}\Big| L = t\right). \tag{24}
$$

Now,

$$
f_C(t) E\left(h^*(L) E\left(\frac{\dot{Q}_c \dot{Q}_l}{Q_\beta(1 - Q_\beta)}\Big| L, C\right)\Big| C = t\right)
$$

$$
= f_C(t) E\left(h^*(s) E\left(\frac{\dot{Q}_c \dot{Q}_l}{Q_\beta(1 - Q_\beta)} | L = s, C = t\right)| C = t\right)
$$

$$
= f_C(t) \int h^*(s) E\left(\frac{\dot{Q}_c \dot{Q}_l}{Q_\beta(1 - Q_\beta)} | L = s, C = t\right) f_{L|C}(s|t) ds
$$

$$
= \int h^*(s) E\left(\frac{\dot{Q}_c \dot{Q}_l}{Q_\beta(1 - Q_\beta)} | L = s, C = t\right) f_{L,C}(s, t) ds
$$

and

$$
f_L(t) E\left(h^*(C) E\left(\frac{\dot{Q}_c \dot{Q}_l}{Q_\beta(1 - Q_\beta)}\Big| L, C\right)\Big| L = t\right)
$$

$$
= f_L(t) E\left(h^*(s) E\left(\frac{\dot{Q}_c \dot{Q}_l}{Q(1 - Q)}\Big| L = t, C = s\right)\Big| L = t\right)
$$

$$
= f_L(t) \int h^*(s) E\left(\frac{\dot{Q}_c \dot{Q}_l}{Q(1 - Q)}\Big| L = t, C = s\right) f_{C|L}(s|t) ds
$$

$$= \int h^*(s) E\left(\frac{\dot{Q}_c \dot{Q}_l}{Q_\beta(1 - Q_\beta)}\Big| L = t, C = s\right) f_{L,C}(t, s) ds,$$

where $f_{L|C}$ and $f_{C|L}$ are the conditional density of L given C and the conditional density of C given L, respectively. Hence

$$f_C(t) E\left(h^*(L) E\left(\frac{\dot{Q}_c \dot{Q}_l}{Q_\beta(1 - Q_\beta)}|L, C\right)|C = t\right)$$

$$+ f_L(t) E\left(h^*(C) E\left(\frac{\dot{Q}_c \dot{Q}_l}{Q_\beta(1 - Q_\beta)}\Big| L, C\right)\Big| L = t\right)$$

$$= \int h^*(s) E\left(\frac{\dot{Q}_c \dot{Q}_l}{Q_\beta(1 - Q_\beta)}|L = s, C = t\right) f_{L,C}(s, t) ds$$

$$+ \int h^*(s) E\left(\frac{\dot{Q}_c \dot{Q}_l}{Q_\beta(1 - Q_\beta)}\Big| L = t, C = s\right) f_{L,C}(t, s) ds. \tag{25}$$

Finally, from (23)–(25), we obtain

$$h^*(t) - \int h^*(s) r(t, s) ds / g(t) = o(t) / g(t), \tag{26}$$

where $g(t), o(t)$, and $r(t, s)$ are given in (11), (12), and (13), respectively. It is easy to see that $g(t) > 0$ for $t \in [\tau_0, \tau_1]$. Define the operator A as $A[h] = -\int h^*(s) r(t, s) ds / g(t)$ and I as the identity operator. Therefore (26) can be written as $(I + A)[h^*] = o(t) / g(t)$. Since h^* is L_2 integrable function and $A[h^*]$ is continuously differentiable function then A is a compact operator on $[\tau_0, \tau_1]$. It is clear that the invertibility of the operator $I + A$ grantees the existence and uniqueness of the solution h^*. Since the kernel function, $r(t, s)$, is L_2 bounded then by Theorem 4.25 of Rudin (1973), it is sufficient to prove that $I + A$ is one-to-one operator that is if $(I + A)[h] = 0$ then $h(t) = 0$ on $[\tau_0, \tau_1]$. Assume $(I + A)[h] = 0$ then $o(t) = 0$. Following Zeng et al. (2006), if $(I + A)[h] = 0$ then for any function h on $[\tau_0, \tau_1]$, we have

$$0 = \int h(t) o(t) dt$$

$$= \int h(t) \left[f_C(t) E\left(\frac{\dot{Q}_c \dot{Q}_\beta Z}{Q_\beta(1 - Q_\beta)}|C = t\right) - f_L(t) E\left(\frac{\dot{Q}_l \dot{Q}_\beta Z}{Q_\beta(1 - Q_\beta)}|L = t\right)\right] dt$$

$$= \int h(t) E\left(\frac{\dot{Q}_c \dot{Q}_\beta Z}{Q_\beta(1 - Q_\beta)}|C = t\right) f_C(t) dt - \int h(t) E\left(\frac{\dot{Q}_l \dot{Q}_\beta Z}{Q_\beta(1 - Q_\beta)}|L = t\right) f_L(t) dt$$

$$= E\left(h(t) E\left(\frac{\dot{Q}_c \dot{Q}_\beta Z}{Q_\beta(1 - Q_\beta)}|C = t\right)\right) - E\left(h(t) E\left(\frac{\dot{Q}_l \dot{Q}_\beta Z}{Q_\beta(1 - Q_\beta)}|L = t\right) f_L(t)\right)$$

$$= E\Big(h(C)\frac{\dot{Q}_c\dot{Q}_\beta Z}{Q_\beta(1-Q_\beta)}\Big) - E\Big(h(L)\frac{\dot{Q}_l\dot{Q}_\beta Z}{Q_\beta(1-Q_\beta)}\Big)$$

$$= E\Big(\frac{\dot{Q}_\beta Z(h(C)\dot{Q}_c - h(L)\dot{Q}_l)}{Q_\beta(1-Q_\beta)}\Big)$$

$$= E(\ell_{\beta,\lambda}\ell_H[h]),$$

which implies that $E(\ell_H[h^*]\ell_H[h]) = 0$ for any h. By taking $h^* = h$, we obtain $E(\ell_H^2[h]) = 0$ and hence $\ell_H[h] = 0$. From (8), we get $h(t) = 0$ for any $t \in [\tau_0, \tau_1]$.
□

Lemma 1 (Covering Number) *Assume the Assumptions C1–C5 hold. The ε-covering number of the class $\mathcal{L}_1$ associated with $L_1(P_n)$ norm, $N(\varepsilon, \mathcal{L}_1, L_1(P_n))$, is bounded by $K(M/\varepsilon)^{d+q+1}$, where $M = \max(M_\beta, M_\gamma)$.*

Proof Let $\theta^{(i)} \equiv (H^{(i)}, \beta_i) \in \mathbb{R}^n$, $i = 1, 2$. Observe that

$$|l_n(\theta^{(1)}|\mathbf{V}) - l_n(\theta^{(2)}|\mathbf{V})| = \Big|\delta \log\Big(\frac{Q_{\theta^{(1)}}}{Q_{\theta^{(2)}}}\Big) + (1-\delta)\log\Big(1 - \frac{Q_{\theta^{(1)}}}{Q_{\theta^{(2)}}}\Big)\Big|$$

$$= \Big|\delta \log\Big(\frac{S_\epsilon(H_n^{(1)}(c) + \beta_1^\mathsf{T} z)}{S_\epsilon(H_n^{(2)}(c) + \beta_2^\mathsf{T} z)}\Big) - \log\Big(\frac{S_\epsilon(H_n^{(1)}(l) + \beta_1^\mathsf{T} z)}{S_\epsilon(H_n^{(2)}(l) + \beta_2^\mathsf{T} z)}\Big)$$

$$+ (1-\delta)\Big(\frac{S_\epsilon(H_n^{(1)}(l) + \beta_1^\mathsf{T} z) - S_\epsilon(H_n^{(1)}(c) + \beta_1^\mathsf{T} z)}{S_\epsilon(H_n^{(2)}(l) + \beta_2^\mathsf{T} z) - S_\epsilon(H_n^{(2)}(c) + \beta_2^\mathsf{T} z)}\Big)\Big|$$

$$\leq |\log(S_\epsilon(H_n^{(1)}(c) + \beta_1^\mathsf{T} z)) - \log(S_\epsilon(H_n^{(2)}(c) + \beta_2^\mathsf{T} z))|$$

$$+ |\log(S_\epsilon(H_n^{(1)}(l) + \beta_1^\mathsf{T} z)) - \log(S_\epsilon(H_n^{(2)}(l) + \beta_2^\mathsf{T} z))|$$

$$+ |\log(S_\epsilon(H_n^{(1)}(l) + \beta_1^\mathsf{T} z) - S_\epsilon(H_n^{(1)}(c) + \beta_1^\mathsf{T} z))$$

$$- \log(S_\epsilon(H_n^{(2)}(l) + \beta_2^\mathsf{T} z) - S_\epsilon(H_n^{(2)}(c) + \beta_1^\mathsf{T} z))|.$$

By mean-value theorem and Assumptions **C1–C5**, we can obtain

$$|l_n(\theta^{(1)}|\mathbf{V}) - l_n(\theta^{(2)}|\mathbf{V})| \leq K|S_\epsilon(H^{(1)}(c) + \beta_1^\mathsf{T} z) - S_\epsilon(H^{(2)}(c) + \beta_2^\mathsf{T} z)|$$

$$+ K|S_\epsilon(H_n^{(1)}(l) + \beta_1^\mathsf{T} z) - S_\epsilon(H_n^{(2)}(l) + \beta_2^\mathsf{T} z)|$$

$$\leq K(|\beta_1 - \beta_2|Z + |H_n^{(1)}(l) - H_n^{(2)}(l)| + |H_n^{(1)}(c) - H_n^{(2)}(c)|).$$

Since $H_n \in \mathbb{H}_n$, then it can be represented by $H_n^{(j)}(t) = \sum_{k=0}^q \gamma_k^{(j)} A_k(t)$, for $j = 1, 2$. Then

$$|H_n^{(t)}(t) - H_n^{(2)}(t)| = \left|\sum_{k=0}^{q}(\gamma_k^{(1)} - \gamma_k^{(2)})A_k(t)\right| < \left|\sum_{k=0}^{q}(\gamma_k^{(1)} - \gamma_k^{(2)})\right| \le \sum_{k=0}^{q}\left|\gamma_k^{(1)} - \gamma_k^{(2)}\right|$$

$$\le \max_{0\le k\le q}|\gamma_k^{(1)} - \gamma_k^{(2)}| = \|\gamma^{(1)} - \gamma^{(2)}\|_\infty.$$

It follows that for any $\theta_n \in \Theta$, we have

$$P_n|l_n(\theta^{(1)}|\mathbf{V}) - l_n(\theta^{(2)}|\mathbf{V})| = K\|\beta_1 - \beta_2\| + K\|\gamma^{(1)} - \gamma^{(2)}\|_\infty.$$

Now, by Assumption **C1**, $\mathbb{B}$ is a compact subset of $\mathbb{R}^d$, then using Lemma 2.5 of Geer and van de Geer (2000), $\{\beta \in \mathbb{R}^d, \|\beta\| \le M_\beta\}$ it is covered by $(20KM_\beta/\varepsilon)^d$ balls with radius $\varepsilon/4k$ and consequently, the class $\{\beta^\mathsf{T}Z : \beta \in \mathbb{B}\}$ is covered by $(20KM_\beta/\varepsilon)^d$ balls with radius $\varepsilon/4k$ due to the bounded Assumption **C4**. Similarly, the class $\{\gamma \in \mathbb{R}^{q+1}, \sum_{j=0}^{q}|\gamma_j| \le M_\gamma\}$ is covered by $(20KM_\gamma/\varepsilon)^{q+1}$ balls with radius $\varepsilon/4k$. Hence

$$N(\varepsilon, \mathcal{L}_1, L_1(P_n)) \le (20KM_\beta/\varepsilon)^d(20KM_\gamma/\varepsilon)^{q+1} \le K(M/\varepsilon)^{d+q+1}. \qquad \Box$$

Lemma 2 (Bracketing Number) *Assume the Assumptions **C1**–**C5** hold. The ε-bracketing number of the class $\mathcal{L}_1$ associated with $L_2(P)$ norm, $N(\varepsilon, \mathcal{L}_1, L_2(P))$, is bounded by $K(M/\varepsilon)^{d+q+1}$, where $M = \max(M_\beta, M_\gamma)$.*

Proof For $\theta^{(j)} = (\beta_j, H_n^{(j)}) \in \Theta_n$, $j = 1, 2$, define the distance $\tilde{d}(\theta^{(1)}, \theta^{(2)}) = \|\beta^{(1)} - \beta^{(2)}\| + \|H_n^{(1)} - H_n^{(2)}\|_\infty$. From the proof of Lemma 1, we have

$$|l_n(\theta^{(1)}|\mathbf{V}) - l_n(\theta^{(2)}|\mathbf{V})| \le K(\|\beta_1 - \beta_2\| + \|\gamma^{(1)} - \gamma^{(2)}\|_\infty) = K\tilde{d}(\theta^{(1)}, \theta^{(2)}).$$
$$\Box$$

By Theorem 2.7.11 of van der Vaart and Wellner (1996), we have

$$N_{[]}(2K\varepsilon, \mathcal{L}_1, L_2(P) \le N(\varepsilon, \Theta_n, \tilde{d}),$$

where $N_{[]}(2K\varepsilon, \mathcal{L}_1, L_2(P)$ is the bracketing number associated with $L_2(P)$ norm of the class $\mathcal{L}_1$ and $N(\varepsilon, \Theta_n, \tilde{d})$ is the covering number of Θ_n associated with distance $\tilde{d}$. The definitions of the bracketing number and covering number are given in the Definitions 2.1.5 and 2.1.6 of van der Vaart and Wellner (1996), respectively. From Lemma 8 of Hu et al. (2017), we have $N(\varepsilon, \Theta_n, \tilde{d}) = K(\eta/\varepsilon)^{q+1}$. By Theorem 2.7.11 of van der Vaart and Wellner (1996), the bracketing number associated with $L_2(P)$ of the class $\mathcal{L}_1$,

$$N_{[]}(2K\varepsilon, \mathcal{L}_1, L_2(P)) = K(\eta/\varepsilon)^{q+1}.$$

Lemma 3 (Uniform Convergence) *Assume that the Assumptions **C1–C4** hold. Then we have*

$$\|\mathbb{M}_n - \mathbb{M}\|_{\Theta_n} \to_{a.s.} 0.$$

Proof By Assumptions **C1–C4**, we conclude that $l_n(\theta|\mathbf{V})$ is bounded, so without loss of generality, let $|l_n(\theta|\mathbf{V})| \leq 1$. Define $\delta_n = \varepsilon n^{-1/2+\alpha}(\log(n))^{1/2}$ as a non-increasing sequence of positive numbers with $0 < \alpha < 1/2$ and $\varepsilon > 0$. It can be seen that for every $l_n(\theta|\mathbb{V}) \in \mathcal{L}_1$ and for large n, we have

$$\frac{var(P_n l_n(\theta|\mathbf{V}))}{(4\delta_n)^2} \leq \frac{\frac{1}{n}var(l^2(\theta|\mathbf{V}))}{16n^{2\alpha}\log(n)} \leq \frac{Pl^2(\theta|\mathbf{V})}{16n^{2\alpha}\log(n)} \leq \frac{1}{16n^{2\alpha}\log(n)} \leq \frac{1}{2},$$

since $|l_n(\theta|\mathbf{V})| \leq 1$ and using the i.i.d property of $V_1, \cdots, V_n$. Let $\sigma^{\mathsf{T}} = (\sigma_1, \cdots, \sigma_n)$ be a sequence of independent random variables with $P_r(\sigma_i = 1) = P_r(\sigma_i = -1) = \frac{1}{2}$, for every $i = 1, 2, \cdots, n$. Assume also σ is independent of $\mathbf{V}$. Define the symmetrized empirical measure

$$\mathbb{M}^{\sigma}(\theta) := P_n^{\sigma}(l_n(\theta|\mathbf{V})) = \frac{1}{n}\sum_{i=1}^{n}\sigma_i l_n(\theta|V_i), \ \theta \in \Theta_n.$$

By Equation (31) of Pollard (1984) we have

$$P_r\left(\sup_{\theta \in \Theta_n} |\mathbb{M}_n^{\sigma}(\theta)| > 2\delta_n \Big| \mathbf{V}\right) \leq 2N(\delta_n, \mathcal{L}_1, L_1(P_n)) \exp\left\{-\frac{1}{2}n\delta_n^2 / \max_j P_n g_j\right\},$$

where the maximum runs over of all functions with covering number $N(\delta_n, \mathcal{L}_1, L_1(P_n))$ in the class $\mathcal{L}_1$. Using the fact that the class $\mathcal{L}_1$ is uniformly bounded by 1, and after taking expectations over $\mathbf{V}$, we obtain

$$P_r\left(\sup_{\theta \in \Theta_n} |\mathbb{M}_n^{\sigma}(\theta)| > 2\delta_n\right) \leq 2N(\delta_n, \mathcal{L}_1, L_1(P_n)) \exp\left\{-\frac{1}{2}n\delta_n^2\right\}. \qquad (27)$$

Hence, from Equation (31) (Pollard 1984), Eq. (27) and Lemma 1, we can deduce that

$$P_r\left(\sup_{\theta \in \Theta_n} |\mathbb{M}_n(\theta)) - \mathbb{M}(\theta))| > 8\delta_n\right) \leq 4P_r\left(\sup_{\theta \in \Theta_n} |\mathbb{M}_n^{\sigma}(\theta)| > 2\delta_n\right)$$

$$\leq 8N(\delta_n, \mathcal{L}_1, L_1(P_n)) \exp\left\{-\frac{1}{2}n\delta_n^2\right\}$$

$$\leq K(M/\delta_n)^{d+q+1} \exp\left\{-\frac{1}{2}n\delta_n^2\right\}$$

$$= K \exp\left\{(1/2 - \alpha)(d + q + 1)\log(n) - (d + q + 1)(\log M)\right.$$

$$-(d+q+1)(\log \varepsilon) - \frac{1}{2}(d+q+1)\log\log(n) - \frac{1}{2}\epsilon^2 n^{2\alpha}\log(n)\Big\}$$

$$\leq K_1 e^{-K_2 n^{2\alpha}\log(n)} \to 0 \text{ as } n \to 0.$$

Hence, $\sum_{n=1}^{\infty} P(\sup_{\theta \in \Theta_n} |\mathbb{M}_n(\theta) - \mathbb{M}(\theta)| > 8\delta_n) < \infty$. By the Borel–Cantelli lemma,

$$\sup_{\theta \in \Theta_n} |\mathbb{M}_n(\theta) - \mathbb{M}(\theta)| \to 0, \, a.s. P_{\theta_0}.$$

□

Lemma 4 Let $g_1(Z) = (\beta - \beta_0)^\mathsf{T} Z$, $g_2(C) = H(C) - H_0(C)$ and $g_3(L) = H(L) - H_0(L)$. Let $K < 1$. Then, we have

(1) $(E(g_1(g_2 + g_3)))^2 \leq K E(g_1^2) E(g_2 + g_3)^2.$
(2) $(E(g_2 g_3))^2 \leq K E(g_2^2) E(g_3^2).$

Proof By iterative expectation and Cauchy-Schwarz inequality, we get

$$[E(g_1(g_2 + g_3))]^2 = [E((g_2 + g_3)E(g_1|L, C))]^2$$
$$\leq E(g_2 + g_3)^2 E[E(g_1|L, C)]^2$$
$$= E(g_2 + g_3)^2 E(E([E(g_1|L, C)]^2|L, C)).$$

Observe that

$$E([E(Z|L, C)]^{\otimes 2}|L, C)$$
$$= E([Z - (Z - E(Z|L, C))]^{\otimes 2}|L, C)$$
$$= E(Z^{\otimes 2} + (Z - E(Z|L, C))^{\otimes 2} - 2Z(Z - E(Z|L, C))^\mathsf{T})|L, C)$$
$$= E(Z^{\otimes 2}|L, C) + var(Z|L, C) - 2E(Z^{\otimes 2}|L, C) + 2[E(Z|L, C)]^{\otimes 2}$$
$$= E(Z^{\otimes 2}|L, C) + var(Z|L, C) - 2var(Z|L, C)$$
$$= E(Z^{\otimes 2}|L, C) - var(Z|L, C)$$
$$\leq (1 - \varpi_1)E(Z^{\otimes 2}|L, C) \tag{28}$$

by Assumption C7(i). Then

$$E(E([E(g_1|L, C)]^2|L, C)) = E((\beta - \beta_0)^\mathsf{T} E([E(Z|L, C)]^{\otimes 2}|L, C)(\beta - \beta_0))$$
$$\leq (1 - \varpi_1)E((\beta - \beta_0)^\mathsf{T} E(Z^{\otimes 2}|L, C)(\beta - \beta_0))$$
$$= (1 - \varpi_1)E((\beta - \beta_0)^\mathsf{T} Z)^2$$
$$= (1 - \varpi_1)E(g_1(Z))^2$$

using (28). This completes the proof (1). Similarly, for (2), we have

$$
\begin{aligned}
[E(g_2 g_3)]^2 &= [E(g_3)E(g_2|L))]^2 \\
&\leq E(g_3)^2 E[E(g_2|L)]^2 \\
&= E(g_3)^2 E(E([E(g_2|L)]^2|L)).
\end{aligned}
$$

Note that

$$
\begin{aligned}
E([\ E\ (H(C) &- H_0(C)|L)]^2|X, W) \qquad\qquad\qquad\qquad\qquad (29)\\
&= E([H(C) - H_0(C) - (H(C) - H_0(C) - E(H(C) - H_0(C)|L))]^2|L) \\
&= E((H(C) - H_0(C))^2 + (H(C) - H_0(C) - E(H(C) - H_0(C)|L))^2 \\
&\quad -2(H(C) - H_0(C))(H(C) - H_0(C) - E(H(C) - H_0(C)|L)))|L) \\
&= E((H(C) - H_0(C))^2|L) + var(H(C) - H_0(C)|L) \\
&\quad -2E((H(C) - H_0(C))^2|L) + 2(E(H(C) - H_0(C)|L))^2 \\
&= E((H(C) - H_0(C))^2|L) - var(H(C) - H_0(C)|L) \\
&\leq (1 - \varpi_2)E((H(C) - H_0(C))^2|L) \qquad\qquad\qquad\qquad (30)
\end{aligned}
$$

using condition **C7**(ii). Then

$$
\begin{aligned}
E(E([E(g_2|L)]^2|L)) &= E(E([E(H(C) - H_0(C)|L)]^2|L)) \\
&\leq (1 - \varpi_2)E(E((H(C) - H_0(C))^2|L)) \\
&\leq (1 - \varpi_2)E(H(C) - H_0(C))^2 \\
&= (1 - \varpi_2)E(g_2(C))^2
\end{aligned}
$$

using (29). This completes the proof.   □

Lemma 5 *Assume the assumptions **C1–C5** hold. For $\theta \in \Theta_n$, we have*

$$
K_1 d^2(\theta, \theta_0) \leq \mathbb{M}(\theta_0) - \mathbb{M}(\theta) \leq K_2 d^2(\theta, \theta_0)
$$

for some real constants $K_1 < K_2$.

Proof First, note that, by assumptions **C1–C3**, $Q_\theta = S_\epsilon(H(c) + \beta^\mathsf{T} z)/S_\epsilon(H(l) + \beta^\mathsf{T} z)$ is bounded away from 0 and 1. Define $L(\theta|\mathbf{V})$ to be the likelihood function corresponding to $l_n(\theta|\mathbf{V})$ and P is the probability measure of $\mathbf{V}$. Note that P is closely related to $L(\theta_0|\mathbf{V})$. Similar to the proof of Lemma 25.85 of van der Vaart (1998)

$$
\mathbb{M}(\theta_0) - \mathbb{M}(\theta) = P(\log(L(\theta_0|\mathbf{V})) - \log(L(\theta|\mathbf{V})))
$$

$$= P\left(\log \frac{L(\theta_0|\mathbf{V})}{L(\theta|\mathbf{V})}\right)$$

$$\geq K \int \left(\sqrt{L(\theta_0|\mathbf{V})} - \sqrt{L(\theta|\mathbf{V})}\right)^2 d\mu$$

$$= K \int \frac{\left(L(\theta_0|\mathbf{V}) - L(\theta|\mathbf{V})\right)^2}{L(\theta_0|\mathbf{V})\left(\sqrt{L(\theta_0|\mathbf{V})} + \sqrt{L(\theta|\mathbf{V})}\right)^2} L(\theta_0|\mathbf{V})d\mu$$

$$\geq K \int \left(L(\theta_0|\mathbf{V}) - L(\theta|\mathbf{V})\right)^2 dP$$

$$= K P\left(L(\theta_0|\mathbf{V}) - L(\theta|\mathbf{V})\right)^2$$

$$= K P\left(\Delta(Q_{\theta_0} - Q_\theta) + (1 - \Delta)(Q_{\theta_0} - Q_\theta)\right)^2$$

$$= K P\left(\Delta(Q_{\theta_0} - Q_\theta)^2 + (1 - \Delta)(Q_{\theta_0} - Q_\theta)^2\right)$$

$$= K P(Q_{\theta_0} - Q_\theta)^2$$

$$\geq K P((\beta - \beta_0)^\mathsf{T} Z + (H(C) - H_0(C)) + (H(L) - H_0(L)))^2,$$

by Taylor series. By Assumptions **C1–C4**, Lemma 4 and Lemma A6 of Murphy and van der Vaart (1997), we get

$$\mathbb{M}(\theta_0) - \mathbb{M}(\theta) \geq K(P((\beta - \beta_0)^\mathsf{T} Z)^2 + P(H(C) - H_0(C))^2 + P(H(L) - H_0(L))^2)$$

$$\geq K_1(\|\beta - \beta_0\|^2 + P(H(C) - H_0(C))^2 + P(H(L) - H_0(L))^2)$$

$$= K_1 d^2(\theta, \theta_0).$$

Next, we consider the right-hand inequality. Notice that Since

$$E(\Delta|T > L, C, Z) = P(T \geq C|T > L, C, Z) = Q_{\theta_0}.$$

Observe that

$$\mathbb{M}(\theta_0) - \mathbb{M}(\theta) = P(l_n(\theta_0|\mathbf{V}) - l_n(\theta|\mathbf{V}))$$

$$= P\left(\Delta \log\left(\frac{Q_{\theta_0}}{Q_\theta}\right) + (1 - \Delta) \log\left(\frac{1 - Q_{\theta_0}}{1 - Q_\theta}\right)\right)$$

$$= P\left(Q_{\theta_0} \log\left(\frac{Q_{\theta_0}}{Q_\theta}\right) + (1 - Q_{\theta_0}) \log\left(\frac{1 - Q_{\theta_0}}{1 - Q_\theta}\right)\right)$$

$$= P\left(Q_\theta\left[\frac{Q_{\theta_0}}{Q_\theta} \log\left(\frac{Q_{\theta_0}}{Q_\theta}\right) - \frac{Q_{\theta_0}}{Q_\theta} + 1\right]\right)$$

$$+(1 - Q_\theta)\left[\frac{(1 - Q_{\theta_0})}{(1 - Q_\theta)} \log\left(\frac{1 - Q_{\theta_0}}{1 - Q_\theta}\right) - \frac{1 - Q_{\theta_0}}{1 - Q_\theta} + 1\right]\right)$$

$$= P\left(Q_\theta D\left[\frac{Q_{\theta_0}}{Q_\theta}\right] + (1 - Q_\theta)D\left[\frac{1 - Q_{\theta_0}}{1 - Q_\theta}\right]\right),$$

where $D(t) = t \log(t) - t + 1$. It is easy to see that $D(t) \leq (t - 1)^2$ for t in a neighborhood of $t = 1$. By assumptions **C1–C5**, it follows that

$$\mathbb{M}(\theta_0) - \mathbb{M}(\theta) \leq P\left(\frac{[Q_\theta - Q_{\theta_0}]^2}{Q_\theta(1 - Q_\theta)}\right)$$

$$\leq K P[Q_\theta - Q_{\theta_0}]^2$$

$$\leq K P((\beta - \beta_0)^\mathsf{T} Z + H(C) - H_0(C) + H(L) - H_0(L))^2$$

$$\leq K(\beta - \beta_0)^\mathsf{T} P(ZZ^\mathsf{T})(\beta - \beta_0) + P(H(C) - H_0(C))^2 + P(H(L) - H_0(L))^2$$

$$\leq K_2(\beta - \beta_0)^\mathsf{T}(\beta - \beta_0) + P(H(C) - H_0(C))^2 + P(H(L) - H_0(L))^2$$

$$= K_2(\|\beta - \beta_0\|^2 + \|H(C) - H_0(C)\|_2^2 + \|H(L) - H_0(L)\|_2^2)$$

$$= K_2 d^2(\theta, \theta_0).$$

This completes the proof.   □

Proof of Theorem 2 *(Consistency)* The proof is accomplished by verifying the conditions of Theorem 5.7 of van der Vaart (1998). First, the proof of the uniform convergence condition of the theorem is established in Lemma 3. From Lemma 5,

$$\mathbb{M}(\theta_0) - \mathbb{M}(\theta) \geq K d^2(\theta, \theta_0).$$

Then, it implies that

$$\sup_{\theta:d(\theta,\theta_0)>\epsilon} \mathbb{M}(\theta) \leq \mathbb{M}(\theta_0) - K\epsilon^2 \leq \mathbb{M}(\theta_0).$$

Finally, we prove the nearly maximization condition of the theorem. From Lu et al. (2007), there exists a projection $H_{0,n}$ of the true value H_0 on the space $\mathbb{H}_n$ such that $\|H_{0,n} - H_0\|_\infty \leq O(n^{-rv})$. This also implies that $\|H_{0,n} - H_0\|_2 = O(n^{-rv})$. Let $\theta_{0,n} = (\beta_0, H_{0,n})$. Observe that

$$\mathbb{M}_n(\hat{\theta}_n) - \mathbb{M}_n(\theta_0) = \mathbb{M}_n(\hat{\theta}_n) - \mathbb{M}_n(\theta_{0,n}) + \mathbb{M}_n(\theta_{0,n}) - \mathbb{M}_n(\theta_0)$$

$$\geq \mathbb{M}_n(\theta_{0,n}) - \mathbb{M}_n(\theta_0)$$

$$\geq (P_n - P)(l_n(\theta_{0,n}|\mathbf{V}) - l_n(\theta_0|\mathbf{V})) + P(l_n(\theta_{0,n}|\mathbf{V}) - l_n(\theta_0|\mathbf{V})),$$

since $\hat{\theta}_n$ is the sieve maximum likelihood estimator of θ. First, we consider the first term. Let $\mathcal{L}_2(\eta) = \{l_n(\theta_0|\mathbf{V}) - l_n(\theta_{0,n}|\mathbf{V}) : H \in \mathbb{H}_n, \|H - H_0\| < \eta\}$. Let

$\theta^{(j)} = (\beta_0, H^{(j)}) \in \Theta_n, j = 1, 2$ such that $\|H^{(j)} - H_0\| \leq \eta$. From Lemma 2, the ε-bracketing number associated with $L_2(P)$ of the class $\mathcal{L}_2(\eta)$,

$$N_{[]}(2K\varepsilon, \mathcal{L}_2(\eta), L_2(P)) = K(\eta/\varepsilon)^{q+1}.$$

Then the bracketing integral of the class $\mathcal{L}_2$ is

$$J_{[]}(\zeta, \mathcal{L}_2(\eta), L_2(P)) = \int_0^\zeta \sqrt{\log N_{[]}(2K\varepsilon, \mathcal{L}_2(\eta), L_2(P))} d\varepsilon$$

$$= \int_0^\zeta \sqrt{\log(K(\eta/\varepsilon)^{q+1})} d\varepsilon \leq K\eta\sqrt{q+1} < \infty.$$

Therefore, the class $\mathcal{L}_2(\eta)$ is P-Donsker class by Theorem 19.5 of van der Vaart (1998). Moreover, form the Assumptions **C1–C4** and using the dominated convergence theorem, one can show that $P(l_n(\theta_{0,n}|\mathbf{V}) - l_n(\theta_0|\mathbf{V}))^2 \rightarrow 0$ and $n \rightarrow \infty$. Hence, by Lemma 19.24 of van der Vaart (1998), we conclude that $(P_n - P)(l_n(\theta_{0,n}|\mathbf{V}) - l_n(\theta_0|\mathbf{V})) = o_P(n^{-1/2})$. For the second term, using the Taylor expansion with Assumptions **C1–C5**, we obtain

$$P(l_n(\theta_{0,n}|\mathbf{V}) - l_n(\theta_0|\mathbf{V})) = -k(\theta_{0,n} - \theta_0)^2 \geq -O(n^{-2rv}) = -o(1).$$

Therefore,

$$\mathbb{M}_n(\hat{\theta}_n) - \mathbb{M}_n(\theta_0) \geq o_P(n^{-1/2}) - o(1) = -o_P(1).$$

This completes the proof of $d(\hat{\theta}_n, \theta_0) \rightarrow_P 0$.   □

Proof of Theorem 3 *(Rate of Convergence)* We apply Theorem 3.2.5 of van der Vaart and Wellner (1996) page 289 to prove this theorem. The first condition of Theorem 3.2.5 of van der Vaart and Wellner (1996) is already proved in the proof of Theorem 2. From Lemma 3, the ε-bracketing number of the class $\mathcal{L}_3(\eta) = \{l_n(\theta|\mathbf{V}) - l_n(\theta_0|\mathbf{V}) : d(\theta, \theta_0) < \eta, \theta \in \Theta_n\}$ with respect to $L_2(P)$ norm is bounded by $K(\eta/\varepsilon)^{q+1}$ and this leads to the bracketing integral $J_{[]}(\eta, \mathcal{L}_3(\eta), L_2(P)) \leq K\eta\sqrt{q+1}$. By using the Assumptions **C1–C4** and Lemma 3.4.2 of van der Vaart and Wellner (1996) and the fact that $q = O(n^v)$, we get

$$\phi_n(\eta) = J_{[]}(\eta, \mathcal{L}_3(\eta), L_2(P))\left(1 + \frac{J_{[]}(\eta, \mathcal{L}_3(\eta), L_2(P))K}{\eta^2\sqrt{n}}\right)$$

$$= \eta\sqrt{q+1} + (q+1)n^{-1/2}$$

$$= n^{v/2}\eta + n^{v-1/2}.$$

Notice that, if $rv > (1-v)/2$, then, for $r_n = n^{(1-v)/2}$, we have

$$r_n^2 \phi_n(r_n^{-1}) = n^{1-v}[n^{v-1/2} + n^{v-1/2}] = O(n^{1/2}),$$

and if $rv < (1-v)/2$, then for $r_n = n^{rv}$, we have

$$\begin{aligned}
r_n^2 \phi_n(r_n^{-1}) &= n^{2rv} \phi_n(n^{-rv}) \\
&= n^{2rv}[n^{v/2}n^{-rv} + n^{v-1/2}] \\
&= n^{v/2+rv} + n^{2rv+v-1/2} \\
&= n^{1/2}[n^{rv-(1-v)/2} + n^{2rv-(1-v)}] < n^{1/2}.
\end{aligned}$$

Hence we get $r_n = n^{\min(pv,(1-v)/2)}$. This establishes the second condition of Theorem 3.2.5 of van der Vaart and Wellner (1996). From the proof of consistency, we have shown that

$$\begin{aligned}
\mathbb{M}_n(\hat{\theta}_n) - \mathbb{M}_n(\theta_0) &\geq (P_n - P)(l_n(\theta_{0,n}|\mathbf{V}) - l_n(\theta_0|\mathbf{V})) \\
&\quad + P(l_n(\theta_{0,n}|\mathbf{V}) - l_n(\theta_0|\mathbf{V})). \tag{31}
\end{aligned}$$

First, we consider the first term of (31). From the proof of Theorem 2, we have proved that the class $\{l_n(\beta_0, H_n|\mathbf{V}) - l_n(\theta_0, H_0|\mathbf{V}) : H_n \in \mathbb{H}_n, \|H_n - H\|_2 \leq \eta\}$ is P-Donsker. Because of $\|H_{0,n} - H_0\|_\infty = O(n^{-rv})$ which implies that $\|H_{0,n} - H_0\|_2 = O(n^{-rv})$ and using Assumptions C1–C4, the mean-value theorem and the bounded convergence theorem, we obtain

$$P\left(\frac{l_n(\theta_{0,n}|\mathbf{V}) - l_n(\theta_0|\mathbf{V})}{n^{-rv+\varepsilon}}\right)^2 \to 0,$$

for $0 < \varepsilon < 1/2 - rv$. Therefore, by Lemma 19.24 of van der Vaart (1998), we get

$$(P_n - P)\left(\frac{l_n(\theta_{0,n}|\mathbf{V}) - l_n(\theta_0|\mathbf{V})}{n^{-rv+\varepsilon}}\right) = o_p(n^{-1/2}),$$

and consequently, this gives

$$(P_n - P)(l_n(\theta_{0,n}|\mathbf{V}) - l_n(\theta_0|\mathbf{V})) = o_p(n^{-rv+\varepsilon}n^{-1/2}) = o_p(n^{-2rv}),$$

by choosing $\varepsilon = 1/2 - rv$. Next, consider the second term of (31). Using Taylor series, Assumptions C1–C5, Lemmas 4 and 5, we can show that

$$\begin{aligned}
\mathbb{M}(\theta_{0,n}) - \mathbb{M}(\theta_0) &\geq -K(P(H_{0,n}(C) - H_0(C))^2 + P(H_{0,n}(L) - H_0(L))^2) \\
&= -Kd^2(\theta_{0,n}, \theta_0) = -O(n^{-2vr}).
\end{aligned}$$

Therefore,

$$\mathbb{M}_n(\hat{\theta}_n) - \mathbb{M}(\theta_0) \geq -O_p(n^{-2rv}) = O_p(n^{-2\min(rv,(1-v)/2)}) = -O_p(r_n^{-2}).$$

This completes the proof.   □

Proof of Theorem 4 *(Normality)* The proof of this theorem is established by utilizing the ideas of Shen (1997) and Chen et al. (2006). Let $\delta_n = n^{-1/4}$. By Lu et al. (2007), for every $w^* \in \overline{\mathbb{V}}$, there exists projection, w_n^* on the space $\Theta_n - \theta$ such that $\|w^* - w_n^*\| = O(n^{-rv})$. For $v > 1/4$, it follows that $\delta_n \|w^* - w_n^*\| = o(n^{-1/2})$. Let ϵ_n by any positive sequence such that $\epsilon_n = o(n^{-1/2})$. Define $\rho(\theta - \theta_0|\mathbf{V}) = l_n(\theta|\mathbf{V}) - l_n(\theta_0|\mathbf{V}) - \dot{l}_n(\theta_0|\mathbf{V})[\theta - \theta_0]$. Let $\theta^* \in \{\theta \in \Theta_n : |\hat{\theta} - \theta| = \epsilon_n w_n^*\}$. Without loss of generality, we assume $\hat{\theta} > \theta^*$. Now, since $\hat{\theta}$ maximizes the log-likelihood over Θ, then, using Taylor expansion and the fact that $P(\dot{l}_n(\theta_0|\mathbf{V})[w^*] = 0$, we have

$$\begin{aligned}
0 \leq\ & P_n\{l_n(\hat{\theta}|\mathbf{V}) - l_n(\theta^*|\mathbf{V})\} \\
=\ & (P_n - P)\{l_n(\hat{\theta}|\mathbf{V}) - l_n(\theta^*|\mathbf{V})\} + P\{l_n(\hat{\theta}|\mathbf{V}) - l_n(\theta^*|\mathbf{V})\} \\
=\ & (P_n - P)\{l_n(\hat{\theta}|\mathbf{V}) - l_n(\theta_0|\mathbf{V}) - \dot{l}_n(\theta_0|\mathbf{V})[\hat{\theta} - \theta_0] - l_n(\theta^*|\mathbf{V}) + l_n(\theta_0|\mathbf{V}) \\
& +\dot{l}_n(\theta_0|\mathbf{V})[\theta^* - \theta_0]\} + P\{l_n(\hat{\theta}|\mathbf{V}) - l_n(\theta_0|\mathbf{V}) - \dot{l}_n(\theta_0|\mathbf{V})[\hat{\theta} - \theta_0] \\
& -l_n(\theta^*|\mathbf{V}) + l_n(\theta_0|\mathbf{V}) + \dot{l}_n(\theta_0|\mathbf{V})[\theta^* - \theta_0]\} \\
& +(P_n - P)\dot{l}_n(\theta_0|\mathbf{V})[\hat{\theta} - \theta^*] + P\dot{l}_n(\theta_0|\mathbf{V})[\hat{\theta} - \theta^*] \\
=\ & (P_n - P)\{\rho(\hat{\theta} - \theta_0|\mathbf{V}) - \rho(\theta^* - \theta_0|\mathbf{V})\} + P\{\rho(\hat{\theta} - \theta_0|\mathbf{V}) - \rho(\theta^* - \theta_0|\mathbf{V})\} \\
& +\epsilon_n P_n \dot{l}_n(\theta_0|\mathbf{V})[w_n^* - w^*] + \epsilon_n P_n \dot{l}_n(\theta_0|\mathbf{V})[w^*] \\
:=\ & I_1 + I_2 + I_3 + \epsilon_n(P_n - P)\dot{l}_n(\theta_0|\mathbf{V})[w^*].
\end{aligned} \tag{32}$$

First, we prove

$$I_1 = (P_n - P)\{\rho(\hat{\theta} - \theta_0|\mathbf{V}) - \rho(\theta^* - \theta_0|\mathbf{V})\} = \epsilon_n o_p(n^{-1/2}). \tag{33}$$

Using Taylor expansion, we get

$$\begin{aligned}
I_1 &= (P_n - P)\{l_n(\hat{\theta}|\mathbf{V}) - l_n(\theta^*|\mathbf{V}) - \dot{l}_n(\theta_0|\mathbf{V})[\hat{\theta} - \theta^*]\} \\
&= (P_n - P)\{l_n(\hat{\theta}|\mathbf{V}) - l_n(\theta^*|\mathbf{V}) - \epsilon_n \dot{l}_n(\theta_0|\mathbf{V})w_n^*\} \\
&= \epsilon_n(P_n - P)\{\dot{l}(\tilde{\theta}|\mathbf{V})[w_n^*] - \dot{l}_n(\theta_0|\mathbf{V})[w_n^*]\},
\end{aligned}$$

where $\tilde{\theta} \in \Theta_n$ lies between $\hat{\theta}$ and θ^*. Let $\mathcal{L}_4 = \{\dot{l}_n(\theta|\mathbf{V})[w_n^*] - \dot{l}_n(\theta_0|\mathbf{V})[w_n^*]; \theta \in \Theta_n; d(\theta; \theta_0) < \delta_n, \|w_n^*\| < \delta_n\}$. Note that w_n^* is bonded due to the boundedness of the space $\Theta_n - \theta$. Similar to Lemma 2, one can show that that the ε-bracketing number of the class $\mathcal{L}_4$ associated with $L_2(P)$ norm is bounded by $K(M/\varepsilon)^{d+q+1}$. This implies that the class $\mathcal{L}_4$ is P-Donsker class due to the Theorem 19.5 of van der Vaart (1998). Then

$$P((\dot{l}_n(\theta|\mathbf{V}) - \dot{l}_n(\theta_0|\mathbf{V}))w_n^*)^2 = P(\ddot{l}_n(\tilde{\theta}|\mathbf{V})(\theta - \theta_0)w_n^*)^2 \leq \delta_n^2 K \to 0,$$

due to the Assumptions **C1–C5**. Hence by Lemma 19.24 and Corollary 2.3.12 of van der Vaart and Wellner (1996), we conclude that $I_1 = o_P(n^{-1/2})$. Next, the proof of

$$I_2 = P\{\rho(\hat{\theta} - \theta_0|\mathbf{V}) - \rho(\theta^* - \theta_0|\mathbf{V})\} = -\epsilon_n\langle\hat{\theta} - \theta_0, w^*\rangle + \epsilon_n o_p(n^{-1/2}) \quad (34)$$

is similar to that of Hu et al. (2017), so it is omitted. Finally, we prove

$$I_3 = P_n\dot{l}_n(\theta_0|\mathbf{V})[w_n^* - w^*] = \epsilon_n o_p(n^{-1/2}). \quad (35)$$

Utilizing the fact $\|w_n^* - w^*\| = o(1)$, and the i.i.d. data, $V_1, \cdots, V_n$, then using the Chebyshev's inequality, for any $\eta > 0$, we have

$$Pr(\sqrt{n}P_n\dot{l}_n(\theta_0|\mathbf{V})[w_n^* - w^*] > \eta) \leq \sqrt{n}E(P_n\dot{l}_n(\theta_0|\mathbf{V})[w_n^* - w^*])/\eta$$

$$\leq \sqrt{n}\sqrt{E(P_n\dot{l}_n(\theta_0|\mathbf{V})[w_n^* - w^*])^2}/\eta$$

$$= \sqrt{E(\dot{l}_n(\theta_0|\mathbf{V})[w_n^* - w^*])^2}/\eta$$

$$= \|w_n^* - w^*\|/\eta \to_P 0,$$

as $n \to \infty$, where $\to_P$ denotes the convergence in probability. By substituting (33), (34) and (35) in (32), and using the central limit theorem, we obtain

$$\sqrt{n}\langle\hat{\theta} - \theta_0, w^*\rangle = \sqrt{n}(P_n - P)\dot{l}_n(\theta_0|\mathbf{V})[w^*] + o_p(1) \to_d N(0, \|w^*\|^2), (36)$$

where $\|w^*\|^2 = P(\dot{l}_n(\theta_0|\mathbf{V})[w^*])^2 = \|\dot{\mathcal{Q}}(\theta_0)\|^2$. By (14) and (15), we get

$$\sqrt{n}(\mathcal{Q}(\hat{\theta}) - \mathcal{Q}(\theta_0)) = \sqrt{n}\dot{\mathcal{Q}}(\theta_0)[\hat{\theta} - \theta_0] = \sqrt{n}\langle\hat{\theta} - \theta_0, w^*\rangle \to_d N(0, \|\dot{\mathcal{Q}}(\theta_0)\|^2).$$

□

References

Bickel, P. J., Klaassen, C. A., Bickel, P. J., Ritov, Y., Klaassen, J., Wellner, J. A., & Ritov, Y. (1993). *Efficient and adaptive estimation for semiparametric models* (Vol. 4). Baltimore: Johns Hopkins University Press.

Chen, K., Jin, Z., & Ying, Z. (2002). Semiparametric analysis of transformation models with censored data. *Biometrika, 89*(3), 659–668.

Chen, X., Fan, Y., & Tsyrennikov, V. (2006). Efficient estimation of semiparametric multivariate copula models. *Journal of the American Statistical Association, 101*(475), 1228–1240.

Cheng, S., Wei, L., & Ying, Z. (1995). Analysis of transformation models with censored data. *Biometrika, 82*(4), 835–845.

De Gruttola, V., & Lagakos, S. W. (1989). Analysis of doubly-censored survival data, with application to aids. *Biometrics, 45*, 1–11.

Fang, H.-B., & Sun, J. (2001). Consistency of nonparametric maximum likelihood estimation of a distribution function based on doubly interval-censored failure time data. *Statistics and Probability Letters, 55*(3), 311–318.

Geer, S. A., & van de Geer, S. (2000). *Empirical Processes in M-estimation* (Vol. 6). Cambridge: Cambridge University Press.

Hu, T., & Xiang, L. (2016). Partially linear transformation cure models for interval-censored data. *Computational Statistics and Data Analysis, 93*, 257–269.

Hu, T., Zhou, Q., & Sun, J. (2017). Regression analysis of bivariate current status data under the proportional hazards model. *Canadian Journal of Statistics, 45*(4), 410–424.

Huang, J., & Rossini, A. (1997). Sieve estimation for the proportional-odds failure-time regression model with interval censoring. *Journal of the American Statistical Association, 92*(439), 960–967.

Huang, J., & Wellner, J. A. (1997). Interval censored survival data: a review of recent progress. In *Proceedings of the First Seattle Symposium in Biostatistics* (pp. 123–169). Berlin: Springer.

Keiding, N. (1991). Age-specific incidence and prevalence: a statistical perspective. *Journal of the Royal Statistical Society: Series A (Statistics in Society), 154*(3), 371–396.

Kim, J. S. (2003). Efficient estimation for the proportional hazards model with left-truncated and case 1 interval-censored data. *Statistica Sinica, 13*(2), 519–537.

Kim, M. Y., De Gruttola, V. G., & Lagakos, S. W. (1993). Analyzing doubly censored data with covariates, with application to aids. *Biometrics, 49*(1), 13–22.

Lange, K. (1994). An adaptive barrier method for convex programming. *Methods and Applications of Analysis, 1*(4), 392–402.

Lorentz, G. G. (2013). *Bernstein polynomials* (2nd ed.). New York: American Mathematical Society.

Lu, M., Zhang, Y., & Huang, J. (2007). Estimation of the mean function with panel count data using monotone polynomial splines. *Biometrika, 94*(3), 705–718.

Lu, S., Wu, J., & Lu, X. (2019). Efficient estimation of the varying-coefficient partially linear proportional odds model with current status data. *Metrika, 82*(2), 173–194.

McLain, A. C., & Ghosh, S. K. (2013). Efficient sieve maximum likelihood estimation of time-transformation models. *Journal of Statistical Theory and Practice, 7*(2), 285–303.

Murphy, S. A., & van der Vaart, A. W. (1997). Semiparametric likelihood ratio inference. *The Annals of Statistics, 25*(4), 1471–1509.

Murphy, S. A., & Van der Vaart, A. W. (2000). On profile likelihood. *Journal of the American Statistical Association, 95*(450), 449–465.

Pan, W., & Chappell, R. (2002). Estimation in the cox proportional hazards model with left-truncated and interval-censored data. *Biometrics, 58*(1), 64–70.

Pollard, D. (1984). *Convergence of Stochastic Processes (Springer Series in Statistics)*. Springer Series in Statistics. New York: Springer.

Rudin, W. (1973). *Functional analysis*. New York: McGraw-Hill.

Shen, P.-S. (2014). Proportional hazards regression with interval-censored and left-truncated data. *Journal of Statistical Computation and Simulation, 84*(2), 264–272.

Shen, P.-S., Chen, H.-J., Pan, W.-H., & Chen, C.-M. (2019). Semiparametric regression analysis for left-truncated and interval-censored data without or with a cure fraction. *Computational Statistics and Data Analysis, 140*, 74–87.

Shen, X. (1997). On methods of sieves and penalization. *The Annals of Statistics, 25*(6), 2555–2591.

Sun, J. (1995). Empirical estimation of a distribution function with truncated and doubly interval-censored data and its application to aids studies. *Biometrics, 51*(3), 1096–1104.

Sun, J. (1997). Self-consistency estimation of distributions based on truncated and doubly censored survival data with applications to aids cohort studies. *Lifetime Data Analysis, 3*(4), 305–313.

Sun, J. (2006). *The Statistical Analysis of Interval-Censored Failure Time Data*. New York: Springer.

Sun, J., & Kalbfleisch, J. D. (1996). Nonparametric tests of tumor prevalence data. *Biometrics, 52*(2), 726–731.

van der Vaart, A. (1998). *Asymptotic Statistics*. Cambridge: Cambridge University Press.

van der Vaart, A., & Wellner, J. A. (1996). *Weak convergence and empirical processes*. New York: Springer.

Wang, P., Li, D., & Sun, J. (2020). A pairwise pseudo-likelihood approach for left-truncated and interval-censored data under the cox model. *Biometrics,77*(4), 1303–1314 (2021). DOI: 10.1111/biom.13394.

Wang, P., Tong, X., Zhao, S., & Sun, J. (2015). Regression analysis of left-truncated and case i interval-censored data with the additive hazards model. *Communications in Statistics-Theory and Methods, 44*(8), 1537–1551.

Wang, P., Zhao, H., & Sun, J. (2016). Regression analysis of case k interval-censored failure time data in the presence of informative censoring. *Biometrics, 72*(4), 1103–1112.

Wellner, J. A., Zhang, Y., et al. (2007). Two likelihood-based semiparametric estimation methods for panel count data with covariates. *The Annals of Statistics, 35*(5), 2106–2142.

Zeng, D., Cai, J., & Shen, Y. (2006). Semiparametric additive risks model for interval-censored data. *Statistica Sinica, 16*(1), 287–302.

Zhang, B., Tong, X., Zhang, J., Wang, C., & Sun, J. (2013). Efficient estimation for linear transformation models with current status data. *Communications in Statistics-Theory and Methods, 42*(17), 3191–3203.

Zhang, Y., Hua, L., & Huang, J. (2010). A spline-based semiparametric maximum likelihood estimation method for the cox model with interval-censored data. *Scandinavian Journal of Statistics, 37*(2), 338–354.

A Review of Flexible Transformations for Modeling Compositional Data

Michail Tsagris and Connie Stewart

Abstract Vectors of non-negative components carrying only relative information, and often normalized to sum to one, are referred to as compositional data and their sample space is the simplex. Compositional data arise in many applications across a variety of disciplines such as ecology, geology, demography, and economics to name a few. For some time, log-ratio methods have been a popular approach for analyzing compositional data and have motivated much of the recent research in the area. In this paper, we consider two recently proposed transformations for data defined on the simplex. The first, referred to as the α-transformation, transforms the data from the simplex to a subset of Euclidean space while a more complex transformation, involving folding, results in data with Euclidean sample space. In both cases, the transformed data are assumed to follow a multivariate normal distribution and the parameter α provides flexibility compared to the traditional log-ratio transformations. Through an empirical study using several real-life data sets we illustrate that the α-transformation may be sufficient and preferred in practice compared to the α-folded model, and further that it is often needed over the log-ratio transformation.

Keywords α-folding transformation · α-transformation · Compositional data · Isometric log-ratio transformation

1 Introduction

In many multivariate data analysis applications, the variables carry only relative information and the data are then commonly normalized to sum to one. Such data are

M. Tsagris
Department of Economics, University of Crete, Rethymnon, Greece
e-mail: mtsagris@uoc.gr

C. Stewart (✉)
Department of Mathematics and Statistics, University of New Brunswick, Saint John, NB, Canada
e-mail: cstewart@unb.ca

© The Author(s), under exclusive license to Springer Nature Switzerland AG 2022   225
W. He et al. (eds.), *Advances and Innovations in Statistics and Data Science*, ICSA
Book Series in Statistics, https://doi.org/10.1007/978-3-031-08329-7_10

referred to as compositional data and the corresponding variables as components. Numerous examples of compositional data arising in practice are cited in Tsagris and Stewart (2020) and, in Sect. 3, additional examples of compositional data from a variety of disciplines are presented. While examples of compositional data are widespread, modeling compositional data presents some statistical challenges due, predominantly, to their restricted sample space. More specifically, the corresponding sample space for a D-part composition, $\mathbf{x} = (x_1, x_2, \ldots, x_D)$, is the simplex, defined as

$$
\mathcal{S}^{D-1} = \left\{ \mathbf{x} = (x_1, x_2, \ldots, x_D) : x_i > 0,\ i = 1, 2, \ldots D,\ \sum_{i=1}^{D} x_i = 1 \right\}.
$$

Note that due to the constraint, $\sum_{i=1}^{D} x_i = 1$, only $D - 1$ components are needed to determine the composition.

The analysis of compositional data relies on the availability of appropriate models. Although the Dirichlet distribution, with its support the simplex, may, in some applications, be sufficient to model compositional data directly (that is, without transforming the data), some of its properties limit its flexibility (see Aitchison 2003). Alternatively, common practice to modeling compositional data, originating from Aitchison (2003), involves transforming the data from the simplex ($\mathcal{S}^{D-1}$) to Euclidean space ($\mathcal{R}^{D-1}$) using a log-ratio transformation so that standard multivariate procedures may then be applicable. The isometric log-ratio transformation (Egozcuef et al. 2003) is one such popular transformation and is defined in Sect. 2. One issue with any log-ratio transformation approach, however, is that there is no guarantee that the transformed data are multivariate normally distributed, a requirement for many conventional multivariate procedures. Another difficulty is that a log-ratio transformation cannot be applied to data sets containing zeros, at least without first modifying the zeros. While several imputation approaches have been proposed (see, for instance, Palarea-Albaladejo et al. (2007) and Palarea-Albaladejo and Martín-Fernández (2008)), these methods are not ideal when there are a significant number of zeros in the data or the zeros are legitimately zero (that is, not due to rounding). As a means of handling the problem of modeling zeros in the compositional data directly, Stephens (1982) and Scealy and Welsh (2011,b) made use of the square root transformation. Another approach developed by Stewart and Field (2011) involves dividing the data according to where the zeros occur and, within each group, modeling the nonzero components in the compositions using a log-ratio transformation. A mixture model is then used to describe the data.

The α-transformation, analogous to the Box-Cox transformation, was proposed by Tsagris et al. (2011) and includes the isometric log-ratio transformation as α converges to 0. While this transformation (defined in Sect. 2) provides flexibility and has been used effectively in a variety of situations (Tsagris 2015; Scealy et al. 2015; Tsagris et al. 2016, 2017; Ankam and Bouguila 2018), a theoretical drawback is that it transforms the compositional data from $\mathcal{S}^{D-1}$ to a subset of $\mathcal{R}^{D-1}$. In Tsagris and Stewart (2020), the α-folding transformation was introduced as an extension to the α-transformation with the purpose of ensuring a transformation from $\mathcal{S}^{D-1}$ to $\mathcal{R}^{D-1}$. This desirable property, however, is accompanied by added complexity. Note that an alternative folding model for compositional data was proposed by Scealy and Welsh (2014b) as a means of dealing with the same issue that arises with the square root transformation of Scealy and Welsh (2011,b).

In this paper, several data sets are examined to evaluate empirically how frequently the folding is indeed needed in practice. In addition, the value of using the α parameter over its competitor, the isometric log-ratio transformation is considered. The findings in this paper will inform (1) researchers who are working on extending and developing new methodology for the analysis of compositional data and (2) practitioners seeking suitable, but unnecessarily complicated, models.

2 Transformations for Compositional Data

2.1 Isometric Log-Ratio Transformation

Conventionally, Aitchison's log-ratio transformation methodology has been used to transform compositional data to multivariate normality (Aitchison 2003). Arising from this work is the so-called isometric log-ratio (ilr) transformation approach (Egozcuef et al. 2003) which, based heavily on its mathematical properties, has been promoted in the compositional data literature.

For a composition $\mathbf{x} = (x_1, x_2, \ldots, x_D)$, we define the ilr transformation as

$$\mathbf{z}(\mathbf{x}) = \mathbf{H}\mathbf{w}_0(\mathbf{x}), \tag{1}$$

where

$$\mathbf{w}_0(\mathbf{x}) = \log\left(\frac{x_i}{\prod_{j=1}^{D} x_j^{1/D}}\right), \quad \text{for } i = 1, \ldots, D$$

and $\mathbf{H}$ is the Helmert matrix (an orthonormal $D \times D$ matrix) after deletion of the first row (Lancaster 1965). The transformation $\mathbf{w}_0(\mathbf{x})$ is the centered log ratio (clr) transformation defined in Aitchison (1983). The D clr transformed components sum to 0 and, with this transformation, the issue of the unit sum constraint is simply replaced by a zero sum constraint. Multiplication by $\mathbf{H}$ results in a transformation from $\mathcal{S}^{D-1}$ to $\mathcal{R}^{D-1}$ and the transformed data are no longer constrained. The function call *alfa(x,0)* in the R package *Compositional* (Tsagris et al. 2020) can be used to transform nonzero compositional data using the above ilr transformation.

2.2 α-transformation

A more general Box-Cox type transformation involving a power transformation α was developed by Tsagris et al. (2011), and termed the α-transformation, defined as

$$\mathbf{z}_\alpha(\mathbf{x}) = \mathbf{H}\mathbf{w}_\alpha(\mathbf{x}), \tag{2}$$

where

$$\mathbf{w}_\alpha(\mathbf{x}) = \frac{D\mathbf{u}_\alpha - 1}{\alpha}$$

and

$$\mathbf{u}_\alpha(\mathbf{x}) = \left(\frac{x_1^\alpha}{\sum_{j=1}^D x_j^\alpha}, \ldots, \frac{x_D^\alpha}{\sum_{j=1}^D x_j^\alpha} \right)^T .$$

As $\alpha \to 0$, the α-transformation in Eq. (2) converges to the ilr transformation. For convenience purposes, α is generally restricted to the interval $[-1, 1]$, but this interval can be reduced to $(0, 1]$ if there are zeros in the data. The parameter α can be estimated via maximum likelihood estimation, assuming the α-transformed data follow a multivariate normal distribution, with the resulting distribution called the α-normal distribution (Tsagris et al. 2011). In the *R* package *Compositional*, the optimal value of α is chosen via the function *alfa.tune* and function *alfa(x, a)* transforms the data.

The α-transformation is one-to-one and maps the data inside $\mathcal{S}^{D-1}$ to a **subset** of $(D-1)$-dimensional real space, $\mathbb{A}^{D-1}$, given by

$$\mathbb{A}^{D-1} = \left\{ \mathbf{H}\mathbf{w}_\alpha \left| -\frac{1}{\alpha} \leq w_{i,\alpha} \leq \frac{D-1}{\alpha}, \sum_{i=1}^D w_{i,\alpha} = 0 \right. \right\} .$$

In theory, using this transformation approach may neglect an important amount of probability of the multivariate normal distribution. This potential shortcoming motivated the development of the α-folding transformation recently introduced in Tsagris and Stewart (2020) and defined below in Sect. 2.3.

2.3 α-Folding Transformation

The following extension to the α-transformation in Eq. (2) was shown by Tsagris and Stewart (2020) to be a one-to-one transformation from the simplex to $(D-1)$-dimensional real space:

$$y = \begin{cases} z_\alpha(x) & \text{with probability } p \\ \dfrac{z_\alpha(x)}{w_\alpha^{*2}(x)} & \text{with probability } 1 - p, \end{cases} \qquad (3)$$

where $w_\alpha^*(x) = \alpha \min \{w_{1,\alpha}(x), \ldots, w_{D,\alpha}(x)\}$ and $z_\alpha(x) = Hw_\alpha(x)$.

The inverse of Eq. (3) is referred to as the α-**folding transformation** and is as follows

$$x = \begin{cases} z_\alpha^{-1}(y) & \text{if } y \in \mathbb{A}^{D-1} \\ w_\alpha^{-1}\left(\dfrac{H^T y}{q_\alpha^{*2}(y)}\right) & \text{if } y \in \mathbb{R}^{D-1} \setminus \mathbb{A}^{D-1}, \end{cases} \qquad (4)$$

where $q_\alpha^*(y) = \alpha \min \{H^T y\}$.

If $y \sim N_{D-1}(\mu_\alpha, \Sigma_\alpha)$ then (Tsagris and Stewart 2020) showed that the distribution of x, defined as in Eq. (4), is given below

$$f(x|\alpha, p, \mu_\alpha, \Sigma_\alpha) = p \frac{|J_\alpha^0|}{|2\pi \Sigma_\alpha|^{1/2}} \times \exp\left[-\frac{1}{2}(z_\alpha(x) - \mu_\alpha)^T \Sigma_\alpha^{-1}(z_\alpha(x) - \mu_\alpha)\right]$$

$$+ (1 - p) \frac{|J_\alpha^1|}{|2\pi \Sigma_\alpha|^{1/2}}$$

$$\times \exp\left[-\frac{1}{2}\left(\frac{z_\alpha(x)}{w_\alpha^{*2}(x)} - \mu_\alpha\right)^T \Sigma_\alpha^{-1}\left(\frac{z_\alpha(x)}{w_\alpha^{*2}(x)} - \mu_\alpha\right)\right], \quad (5)$$

where $x \in S^{D-1}$, $\alpha \in [-1, 1]$, $0 \leq p \leq 1$. Also, $|J_\alpha^0| = D^{D-1+\frac{1}{2}} \prod_{i=1}^{D} \frac{x_i^{\alpha-1}}{\sum_{j=1}^{D} x_j^\alpha}$ and $|J_\alpha^1| = \left(\frac{1}{\alpha w^*(x)}\right)^{2(D-1)}$.

Note that compositional data with zeros cannot be directly modeled by this distribution due to the product in $|J_\alpha^0|$. The authors of Tsagris and Stewart (2020) used the EM algorithm for parameter estimation and this may be carried out using the function *alpha.mle* in the package *R* package *Compositional*, while the function *a.est* selects the optimal value of α.

In this paper, we are specifically interested in the parameters α and p. If the estimate of α is close to zero, then this suggests that the α-transformation in Eq. (2) is not needed and that the ilr transformation in Eq. (1) may be sufficient for the data set at hand. With respect to p, note that $1-p$ can be interpreted as the probability that a vector y is outside of $\mathbb{A}^{D-1}$ (or equivalently that a composition x needs to be folded into the simplex). If $p = 1$ (and $1 - p = 0$), then the density in Eq. (5), reduces to the α-normal distribution in Tsagris et al. (2011). Therefore, in practice, if $1 - p$ is estimated to be close to zero, then the sample space of $z_\alpha(x)$ will be approximately equal to $\mathbb{R}^{D-1}$ and the α-transformation should suffice without the need for folding. Several real-life data sets are explored in Sect. 3 to determine how often the α-transformation tends to be advantageous compared to the ilr transformation, as well as whether folding is typically needed in practice.

3 Real-life Data Applications

To investigate the applicability of the two α-transformations and the ilr transformation in practice, 44 real-life data sets obtained from books, papers, websites, and R packages were examined. Details on the source of the data sets may be found in Table 1. For each data set, the data were first transformed using the α-transformation in Eq. (2) and then a multivariate normal distribution was fit to the transformed data. Using the resulting optimal parameters, 40 million observations were generated from the fitted distribution and the probability left outside the simplex (that is, an estimate of $1 - p$) was computed by determining the proportion of observations that belong to $\mathbb{R}^{D-1} \setminus \mathbb{A}^{D-1}$.

The results appear in Table 2. The sample sizes range from 20 to 485 and the number of components, D, from 3 to 14. The optimal value of the α-transformation in Eq. (2) is reported along with the relevant 95% confidence intervals which reveal whether a value other than 0 yields better results. The confidence intervals were obtained assuming asymptotic normality and the observed Fisher's information (see Tsagris and Stewart 2020). If the 95% confidence interval for the true value of α does not include 0, then this is evidence that the ilr transformation in Eq. (1) is not

Table 1 Data references

Data set	Reference	Data set	Reference
activity10	Aitchison (2003)	juraset	Atteia et al. (1994)
activity31	Aitchison (2003)	lake	Aitchison (2003)
animal	Aitchison (2003)	mn	Greenacre (2009)
buxeda	Buxeda i Garrigós (2008)	mammals	Hartigan (1975)
catalan	Greenacre (2002)	metabolites	Aitchison (2003)
cleameast	Aitchison (2003)	pottery	Baxter et al. (2005)
clamwest	Aitchison (2003)	qrf	Skilbeck (1985)
coffee	Templ et al. (2010)	serum	Aitchison (2003)
diagnosticprob	Aitchison (2003)	shift	Aitchison (2003)
economics	Larrosa (2003)	skulls	Aitchison (2003)
eu04	Eurostat	skyAFM	Aitchison (2003)
eu05	Eurostat	students	DASL library
eu06	Eurostat	twins$_1$	Aitchison (2003)
eu07	Eurostat	twins$_2$	Aitchison (2003)
geochem	compositional.data.com	volley	Louzada et al. (2018)
gdpreg	Eurostat	whitecells$_1$	Aitchison (2003)
glass	Baxter et al. (1990)	whitecells$_2$	Aitchison (2003)
halimba	compositional.data.com	wines	Hron et al. (2012)
household	Aitchison (2003)	yatquat1	Aitchison (2003)
hydrochem	Otero et al. (2005)	yatquat2	Aitchison (2003)
jobs	DASL library	carseg	Graf (2020)
serumprotein	Aitchison (2003)	oecd	DASL library

Table 2 Comparison of the α and the α-folding transformations to 44 data sets. The columns n and D contain the sample size the number of components, respectively. The column $\hat{\alpha}$ contains the optimal value of the α-transformation and the next two column its relevant 95% confidence interval. The values of α that are statistically significantly different from 0 are denoted by an asterisk. The column $1 - \hat{p}$ contains the estimated probability left outside $\mathcal{S}^{D-1}$

Name	n	D	$\hat{\alpha}$	95% CI	$1 - \hat{p}$	Name	n	D	$\hat{\alpha}$	95% CI	$1 - \hat{p}$
activity10	20	6	0.12	(−1.00, 1.00)	0.00	juraset	359	7	−0.01	(−0.11, 0.09)	0.00
activity31	20	6	0.76	(−0.55, 1.00)	0.00	lake	39	3	0.36*	(0.20, 0.52)	0.01
animal	100	4	0.05	(−0.16, 0.25)	0.00	mn	24	3	−0.05	(−0.23, 0.13)	0.00
buxeda	43	5	0.66	(−1.00, 1.00)	0.00	mammals	24	5	0.29*	(0.05, 0.52)	0.00
catalan	41	9	1.00*	(1.00, 1.00)	0.26*	metabolites	67	3	0.49*	(0.22, 0.72)	0.00
cleameast	20	6	0.43	(−0.39, 1.00)	0.00	pottery	45	9	0.22*	(0.04, 0.35)	0.00
clamwest	20	6	0.09	(−0.81, 0.89)	0.00	qrf	75	3	0.46*	(0.20, 0.69)	0.00
coffee	27	3	0.48	(−0.05, 0.98)	0.00	serum	23	3	0.51	(−0.69, 1.00)	0.00
diagnosticprob	30	4	−0.09	(−0.51, 0.32)	0.00	shift	27	4	−0.09	(−0.72, 0.50)	0.00
economics	56	5	0.32*	(0.15, 0.48)	0.00	skulls	102	3	−1.00*	(−1.00, −0.27)	0.00
eu04	34	6	0.63	(−0.10, 1.00)	0.00	skyAFM	23	3	−0.06	(−0.41, 0.26)	0.00
eu05	34	6	0.52	(−0.29, 1.00)	0.00	students	50	3	−0.26	(−0.48, 0.00)	0.00
eu06	34	6	0.53	(−0.35, 1.00)	0.00	twins$_1$	33	5	0.83	(−1.00, 1.00)	0.00
eu07	34	6	0.60	(−0.27, 1.00)	0.00	twins$_2$	33	4	0.91	(−0.05, 1.00)	0.00
geochem	87	10	0.05	(−0.05, 0.15)	0.00	volley	127	3	0.18*	(0.03, 0.31)	0.00
gdpreg	27	13	0.27*	(0.09, 0.45)	0.00	whitecells$_1$	30	3	−0.34*	(−0.61, −0.06)	0.03
glass	47	11	−0.51*	(−0.84, −0.03)	1.00*	whitecells$_2$	30	3	−0.31*	(−0.57, −0.04)	0.01
halimba	332	6	0.45*	(0.38, 0.52)	0.00	wines	30	8	0.26*	(0.14, 0.38)	0.00
household	40	4	−0.04	(−0.14, 0.05)	0.00	yatquat1	40	3	0.37	(−1.00, 1.00)	0.00
hydrochem	485	14	0.02*	(0.01, 0.04)	0.00	yatquat2	40	3	−0.64	(−1.00, 0.83)	0.00
jobs	26	9	0.17	(−0.04, 0.38)	0.00	carseg	152	5	−0.49*	(−0.70, −0.26)	0.12*
serumprotein	36	4	0.21	(−0.52, 0.92)	0.00	oecd	20	4	−0.04	(−0.41, 0.29)	0.00

sufficient. The α-transformation showed that a value other than 0 was statistically significant (using a 5% significance level) in 17 out of the 44 data sets (or almost 39% of the data sets), providing evidence that the α-transformation (over the ilr transformation) should be used in these cases. The statistically significant results are denoted by an asterisk.

In terms of the necessity of folding, the column $1 - \hat{p}$, provides the estimated probability left outside the simplex when the α-normal model is used. In only 6 of the data sets is the probability left outside the simplex nonzero. Furthermore, in three of these cases, the probability may be considered to be inconsequential (since $1 - \hat{p}$ is less than or equal to 0.03). Probabilities greater than 0.03 are denoted by * in Table 2.

4 Conclusion

The prevailing recommended approach for modeling compositional data is to log-transform the data (using the ilr transformation) from the simplex to Euclidean space, and then to assume multivariate normality in order to subsequently apply standard multivariate procedures. Akin to the well-known Box-Cox transformation, the α-transformation, with the corresponding α-normal distribution, has the potential to provide a better fit over the ilr transformation. This transformation, when the range of possible α values is restricted to be greater than zero, also allows problematic zeros in the data to be modeled without any modifications. A downside, however, is that the sample space of the transformed data is a subset of Euclidean space. Theoretically speaking, this could mean that some probability is omitted with the assumption of multivariate normality. Furthermore, in Tsagris and Stewart (2020), it was shown through simulations that, not surprisingly, when this probability is large, parameter estimates based on the α-transformation may be substantially biased compared to those obtained using the α-folded transformation, which was developed to account for this potentially missing probability. For additional simulation study results regarding parameter estimation, as well as computational costs, of the folded model, see Tsagris and Stewart (2020).

The purpose of this work was to review and compare transformations to multivariate normality for compositional data from a practical point of view. In particular, we wanted to address, using a diverse set of examples whether the α-transformation tends to be advantageous over the ilr transformation and whether the more complex (but theoretically sound) α-folding transformation should be commonplace over the α-transformation. While we did identify that, in the majority of the cases (61% of the 44 data sets) the α-transformation favored a value of $\alpha = 0$ (indicating that the ilr transformation is more suitable in these cases), the ilr transformation is clearly not the panacea transformation for all compositional data. Among the data sets, in only 3 cases was the α-folding transformation preferred as the probability left outside the simplex when using the α-transformation was substantial. This in turn reveals that, in practice, the simpler α-transformation may suffice.

It should be emphasized that the choice of α was based on maximum likelihood estimation. In the regression and classification settings, α has been estimated using cross-validation methods (Tsagris 2014, 2015; Tsagris et al. 2016) and therefore our conclusions cannot be extended to these frameworks where no such large empirical study has been conducted. Note, however, that an advantage of the α-transformation in these settings, in contrast to the ilr transformation, is that it is unaffected by the presence of zeros, thus treating this problem naturally.

References

Aitchison, J. (1983). Principal component analysis of compositional data. *Biometrika 70*(1), 57–65.

Aitchison, J. (2003). *The statistical analysis of compositional data*. New Jersey: The Blackburn Press.

Ankam, D., & Bouguila, N. (2018). Compositional data analysis with PLS-DA and security applications. In: *Proceedings of the 2018 IEEE International Conference on Information Reuse and Integration (IRI)* (pp. 338–345).

Atteia, O., Dubois, J., & Webster, R. (1994). Geostatistical analysis of soil contamination in the Swiss Jura. *Environmental Pollution, 86*(3), 315–327.

Baxter, M., Cool, H., & Heyworth, M. (1990). Principal component and correspondence analysis of compositional data: some similarities. *Journal of Applied Statistics, 17*(2), 229–235.

Baxter, M., Beardah, C., Cool, H., & Jackson, C. (2005). Compositional data analysis of some alkaline glasses. *Mathematical Geology, 37*(2), 183–196.

Buxeda i Garrigós, J. (2008). Revisiting the compositional data. Some fundamental questions and new prospects in Archaeometry and Archaeology. In: *Proceedings of the 3rd Compositional Data Analysis Workshop, Girona, Spain*

Egozcue, J., Pawlowsky-Glahn, V., Mateu-Figueras, G., & Barceló-Vidal, C. (2003). Isometric logratio transformations for compositional data analysis. *Mathematical Geology, 35*(3), 279–300.

Graf, M. (2020). SGB: Simplicial Generalized Beta Regression. https://CRAN.R-project.org/package=SGB. R package version 1.0.1.

Greenacre, M. (2002). Ratio maps and correspondence analysis. Tech. rep., Spain: Universitat Pompeu Fabra.

Greenacre, M. (2009). Power transformations in correspondence analysis. *Computational Statistics & Data Analysis, 53*(8), 3107–3116.

Hartigan, J. (1975). *Clustering algorithms*. New York: Willey.

Hron, K., Jelínková, M., Filzmoser, P., Kreuziger, R., Bednář, P., & Barták, P. (2012). Statistical analysis of wines using a robust compositional biplot. *Talanta, 90*, 46–50.

Lancaster, H. (1965). The Helmert matrices. *American Mathematical Monthly, 72*(1), 4–12.

Larrosa, J. (2003). A compositional statistical analysis of capital stock. In: *Proceedings of the 1st Compositional Data Analysis Workshop, Girona, Spain*.

Louzada, F., Shimizu, T.K., Suzuki, A.K., Mazucheli, J., & Ferreira, P.H. (2018). Compositional regression modeling under tilted normal errors: An application to a brazilian super league volleyball data set. *Chilean Journal of Statistics (ChJS), 9*(2), 33–53.

Otero, N., Tolosana-Delgado, R., Soler, A., Pawlowsky-Glahn, V., & Canals, A. (2005). Relative vs. absolute statistical analysis of compositions: A comparative study of surface waters of a Mediterranean river. *Water Research, 39*(7), 1404–1414.

Palarea-Albaladejo, J., Martín-Fernández, J. (2008). A modified EM alr-algorithm for replacing rounded zeros in compositional data sets. *Computers & Geosciences, 34*(8), 902–917.

Palarea-Albaladejo, J., Martín-Fernández, J., & Gómez-García, J. (2007). A parametric approach for dealing with compositional rounded zeros. *Mathematical Geology, 39*(7), 625–645.

Scealy, J., & Welsh, A. (2011). Properties of a square root transformation regression model. In: *Proceedings of the 4rth Compositional Data Analysis Workshop, Girona, Spain.*

Scealy, J., & Welsh, A. (2011). Regression for compositional data by using distributions defined on the hypersphere. *Journal of the Royal Statistical Society. Series B, 73*(3), 351–375.

Scealy, J., Welsh, A. (2014b). Colours and cocktails: Compositional data analysis 2013 Lancaster lecture. *Australian & New Zealand Journal of Statistics, 56*(2), 145–169.

Scealy, J., De Caritat, P., Grunsky, E.C., Tsagris, M.T., & Welsh, A. (2015). Robust principal component analysis for power transformed compositional data. *Journal of the American Statistical Association, 110*(509), 136–148.

Skilbeck, C. (1985). Sedimentological Development of the Myall Trough: Carboniferous Forearc Basin. Ph.D. thesis, Australia: The University of Sydney.

Stephens, M.A.: Use of the von Mises distribution to analyse continuous proportions. *Biometrika, 69*(1), 197–203 (1982).

Stewart, C., & Field, C. (2011). Managing the Essential Zeros in Quantitative Fatty Acid Signature Analysis. *Journal of Agricultural, Biological, and Environmental Statistics, 16*(1), 45–69.

Templ, M., Hron, K., & Filzmoser, P. (2010). robCompositions: Robust Estimation for Compositional Data. R package version, vol. 1(3).

Tsagris, M. (2014). The k-NN algorithm for compositional data: a revised approach with and without zero values present. *Journal of Data Science, 12*(3), 519–534.

Tsagris, M. (2015). Regression analysis with compositional data containing zero values. *Chilean Journal of Statistics, 6*(2), 47–57.

Tsagris, M., Preston, S., & Wood, A. (2011). A data-based power transformation for compositional data. In: *Proceedings of the 4rth Compositional Data Analysis Workshop, Girona, Spain.*

Tsagris, M., Preston, S., & Wood, A. T. (2016). Improved classification for compositional data using the α-transformation. *Journal of Classification, 33*(2), 243–261.

Tsagris, M., Preston, S., & Wood, A.T. (2017). Nonparametric hypothesis testing for equality of means on the simplex. *Journal of Statistical Computation and Simulation, 87*(2), 406–422

Tsagris, M., & Stewart, C. (2020). A folded model for compositional data analysis. *Australian & New Zealand Journal of Statistics, 62*(2), 249–277.

Tsagris, M., Athineou, G., & Alenazi, A. (2020). Compositional: Compositional Data Analysis. https://CRAN.R-project.org/package=Compositional. R package version 4.3.

Identifiability and Estimation of Autoregressive ARCH Models with Measurement Error

Mustafa Salamh and Liqun Wang

Abstract The autoregressive conditional heteroscedasticity (ARCH) model and its various generalizations have been widely used to analyze economic and financial data. Although many variables like GDP, inflation, and commodity prices are imprecisely measured, research focusing on the mismeasured response processes in GARCH models is sparse. We study a dynamic model with ARCH error where the underlying process is latent and subject to additive measurement error. We show that, in contrast to the case of covariate measurement error, this model is identifiable by using the observations of the proxy process only and no extra information is needed. We construct GMM estimators for the unknown parameters which are consistent and asymptotically normally distributed under general conditions. We also propose a procedure to test the presence of measurement error, which avoids the usual boundary problem of testing variance parameters. We carry out Monte Carlo simulations to study the impact of measurement error on the naive maximum likelihood estimators and have found interesting patterns of their biases. Moreover, the proposed estimators have fairly good finite sample properties.

Keywords Dynamic ARCH model · Errors in variables · Generalized method of moments · Measurement error · Semiparametric estimation

1 Introduction

Since the seminal works of Engle (1982) and Bollerslev (1986), the autoregressive conditional heteroscedasticity (ARCH) model and its various generalizations have been widely used to analyze economic and financial data, such as GDP, inflation,

M. Salamh
Department of Statistics, Cairo University, Giza, Egypt
e-mail: Mustafa.Salamh@feps.edu.eg

L. Wang (✉)
Department of Statistics, University of Manitoba, Winnipeg, MB, Canada
e-mail: Liqun.Wang@umanitoba.ca

© The Author(s), under exclusive license to Springer Nature Switzerland AG 2022
W. He et al. (eds.), *Advances and Innovations in Statistics and Data Science*, ICSA
Book Series in Statistics, https://doi.org/10.1007/978-3-031-08329-7_11

stock prices, and interest rates, see, e.g., Grier and Perry (2000), Engle et al. (2008), Fang and Miller (2009), Teräsvirta (2009), Francq and Zakoian (2011), and Caporale et al. (2012). Moreover, there is also a large number of empirical studies of agricultural and industrial commodity prices using ARCH/GARCH models, e.g., Ramirez and Fadiga (2003), Roche and McQuinn (2003), and Reitz and Westerhoff (2007). However, it is well documented in the literature that many economic variables including GDP, inflation and commodity prices are imprecisely measured. For example, Wansbeek and Meijer (2000) and Buonaccorsi (2013) provide broad surveys on the issues of measurement errors and their impacts in econometric models. In particular, Alberini and Filippini (2011) emphasize that the US energy prices are mismeasured, while Fan and Wang (2007) point out that high-frequency financial data are particularly noisy. Furthermore, Handbury et al. (2013) investigate the informativeness and bias of the consumer price index (CPI) as a proxy for the "true" inflation and use a classical measurement error model to test for bias in Japanese CPI. This raises an interesting question whether the "ARCH behavior" is only a manifest phenomenon in empirical (observed) processes, or it is an intrinsic property of the underlying (unobserved) processes. Therefore it is of theoretical and practical interests to investigate the problem and impact of measurement error in ARCH-type models.

The errors-in-variables problem has been extensively studied in statistics and econometrics, see, e.g., Carroll et al. (2006); Chen et al. (2011); Wang and Hsiao (2011); Yi et al. (2021), and the references therein. However, most of the research focuses mainly on the problem of measurement error in covariates in regression models. For dynamic models, Staudenmayer and Buonaccorsi (2005) studied autoregressive (AR) model with white noise errors and mismeasured response process, while Buonaccorsi (2010) gives an overview of estimation in dynamic models. Some researchers, e.g., Harvey et al. (1992), Gourieroux et al. (1993) and Francq and Zakoïan (2000), have considered GARCH models where the innovation term contains an unobserved white noise component. However, research focusing on the mismeasured response processes in GARCH models is sparse and even answers to very basic questions are not known. For example, what is the impact of measurement error on parameter estimation and inference? Under what conditions is the model identifiable? How to quantify and correct the estimation bias caused by measurement error?

In this paper we attempt to address some of these questions. To simplify notation and analysis, we start with an autoregressive model with ARCH innovation where the true latent process is measured with additive white noise error process. In contrast to the models with covariate measurement error, we show that all model parameters are identifiable by the observed proxy process only and no extra information is needed. Moreover, we propose a set of moment conditions that are sufficient for the identifiability and therefore can used to construct GMM estimators for the unknown parameters. We investigate the impact of measurement error on the parameter estimation in dynamic ARCH models through Monte Carlo simulations. In particular, we show that the measurement error induces biases in the naive maximum likelihood estimators and the relative biases have certain functional forms. We also develop a statistical test for the presence of measurement error, which is useful because more efficient GMM or maximum quasi-likelihood estimators can be used if the measurement error is found to be absent or ignorable. Finally, we carry out Monte Carlo simulations to examine the finite sample behavior of our proposed estimators and compare them with the naive maximum likelihood estimators.

The paper is organized as follows. In Sect. 2 we introduce the model and show it is identifiable without extra information. In Sect. 3 we construct the GMM estimators and provide their asymptotic properties. In Sect. 4 we propose a test for the measurement error. Further, we carry out Monte Carlo simulations to study the impact of measurement error on the naive estimators in Sect. 5 and to examine the finite sample properties of the proposed estimators and compare them with the naive MLE in Sect. 6. Finally, conclusions and discussions are given in Sect. 7, while regularity assumptions and mathematical proofs are in the Appendix.

2 The Model and Identifiability

Let $\{X_t\}$ be the unique nonanticipative strictly stationary solution of the following AR(p)-ARCH(q) model (Francq and Zakoian 2011, Ch. 7)

$$_t = \alpha_0(B) X_t + \epsilon_t, \quad t \in \mathbb{Z}, \tag{1}$$

$$\epsilon_t = \sqrt{h_t}\eta_t, \quad h_t = \omega_0 + \beta_0(B)\epsilon_t^2, \tag{2}$$

where $\alpha_0(B) = \sum_{i=1}^{p} \alpha_{0i} B^i$, $\beta_0(B) = \sum_{j=1}^{q} \beta_{0j} B^j$, B is the backshift operator, and $\{\eta_t\}$ is a sequence of iid random variables with $E(\eta_t) = 0$ and $E(\eta_t^2) = 1$. Under this model $\{X_t\}$ is second-order stationary if the unknown parameters satisfy $\omega_0 > 0$, $\beta_{0j} \geq 0$, $j = 1, 2, \ldots, q$, $\sum_{j=1}^{q} \beta_{0j} < 1$ and $\alpha_0(z) \neq 1$ for all $|z| \leq 1$. Moreover, under these conditions $\{X_t\}$ is strictly stationary and ergodic (Francq and Zakoian 2011, Th. 2.5).

Assume that $\{X_t\}$ is not directly observable and instead we observe the proxy process

$$Z_t = X_t + \delta_t, \tag{3}$$

where the measurement error process $\{\delta_t\}$ is iid with $E(\delta_t) = 0$, $E(\delta_t^2) = \sigma_0^2$ and is independent of $\{\eta_t\}$. Note that such a classical measurement error model is commonly used in the literature and is also used by Handbury et al. (2013). Our main interest is consistent estimation of unknown parameters $\theta_0 = (\alpha_0', \beta_0', \omega_0, \sigma_0^2)'$, where $\alpha_0' = (\alpha_{01}, \ldots, \alpha_{0p})$ and $\beta_0' = (\beta_{01}, \ldots, \beta_{0q})$. If $\{X_t\}$ were observable, then this can be done by using standard methods such as least squares or quasi-likelihood methods. However, when only observations on $\{Z_t\}$ are available, several issues arise and one of them is the model identifiability.

It is well-known that in a regression model with covariate measurement error usually extra information such as replicate or instrumental data are needed in order for all parameters to be identifiable. Here we demonstrate that, in contrary, all parameters in model (1)–(3) are identifiable based on the observations on $\{Z_t\}$ only. To simplify notation, we consider the case where $p = q = 1$ and let $Y_t = Z_t - \alpha_0 Z_{t-1}$.

Then under model assumptions we have

$$
\begin{aligned}
E(Y_t|Z_s, s \le t - 2) &= E(Z_t|Z_s, s \le t - 2) - \alpha_0 E(Z_{t-1}|Z_s, s \le t - 2) \\
&= E(\epsilon_t|Z_s, s \le t - 2) + E(\delta_t - \alpha_0 \delta_{t-1}|Z_s, s \le t - 2) \\
&= 0.
\end{aligned}
$$

Since both $E(Z_t|Z_s, s \le t-2)$ and $E(Z_{t-1}|Z_s, s \le t-2)$ are observable functions, α_0 is uniquely identified by the above equation. In order to see the identifiability of other parameters, we consider higher moments. In particular, since

$$
E(Y_t Y_{t-1}) = E(-\alpha_0 \delta_{t-1}^2) = -\alpha_0 \sigma_0^2,
$$

σ_0^2 is identified given that α_0 is identified. Further, from

$$
E(Y_t^2|Z_s, s \le t - 3) = \omega_0 + (1 - \beta_0)(1 + \alpha_0^2)\sigma_0^2 + \beta_0 E(Y_{t-1}^2|Z_s, s \le t - 3),
$$

it is easy to see that β_0 and $\omega_0 + (1 - \beta_0)(1 + \alpha_0^2)\sigma_0^2$ are uniquely determined and hence ω_0 is identified.

3   GMM Estimation

Motivated by the above discussion of identifiability, in this section we propose an estimation procedure based on the following conditional moments. Specifically, let

$$
Y_t(\boldsymbol{\alpha}_0) = [1 - \boldsymbol{\alpha}_0(B)]Z_t. \tag{4}
$$

Then under the model assumptions we have (w.p.1)

$$
\begin{aligned}
E\{Y_t(\boldsymbol{\alpha}_0)|Z_s, s < t - p\} &= E\{\epsilon_t|Z_s, s < t - p\} + E\{[1 - \boldsymbol{\alpha}_0(B)]\delta_t|Z_s, s < t - p\} \\
&= 0
\end{aligned} \tag{5}
$$

and

$$
E\left\{[1 - \boldsymbol{\beta}_0(B)]Y_t^2(\boldsymbol{\alpha}_0)|Z_s, s < t - p - q\right\} = \omega_0 + [1x\boldsymbol{\beta}_0(1)][1 + \alpha_0^2(1)]\sigma_0^2. \tag{6}
$$

where $\boldsymbol{\beta}_0(1) = \sum_{j=1}^q \beta_{0j}$ and $\boldsymbol{\alpha}_0^2(1) = \sum_{j=1}^p \alpha_{0j}^2$. In addition, we have the following unconditional moment condition

$$
E\{Y_t(\boldsymbol{\alpha}_0)Y_{t-1}(\boldsymbol{\alpha}_0)\} = \left[\sum_{j=1}^{p-1} \alpha_{0j}\alpha_{0(j+1)} - \alpha_{01}\right]\sigma_0^2. \tag{7}
$$

Therefore a GMM estimator for $\boldsymbol{\theta}_0$ can be constructed as follows. Denote

$$
\boldsymbol{r}_t(\boldsymbol{\theta}) = \begin{pmatrix} Y_t(\boldsymbol{\alpha}) \\ [1 - \boldsymbol{\beta}(B)]\,Y_t^2(\boldsymbol{\alpha}) - \omega - [1 - \boldsymbol{\beta}(1)][1 + \boldsymbol{\alpha}^2(1)]\sigma^2 \\ Y_t(\boldsymbol{\alpha})Y_{t-1}(\boldsymbol{\alpha}) - [\sum_{j=1}^{p-1}\alpha_j\alpha_{j+1} - \alpha_1]\sigma^2 \end{pmatrix} \tag{8}
$$

and the matrix of instrumental functions

$$
\boldsymbol{G}_t = \begin{pmatrix} f_1(\tilde{Z}_{t-p-1}) & 0 & 0 \\ 0 & f_2(\tilde{Z}_{t-p-q-1}) & 0 \\ 0 & 0 & 1 \end{pmatrix}, \tag{9}
$$

where $f_1(\tilde{Z}_{t-p-1})$ is a k_1-vector of measurable functions of $\tilde{Z}_{t-p-1} = (Z_{t-p-1}, Z_{t-p-2}, \ldots)$, $f_2(\tilde{Z}_{t-p-q-1})$ is a k_2-vector of functions of $\tilde{Z}_{t-p-q-1} = (Z_{t-p-q-1}, Z_{t-p-q-2}, \ldots)$, and $k_1 \geq p, k_2 \geq q+1$ are chosen to achieve identification and efficiency. Then from (5)–(7) we have

$$
E\{\boldsymbol{G}_t\boldsymbol{r}_t(\boldsymbol{\theta}_0)\} = 0. \tag{10}
$$

To simplify notation, in the following we assume that $\tilde{Z}_{t-p-1} = (Z_{t-p-1}, \ldots, Z_{t-p-k_1})$ and $\tilde{Z}_{t-p-q-1} = (Z_{t-p-q-1}, \ldots, Z_{t-p-q-k_2})$. Given the observations $Z_\tau, Z_{\tau+1}, \ldots, Z_n$, $\tau = \min\{1 - p - k_1, 1 - p - q - k_2\}$, the GMM estimator is given by

$$
\hat{\boldsymbol{\theta}}_n = \underset{\boldsymbol{\Theta}}{\operatorname{argmin}}[\sum_{t=1}^n \boldsymbol{G}_t\boldsymbol{r}_t(\boldsymbol{\theta})]'\boldsymbol{\Lambda}_n[\sum_{t=1}^n \boldsymbol{G}_t\boldsymbol{r}_t(\boldsymbol{\theta})], \tag{11}
$$

where $\boldsymbol{\Lambda}_n$ is a nonnegative definite matrix which may depend on the observed data and converges to a positive definite matrix $\boldsymbol{\Lambda}$ as $n \to \infty$. The parameter space $\boldsymbol{\Theta} \subset \mathbb{R}^p \times [0, \infty)^q \times (0, \infty) \times [0, \infty)$ is assumed to be compact and contain $\boldsymbol{\theta}_0$ as an interior point. The asymptotic properties of $\hat{\boldsymbol{\theta}}_n$ can be established in a usual GMM framework. Specifically, denote $\boldsymbol{\Sigma} = E[\boldsymbol{G}_0\boldsymbol{r}_0(\boldsymbol{\theta}_0)\boldsymbol{r}_0'(\boldsymbol{\theta}_0)\boldsymbol{G}_0']$ and $\boldsymbol{\Delta}' = E[\nabla_{\boldsymbol{\theta}}\boldsymbol{r}_0'(\boldsymbol{\theta}_0)\boldsymbol{G}_0']$ where $\nabla_{\boldsymbol{\theta}}\boldsymbol{r}_0'(\boldsymbol{\theta}) = \partial\boldsymbol{r}_0'(\boldsymbol{\theta})/\partial\boldsymbol{\theta}$. Then we have the following asymptotic results for the GMM estimator, the proof of which and further regularity conditions are given in Section 8.

Theorem 1 *The GMM estimator $\hat{\boldsymbol{\theta}}_n$ has the following properties.*

(1) Under Assumption 1–2, $\hat{\boldsymbol{\theta}}_n \overset{a.s.}{\to} \boldsymbol{\theta}_0$ as $n \to \infty$.

(2) Under Assumption 1–6, $\sqrt{n}(\hat{\boldsymbol{\theta}}_n - \boldsymbol{\theta}_0) \overset{d}{\to} N(\boldsymbol{0}, A^{-1}BA^{-1})$ as $n \to \infty$, where $A = \boldsymbol{\Delta}'\boldsymbol{\Lambda}\boldsymbol{\Delta}, B = \boldsymbol{\Delta}'\boldsymbol{\Lambda}\boldsymbol{\Sigma}\boldsymbol{\Lambda}\boldsymbol{\Delta}$.

Given the specified set of instruments, the optimal (efficient) GMM estimator is obtained by taking the weight $\boldsymbol{\Lambda}_n$ to be such that $\boldsymbol{\Lambda}_n^{-1} \overset{p}{\to} \boldsymbol{\Sigma}$ as $n \to \infty$. Then the optimal GMM has asymptotic variance-covariance matrix $A_0^{-1} = (\boldsymbol{\Delta}'\boldsymbol{\Sigma}^{-1}\boldsymbol{\Delta})^{-1}$.

To compute the optimal weight, we propose to use a serial correlation robust estimator of $\boldsymbol{\Sigma}$. Specifically, let $e_t = G_t r_t(\boldsymbol{\theta}_0)$. Then since $E(e_t|\mathcal{F}_{t-p-q-1}) = 0$, we have

$$
\boldsymbol{\Sigma}_n = V \left(n^{-1/2} \sum_{i=1}^{n} e_t \right)
$$

$$
= E(e_0 e_0') + \sum_{i=1}^{p+q} \frac{n-i}{n} [E(e_0 e_{-i}') + E(e_{-i} e_0')].
$$

Similarly to White (2001, p.147) and Wooldridge (1994, Sec.4.5), we can find a positive definite matrix $\boldsymbol{\Lambda}_n$ such that $\boldsymbol{\Lambda}_n^{-1} - \boldsymbol{\Sigma}_n \overset{p}{\to} 0$ as $n \to \infty$, where

$$
\boldsymbol{\Lambda}_n^{-1} = \frac{1}{n} \sum_{t=1}^{n} \hat{e}_t \hat{e}_t' + \sum_{i=1}^{p+q} \frac{m_i(n)}{n} \sum_{t=i+1}^{n} (\hat{e}_t \hat{e}_{t-i}' + \hat{e}_{t-i} \hat{e}_t'),
$$

$\hat{e}_t = G_t r_t(\hat{\boldsymbol{\theta}})$ and $m_i(n) \to 1, i = 1, 2, \ldots, p + q$ are suitably chosen to ensure that $\boldsymbol{\Lambda}_n > 0$. In practice, we can start with $m_i(n) = 1, i = 1, 2, \ldots, p + q$. If $\boldsymbol{\Lambda}_n$ is not positive definite, then we can modify $m_i(n)$ as $m_i(n) = (1 - n^{-1})^i$ or $m_i(n) = \exp(i/n)$ to achieve the desired result.

4   Testing for Measurement Error

Although our GMM framework does not rule out zero measurement error, from practical point of view it is of interest to verify its presence and severity. However, testing for measurement error is generally a challenging task because under the null hypothesis the value of the measurement error variance is on the boundary of the parameter space. The framework in the previous section provides a possibility to construct such a test by applying the similar idea of the incremental Sargan test (Arellano 2003, p.193). Specifically, we construct a test for the following hypotheses on the measurement error variance

$$H_0 : \sigma_0^2 = 0 \quad vs. \quad H_a : \sigma_0^2 > 0. \tag{12}$$

We first consider the problem of estimating a subset of unknown parameters $\boldsymbol{\gamma}_0 = (\boldsymbol{\alpha}_0', \boldsymbol{\beta}_0', \tau_0)'$, where $\boldsymbol{\alpha}_0, \boldsymbol{\beta}_0$ are defined as in the AR(p)-ARCH(q) model (1)–(2) and

$$\tau_0 = \omega_0 + [1 - \beta_0(1)][1 + \alpha_0^2(1)]\sigma_0^2. \tag{13}$$

Then it can be shown that $\boldsymbol{\gamma}_0$ can be identified by the following $k_1 + k_2$ moment conditions

$$E[\boldsymbol{G}_{1t}\tilde{\boldsymbol{r}}_t(\boldsymbol{\gamma}_0)] = 0, \tag{14}$$

where $\tilde{\boldsymbol{r}}_t(\boldsymbol{\gamma}) = (Y_t(\boldsymbol{\alpha}), [1 - \beta(B)]Y_t^2(\boldsymbol{\alpha}) - \tau)'$,

$$\boldsymbol{G}_{1t}' = \begin{pmatrix} Z_{t-p-1} \ Z_{t-p-2} \ \cdots \ Z_{t-p-k_1} & 0 & 0 & \cdots & 0 \\ 0 & 0 & \cdots & 0 & Z_{t-p-q-1} \ Z_{t-p-q-2} \ \cdots \ Z_{t-p-q-k_2} \end{pmatrix}$$

and $k_1 > p, k_2 > q + 1$. Therefore the optimal GMM estimator for $\boldsymbol{\gamma}_0$ is given by

$$\hat{\boldsymbol{\gamma}}_1 = \underset{\Gamma}{\operatorname{argmin}} \, \boldsymbol{b}_{1n}'(\boldsymbol{\gamma}) \boldsymbol{V}_{1n}^{-1} \boldsymbol{b}_{1n}(\boldsymbol{\gamma}), \tag{15}$$

where $\boldsymbol{b}_{1n}(\boldsymbol{\gamma}) = n^{-1} \sum_{t=1}^{n} \boldsymbol{G}_{1t}\tilde{\boldsymbol{r}}_t(\boldsymbol{\gamma})$, $\boldsymbol{V}_{1n}$ is positive definite and $\boldsymbol{V}_{1n} - V[n^{1/2}\boldsymbol{b}_{1n}(\boldsymbol{\gamma}_0)] \xrightarrow{p} 0$, and $\Gamma \subset \mathbb{R}^p \times [0, \infty)^q \times (0, \infty)$ is compact.

Next, under H_0 we consider additional $2p + q$ moment conditions

$$E[\boldsymbol{G}_{2t}\tilde{\boldsymbol{r}}_t(\boldsymbol{\gamma}_0)] = 0, \tag{16}$$

where

$$\boldsymbol{G}_{2t}' = \begin{pmatrix} Z_{t-1} \ Z_{t-2} \ \cdots \ Z_{t-p} & 0 & 0 & \cdots & 0 \\ 0 & 0 & \cdots & 0 & Z_{t-1} \ Z_{t-2} \ \cdots \ Z_{t-p-q} \end{pmatrix}.$$

Similarly, the optimal GMM estimator is given by

$$\hat{\boldsymbol{\gamma}} = \underset{\Gamma}{\operatorname{argmin}} \, \boldsymbol{b}_n'(\boldsymbol{\gamma}) \boldsymbol{V}_n^{-1} \boldsymbol{b}_n(\boldsymbol{\gamma}), \tag{17}$$

where $\boldsymbol{b}_n(\boldsymbol{\gamma}) = n^{-1} \sum_{t=1}^{n} (\boldsymbol{G}_{1t}' \vdots \boldsymbol{G}_{2t}')' \tilde{\boldsymbol{r}}_t(\boldsymbol{\gamma})$, $\boldsymbol{V}_n$ is positive definite and $\boldsymbol{V}_n - V[n^{1/2}\boldsymbol{b}_n(\boldsymbol{\gamma}_0)] \xrightarrow{p} 0$.

Then the test statistic is defined as

$$SW = n\boldsymbol{b}_n'(\hat{\boldsymbol{\gamma}}) \boldsymbol{V}_n^{-1} \boldsymbol{b}_n(\hat{\boldsymbol{\gamma}}) - n\boldsymbol{b}_{1n}'(\hat{\boldsymbol{\gamma}}_1) \boldsymbol{V}_{1n}^{-1} \boldsymbol{b}_{1n}(\hat{\boldsymbol{\gamma}}_1). \tag{18}$$

For this test we have the following result, the proof of which is given in section 8.

Theorem 2 *Under Assumption 1–6 and H_0, $SW \xrightarrow{d} \chi^2_{2p+q}$ as $n \to \infty$.*

5 Impact of Measurement Error

It is well-known that in a linear errors-in-variables model with iid data the usual OLS or ML estimators are attenuated towards zero. The impact of the measurement error in dynamic ARCH models, however, has not been studied before. In this section we carry out Monte Carlo simulations to investigate the behavior of the naive MLE of a Gaussian AR(1)-ARCH(1) model with Gaussian classical additive measurement error. Specifically, we consider the model

$$X_t = \alpha_0 X_{t-1} + \epsilon_t, \tag{19}$$

$$\epsilon_t = \sqrt{h_t}\eta_t, \quad h_t = \omega_0 + \beta_0 \epsilon_{t-1}^2, \tag{20}$$

$$Z_t = X_t + \delta_t, \tag{21}$$

where $\eta_t \sim N(0, 1)$ and $\delta_t \sim N(0, \sigma_0^2)$ are independent and iid sequences. The parameter values are set to $\omega_0 = \sigma_0^2 = 1$, $\alpha_0 \in \{-0.9, -0.8, \ldots, 0.8, 0.9\}$ and $\beta_0 \in \{0.05, 0.1, \ldots, 0.9, 0.95\}$, respectively. In all simulations, 1000 samples of size $n = 10^5$ are generated to accurately estimate the asymptotic bias of ML($\alpha_0, \beta_0, \omega_0$).

We first calculate the relative bias of the ML(α_0) as

$$RB.ML(\alpha_0) = \frac{Bias.ML(\alpha_0)}{\alpha_0} \times 100.$$

Figure 1 shows clearly that the ML(α_0) is biased towards zero, similar to the OLS estimator of the slope parameter in a linear errors-in-variables model. More importantly, the bias has a pattern of a symmetric parabolic function in α_0 and a nearly linear function in β_0. The absolute RB is monotone decreasing in both α_0 and β_0. These observations indicate a similarity between the asymptotic bias of ML(α_0) and OLS(α_0) calculated by regressing Z_t on Z_{t-1}. By direct calculation we can obtain the OLS relative bias as

$$RB.OLS(\alpha_0) = -\frac{1}{1 + \omega_0/(1 - \beta_0)(1 - \alpha_0^2)\sigma_0^2}.$$

This raises an interesting question: To what extend can the OLS(α_0) bias formula be used to approximate and therefore to correct the bias of ML(α_0)? To further investigate this question, we examine the ratio $Bias.OLS(\alpha_0)/Bias.ML(\alpha_0)$ as a function of α_0 and β_0. Figure 2 shows that the formula of Bias.OLS provides good approximation to Bias.ML in a fairly large area of the parameter space. However,

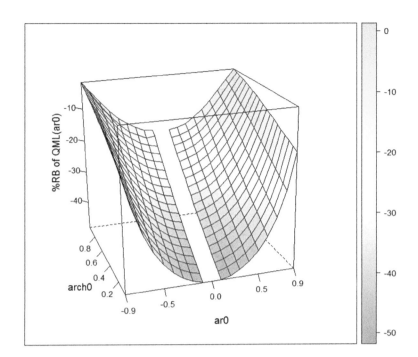

Fig. 1 Relative bias of ML(α_0)

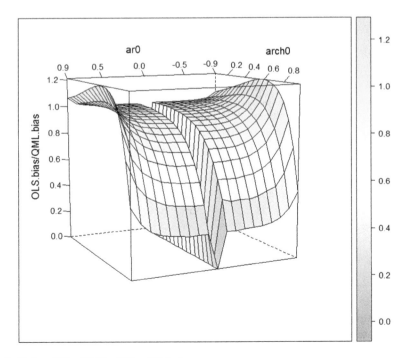

Fig. 2 Ratio of Bias.OLS(α_0)/Bias.ML(α_0)

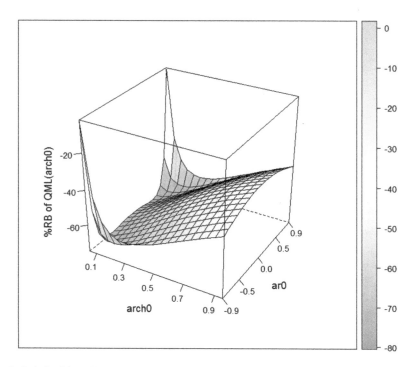

Fig. 3 Relative bias of ML(β_0)

the Bias.OLS formula underestimates the Bias.ML for large values of β_0, which is understandable because the two estimators are more different when β_0 gets larger. Again, it is interesting to see that there is a clear (unknown) functional relationship between Bias.ML and Bias.OLS.

Further, we have also calculated the relative bias of ML(β_0) and ML(ω_0), which are shown in Figs. 3 and 4, respectively. From these figures we can see that the ML(β_0) has downward bias and the absolute relative bias is generally decreasing for $\beta_0 \geq 0.3$ or $|\alpha_0| \leq 0.7$. In contrast, ML(ω_0) has an upward bias pattern, which is similar to the intercept estimator in a linear errors-in-variables model. Again, both Figs. 3 and 4 show clear (but unknown) functional patterns of the asymptotic bias of the MLE. Overall, Figs. 1, 2, 3, and 4 show that the measurement error has more severe effect on the estimate of ω_0 than on α_0 and β_0.

6   Finite Sample Properties

In this section we carry out Monte Carlo simulations to investigate the finite sample properties of the proposed GMM estimator and compare it with the corresponding naive ML estimator. Again we use the model (19)–(21) in the previous section,

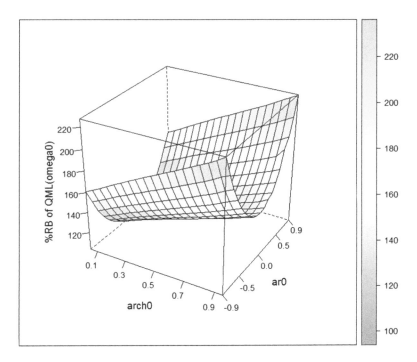

Fig. 4 Relative bias of ML(ω_0)

under which the optimal choice of the instrument matrix G_t depends on the quantities such as $E[Z_{t-h}|\tilde{Z}_{t-p-1}], h = 1, 2, \ldots, p$, $E[Y_{t-h}^2(\alpha_0)|\tilde{Z}_{t-p-q-1}], h = 1, 2, \ldots, q$, and $E[(r_t(\theta_0)r_t'(\theta_0))_{ij}|I_{ij}]$ for some suitably chosen information set I_{ij}. Unfortunately some of these instrumental functions cannot be computed easily without simplification which would require further distributional assumptions on the latent and error processes. Consequently we have attempted with several constructions and found the following procedure to be most practical. Since the number of moment equations used here is the same of the number of unknown parameters, the estimators can be calculated in the following sequential process.

First, compute

$$\hat{\alpha} = \underset{-1 < \alpha < 1}{\text{argmin}} \left[\sum_{t=k_3}^{n} \hat{Z}_{t-1} Y_t(\alpha) \right]^2 , \tag{22}$$

where $k_3 = 4 + k_2$ and $\hat{Z}_{t-1}$ is the linear projection of Z_{t-1} onto $\{Z_{t-2}, Z_{t-3}, \ldots, Z_{t-1-k_1}\}$. Second, let $Y_t = Y_t(\hat{\alpha})$ and compute

$$\hat{\sigma}^2 = \underset{\sigma^2 \geq 0}{\operatorname{argmin}} \left[\sum_{t=k_3}^{n} (Y_t Y_{t-1} + \hat{\alpha}\sigma^2) \right]^2. \tag{23}$$

Third, compute

$$\hat{\beta} = \underset{0 < \beta < 1}{\operatorname{argmin}} \left[\sum_{t=k_3}^{n} \hat{Y}_{t-1}^2 (y_t^2 - \beta y_{t-1}^2) \right]^2, \tag{24}$$

where $\hat{Y}_{t-1}^2$ is the linear projection of Y_{t-1}^2 onto

$$\left\{ \frac{Y_{t-3}^2}{1 + Y_{t-3}^2}, \frac{Y_{t-4}^2}{1 + Y_{t-4}^2}, \dots, \frac{Y_{t-2-k_2}^2}{1 + Y_{t-2-k_2}^2} \right\},$$

and $y_t^2 = Y_t^2 - \overline{Y^2}$, $y_{t-1}^2 = Y_{t-1}^2 - \overline{Y_{-1}^2}$ with

$$\overline{Y^2} = \frac{1}{n - k_3 + 1} \sum_{t=k_3}^{n} Y_t^2, \quad \overline{Y_{-1}^2} = \frac{1}{n - k_3 + 1} \sum_{t=k_3}^{n} Y_{t-1}^2.$$

Finally, compute

$$\hat{\omega} = \underset{\omega > 0}{\operatorname{argmin}} \left[\overline{Y^2} - \hat{\beta}\overline{Y_{-1}^2} - \omega - (1 - \hat{\beta})(1 + \hat{\alpha}^2)\hat{\sigma}^2 \right]^2. \tag{25}$$

It is worthwhile to note that $\hat{Y}_{t-1}^2$ is defined in terms of bounded instruments to guarantee the consistency of the proposed estimator over a wide range of the parameter space.

We generate the data using parameter values $\{0.05, 0.2, 0.35, 0.5, 0.65, 0.8, 0.95\}$ for α_0 and β_0, respectively. In addition, we set $\omega_0 = 1$ and let σ_0^2 vary proportionally to $\sigma_X^2 = \omega_0/(1 - \beta_0)(1 - \alpha_0^2)$ such as $\sigma_0^2 = a\sigma_X^2$, where the noise-to-signal ratio $a \in \{0, 0.25, 0.5, \dots, 1.75, 2\}$, respectively, and $a = 0$ corresponds to the case of no measurement error. Again, we generate 1000 samples for each of the sizes $n = 100, 1000, 10000$ and $n = 100000$ to approximate the asymptotic scenario. In each simulation we compute the naive ML (nML) and two GMM estimators using $k_1 = k_2 = 1$ (GMM1) and $k_1 = k_2 = 5$ (GMM5) instruments, respectively.

The bias and root mean squared error (RMSE) of the estimators are calculated and numerical results for AR and ARCH parameters $\alpha_0, \beta_0, \omega_0$ for some selected cases are reported in Tables 1, 2, and 3. The numerical results for negative α_0 values are similar to those for positive values and therefore are not reported here.

From Tables 1, 2, and 3 we can see that, in the case of no measurement error ($a = 0$), the GMM estimators have both larger bias and RMSE than the naive

Table 1 Bias and **RMSE** of nML, GMM1 and GMM5 estimators for AR parameter α_0 (with $\omega_0 = 1$)

n	α_0	$a = 0.00$			$a = 0.75$			$a = 1.5$		
		nML	GMM1	GMM5	nML	GMM1	GMM5	nML	GMM1	GMM5
		$\beta_0 = 0.2$								
100	0.2	−0.007	−0.022	−0.029	−0.095	0.020	−0.093	−0.120	−0.055	−0.146
		0.109	0.510	0.340	0.142	0.580	0.402	0.159	0.622	0.420
	0.5	−0.011	−0.020	−0.023	−0.227	−0.003	−0.122	−0.304	−0.082	−0.249
		0.094	0.217	0.180	0.254	0.367	0.331	0.323	0.498	0.448
	0.8	−0.015	−0.019	−0.021	−0.359	−0.012	−0.096	−0.489	−0.073	−0.234
		0.067	0.092	0.089	0.382	0.192	0.208	0.505	0.298	0.373
10^5	0.2	−0.000	0.000	0.000	−0.086	−0.001	−0.001	−0.120	−0.002	−0.003
		0.003	0.016	0.016	0.086	0.028	0.028	0.120	0.040	0.039
	0.5	−0.000	0.000	0.000	−0.214	−0.000	−0.000	−0.300	−0.001	−0.001
		0.003	0.005	0.005	0.214	0.010	0.010	0.300	0.016	0.014
	0.8	−0.000	−0.000	−0.000	−0.339	−0.000	−0.000	−0.479	−0.001	−0.001
		0.002	0.002	0.002	0.339	0.005	0.004	0.479	0.009	0.005
		$\beta_0 = 0.5$								
100	0.2	−0.004	−0.063	−0.053	−0.099	−0.010	−0.106	−0.123	−0.086	−0.148
		0.107	0.565	0.353	0.149	0.614	0.409	0.165	0.655	0.418
	0.5	−0.008	−0.025	−0.038	−0.240	−0.034	−0.143	−0.313	−0.118	−0.263
		0.091	0.244	0.207	0.268	0.432	0.351	0.334	0.548	0.464
	0.8	−0.011	−0.021	−0.025	−0.375	−0.022	−0.114	−0.501	−0.094	−0.260
		0.060	0.101	0.098	0.402	0.210	0.235	0.521	0.342	0.406
10^5	0.2	−0.000	0.001	0.001	−0.090	−0.001	−0.002	−0.123	−0.001	−0.002
		0.003	0.026	0.026	0.090	0.037	0.034	0.123	0.044	0.043
	0.5	−0.000	0.000	0.000	−0.222	−0.000	−0.001	−0.307	−0.001	−0.001
		0.003	0.009	0.009	0.222	0.012	0.011	0.307	0.017	0.015
	0.8	−0.000	0.000	0.000	−0.343	−0.000	−0.000	−0.484	−0.000	−0.000
		0.002	0.003	0.003	0.343	0.006	0.004	0.484	0.009	0.005
		$\beta_0 = 0.8$								
100	0.2	−0.003	−0.109	−0.071	−0.120	−0.064	−0.131	−0.138	−0.109	−0.156
		0.107	0.614	0.371	0.169	0.676	0.423	0.180	0.701	0.421
	0.5	−0.006	−0.049	−0.061	−0.290	−0.082	−0.215	−0.350	−0.173	−0.315
		0.093	0.326	0.254	0.320	0.520	0.418	0.373	0.628	0.502
	0.8	−0.009	−0.029	−0.036	−0.452	−0.058	−0.185	−0.559	−0.172	−0.359
		0.053	0.142	0.135	0.483	0.297	0.329	0.581	0.482	0.516
10^5	0.2	−0.000	−0.000	−0.005	−0.105	−0.016	−0.017	−0.136	−0.006	−0.013
		0.003	0.170	0.130	0.105	0.173	0.128	0.137	0.154	0.129
	0.5	−0.000	0.001	−0.001	−0.264	−0.007	−0.008	−0.342	−0.001	−0.003
		0.004	0.059	0.051	0.264	0.093	0.066	0.342	0.053	0.043
	0.8	−0.000	−0.000	−0.001	−0.411	−0.002	−0.003	−0.545	−0.001	−0.001
		0.001	0.020	0.019	0.411	0.032	0.027	0.545	0.018	0.014

Table 2 Bias and **RMSE** of nML, GMM1 and GMM5 estimators for ARCH slope parameter β_0 (with $\omega_0 = 1$)

		$a = 0.00$			$a = 0.75$			$a = 1.5$		
		nML	GMM1	GMM5	nML	GMM1	GMM5	nML	GMM1	GMM5
n	β_0	$\alpha_0 = 0.2$								
100	0.2	−0.030	0.177	0.041	−0.133	0.216	0.039	−0.150	0.225	0.043
		0.146	**0.461**	**0.335**	**0.161**	**0.495**	**0.363**	**0.169**	**0.502**	**0.361**
	0.5	−0.064	−0.044	−0.201	−0.353	−0.079	−0.268	−0.407	−0.074	−0.283
		0.219	**0.424**	**0.388**	**0.385**	**0.447**	**0.429**	**0.425**	**0.451**	**0.431**
	0.8	−0.107	−0.326	−0.460	−0.601	−0.366	−0.580	−0.669	−0.381	−0.615
		0.253	**0.519**	**0.567**	**0.636**	**0.580**	**0.669**	**0.692**	**0.590**	**0.696**
10^5	0.2	−0.000	−0.000	−0.009	−0.134	−0.036	−0.044	−0.167	−0.040	−0.029
		0.005	**0.098**	**0.123**	**0.134**	**0.150**	**0.133**	**0.167**	**0.198**	**0.125**
	0.5	−0.000	−0.002	−0.003	−0.316	−0.005	−0.009	−0.391	−0.003	−0.022
		0.006	**0.032**	**0.035**	**0.316**	**0.064**	**0.064**	**0.391**	**0.125**	**0.108**
	0.8	−0.001	−0.021	−0.024	−0.528	−0.025	−0.036	−0.616	−0.032	−0.051
		0.008	**0.048**	**0.052**	**0.528**	**0.066**	**0.073**	**0.616**	**0.080**	**0.086**
		$\alpha_0 = 0.5$								
100	0.2	−0.028	0.152	0.047	−0.142	0.188	0.021	−0.155	0.219	0.020
		0.145	**0.441**	**0.342**	**0.166**	**0.484**	**0.349**	**0.171**	**0.496**	**0.335**
	0.5	−0.062	−0.041	−0.188	−0.380	−0.103	−0.289	−0.421	−0.071	−0.295
		0.219	**0.417**	**0.384**	**0.405**	**0.448**	**0.435**	**0.436**	**0.452**	**0.432**
	0.8	−0.104	−0.317	−0.449	−0.629	−0.394	−0.612	−0.685	−0.378	−0.615
		0.252	**0.502**	**0.561**	**0.659**	**0.593**	**0.687**	**0.704**	**0.593**	**0.696**
10^5	0.2	−0.000	−0.000	−0.009	−0.150	−0.040	−0.035	−0.175	0.017	0.030
		0.005	**0.098**	**0.123**	**0.150**	**0.175**	**0.121**	**0.175**	**0.290**	**0.218**
	0.5	−0.000	−0.002	−0.003	−0.351	−0.003	−0.014	−0.410	0.004	−0.040
		0.006	**0.032**	**0.035**	**0.351**	**0.091**	**0.087**	**0.411**	**0.204**	**0.185**
	0.8	−0.001	−0.020	−0.022	−0.562	−0.027	−0.041	−0.636	−0.035	−0.059
		0.022	**0.050**	**0.053**	**0.562**	**0.074**	**0.081**	**0.636**	**0.099**	**0.101**
		$\alpha_0 = 0.8$								
100	0.2	−0.024	0.141	0.045	−0.150	0.200	0.029	−0.161	0.230	0.010
		0.145	**0.431**	**0.342**	**0.173**	**0.486**	**0.340**	**0.176**	**0.506**	**0.328**
	0.5	−0.059	−0.041	−0.182	−0.424	−0.113	−0.286	−0.446	−0.089	−0.329
		0.217	**0.411**	**0.380**	**0.439**	**0.455**	**0.439**	**0.454**	**0.460**	**0.448**
	0.8	−0.102	−0.309	−0.429	−0.690	−0.379	−0.635	−0.723	−0.415	−0.670
		0.252	**0.487**	**0.545**	**0.708**	**0.594**	**0.710**	**0.735**	**0.618**	**0.728**
10^5	0.2	−0.000	−0.000	−0.009	−0.170	0.075	0.164	−0.185	0.219	0.393
		0.005	**0.098**	**0.123**	**0.170**	**0.362**	**0.382**	**0.185**	**0.494**	**0.575**
	0.5	−0.000	−0.002	−0.003	−0.410	0.010	−0.053	−0.442	−0.043	0.067
		0.006	**0.032**	**0.035**	**0.410**	**0.286**	**0.266**	**0.442**	**0.417**	**0.396**
	0.8	−0.000	−0.020	−0.022	−0.627	−0.031	−0.063	−0.670	−0.076	−0.108
		0.008	**0.050**	**0.054**	**0.627**	**0.127**	**0.118**	**0.670**	**0.273**	**0.219**

Table 3 Bias and **RMSE** of nML, GMM1 and GMM5 estimators for ARCH intercept parameter ω_0 (with $\omega_0 = 1$)

		$a = 0.00$			$a = 0.75$			$a = 1.5$		
		nML	GMM1	GMM5	nML	GMM1	GMM5	nML	GMM1	GMM5
n	β_0	$\alpha_0 = 0.2$								
100	0.2	0.003	−0.045	0.025	1.043	−0.708	−0.460	1.994	−0.607	−0.343
		0.190	**0.776**	**0.512**	**1.099**	**0.927**	**0.902**	**2.054**	**1.001**	**1.052**
	0.5	0.042	0.361	0.462	1.908	−0.531	−0.139	3.521	−0.420	0.128
		0.240	**1.401**	**0.969**	**1.985**	**1.116**	**1.267**	**3.612**	**1.301**	**1.726**
	0.8	0.110	1.001	1.599	4.802	−0.066	0.917	8.823	0.539	2.016
		0.355	**2.175**	**4.624**	**4.957**	**2.468**	**3.345**	**9.012**	**5.836**	**7.898**
10^5	0.2	−0.000	0.000	0.011	1.101	0.072	0.085	2.127	0.117	0.104
		0.007	**0.122**	**0.153**	**1.101**	**0.269**	**0.258**	**2.127**	**0.410**	**0.338**
	0.5	0.000	0.003	0.005	1.905	0.047	0.059	3.590	0.075	0.116
		0.007	**0.055**	**0.062**	**1.905**	**0.245**	**0.244**	**3.590**	**0.412**	**0.396**
	0.8	0.000	0.054	0.072	4.676	0.103	0.165	8.728	0.209	0.320
		0.008	**0.176**	**0.175**	**4.676**	**0.606**	**0.633**	**8.729**	**0.849**	**0.911**
		$\alpha_0 = 0.5$								
100	0.2	0.001	−0.180	−0.051	1.460	−0.294	0.054	2.714	−0.206	0.313
		0.191	**0.584**	**0.475**	**1.521**	**0.979**	**0.989**	**2.782**	**1.252**	**1.466**
	0.5	0.041	0.108	0.356	2.595	0.062	0.639	4.682	0.148	1.082
		0.241	**0.947**	**0.868**	**2.684**	**1.487**	**1.722**	**4.792**	**1.919**	**2.578**
	0.8	0.113	0.820	1.348	6.366	1.009	2.435	11.536	1.389	3.592
		0.403	**1.938**	**2.657**	**6.559**	**3.708**	**4.954**	**11.784**	**4.891**	**7.102**
10^5	0.2	−0.000	−0.000	0.011	1.545	0.050	0.044	2.900	−0.016	−0.033
		0.007	**0.122**	**0.154**	**1.545**	**0.222**	**0.156**	**2.900**	**0.369**	**0.278**
	0.5	0.000	0.002	0.004	2.617	0.006	0.028	4.809	−0.004	0.086
		0.007	**0.055**	**0.062**	**2.617**	**0.185**	**0.174**	**4.809**	**0.414**	**0.377**
	0.8	0.002	0.042	0.051	6.262	0.085	0.151	11.497	0.121	0.238
		0.053	**0.156**	**0.176**	**6.262**	**0.316**	**0.337**	**11.498**	**0.453**	**0.466**
		$\alpha_0 = 0.8$								
100	0.2	−0.002	−0.188	−0.067	3.453	−0.170	0.222	6.240	0.258	1.096
		0.191	**0.563**	**0.468**	**3.541**	**1.100**	**1.227**	**6.354**	**2.031**	**2.573**
	0.5	0.037	0.062	0.316	5.835	0.452	1.077	10.319	1.187	2.588
		0.241	**0.880**	**0.817**	**5.982**	**2.061**	**2.437**	**10.520**	**3.693**	**4.750**
	0.8	0.107	0.743	1.271	13.969	2.189	4.419	24.908	4.305	7.359
		0.371	**1.664**	**4.663**	**14.324**	**6.165**	**8.307**	**25.415**	**10.275**	**12.976**
10^5	0.2	−0.000	−0.000	0.011	3.663	−0.095	−0.205	6.673	−0.271	−0.489
		0.007	**0.122**	**0.153**	**3.663**	**0.453**	**0.478**	**6.673**	**0.620**	**0.720**
	0.5	0.000	0.002	0.004	5.979	−0.020	0.105	10.721	0.092	−0.129
		0.007	**0.055**	**0.063**	**5.980**	**0.571**	**0.530**	**10.722**	**0.842**	**0.799**
	0.8	0.000	0.039	0.046	13.859	0.087	0.235	24.931	0.306	0.461
		0.008	**0.160**	**0.184**	**13.866**	**0.563**	**0.490**	**24.932**	**1.249**	**1.006**

MLE at sample size $n = 100$, while the bias reduces markedly at sample size $n = 10^5$. However, when the measurement error is present ($a = 0.75$ or $a = 1.5$), the GMMs has significantly smaller bias than the naive MLE at all sample sizes, and significantly smaller RMSE at $n = 10^5$. In particular, while the bias in GMMs reduces significantly at large sample size $n = 10^5$, the bias in naive MLE remains persistently at high level. Overall, the GMM5 using $k_1 = k_2 = 5$ instruments have smaller RMSE but larger bias than the GMM1 using $k_1 = k_2 = 1$ instrument. In general, the AR parameter α_0 has the smallest bias and RMSE, while the ARCH intercept ω_0 has the largest values.

In the following we provide a more detailed summary of findings for each parameter based on over 300 various configurations of parameter values.

AR Parameter α

The nML estimator is clearly downward biased and its absolute relative bias (ARB) is fast increasing (from 20% to 80%) with the noise-to-signal ratio a. The GMM estimators are downward biased in small samples and their ARB are decreasing with α_0 but increasing with β_0. While the ARB of GMM1 has no relation with a that of GMM5 is a fast increasing function of a. The RMSE of the nML estimator has, respectively, a shape of square-root function in a, a clear increasing linear function in α_0, and a slightly increasing linear function of β_0. In contrast, the RMSE of the GMM estimators are decreasing with α_0, but increasing with β_0 and a, respectively. However, the RMSE of GMM5 vanishes in large samples faster than that of GMM1 estimator.

ARCH slope β

Again the nML estimator is clearly downward biased in large samples and most of small sample cases, and its ARB is fast increasing with a (from 40% to 80%). In small samples, the biases of the GMM estimators have a shape of concave function with respect to β_0, while their ARB have a shape of convex function. Furthermore, when the sample size increases the GMM biases vanish very slowly for large α_0 (0.95) and small β_0 (0.05). The RMSE of the nML estimator takes the shape of a square-root function in a, a fast increasing linear function in β_0, has no relation to α_0. The RMSE of the GMM estimators are a convex function of β_0 but have no relation with α_0 or a.

ARCH intercept ω

The nML estimator has an upward bias and the bias is increasing with a, α_0, and β_0, respectively. In small samples the biases of the GMM estimators have, respectively, the shape of a linear function in α_0, an increasing function in β_0, and a fast increasing function in a. However, the bias vanishes slowly when the sample size increases. The RMSE of all three estimators have similar patterns as their respective biases.

7 Conclusions and Discussion

We have studied a dynamic model with autoregressive heteroscedastic error where the underlying process is latent and subject to additive measurement error. We have shown that the model is identifiable by using the observations of a proxy process only. This is in contrast to the case of measurement error in the covariates, where extra information such as external instrumental variables or replicate observations is needed for model identifiability. Moreover, we proposed a set of identifying moment conditions and used them to construct GMM estimators for the unknown parameters. The proposed estimators are consistent and asymptotically normally distributed under usual regularity conditions. As a byproduct, this framework allows us to construct a test for the presence of measurement error. Our Monte Carlo simulation studies show that the measurement error causes downward bias in the naive MLE, and the relative biases have certain functional forms. This is interesting because it provides a possibility to find the formulas that can be used to correct the biases in the naive MLE. Furthermore, the proposed estimators possess fairly good finite sample properties and comparisons with the naive MLE are also presented.

This work attempts to address some basic measurement error problems in dynamic models with ARCH-type errors. There are many more questions and issues remaining to be investigated. For example, it would be interesting to explore other possible moment conditions that can be used to achieve identification and to obtain more efficient estimators. It would also be interesting to study more general measurement error processes. We used a simple ARCH model in order to be able to gain insights of the problem and to obtain some concrete results. From both theoretical and practical point of view, it is important to investigate the measurement error problem in more general GARCH models. Our theoretical framework should apply to GARCH processes as well, but the estimation will be based on a different set of moments than (5)–(7) used here. Another way is to convert the GARCH process to an infinite order ARCH and then truncate it to finite order, so that the estimators based on the moments (5)–(7) can be used directly.

Acknowledgments The research was partially supported by grants from the Natural Sciences and Engineering Research Council of Canada (NSERC).

Appendix

Regularity Assumptions and Mathematical Proofs

In this Appendix we provide the regularity assumptions that are sufficient for the theoretical results in Theorems 1 and 2. We also provide a sketch of the proofs of them, since they follow the general framework of GMM estimation.

Regularity Assumptions

For the asymptotic properties of the GMM estimator $\hat{\theta}_n$ we make the following assumptions, where $\|\cdot\|$ denotes the Euclidean norm.

Assumption 1 *The instrumental functions satisfy* $E\left\|Z_{t-h}f_1(\tilde{Z}_{t-p-1})\right\| < \infty$ *for* $h = 0, 1, \ldots, p$ *and* $E\left\|Z_{t-h}^2 f_2(\tilde{Z}_{t-p-q-1})\right\| < \infty$ *for* $h = 0, 1, \ldots, p + q$.

Assumption 2 θ_0 *is the unique solution to* $E\{G_0 r_0(\theta)\} = 0$ *in* Θ.

Assumption 3 *The covariance matrix* $V[n^{-1/2}\sum_{t=1}^{n} G_t r_t(\theta_0)]$ *is uniformly positive definite.*

Assumption 4 *The instrumental functions satisfy* $E\left\|Z_{t-h}^2 f_1^2(\tilde{Z}_{t-p-1})\right\| < \infty$ *for* $h = 0, 1, 2, \ldots, p$, $E\left\|Z_{t-h}^4 f_2^2(\tilde{Z}_{t-p-q-1})\right\| < \infty$ *for* $h = 0, 1, 2, \ldots, p + q$, *and* $E(Z_0^4) < \infty$.

Assumption 5 $E[\|E(G_0 r_0(\theta_0)|\mathcal{F}_{-j})\|^2] < \infty$, $j = 1, 2, \ldots, p + q$, *where* $\mathcal{F}_t = \sigma(Z_s, s \leq t)$.

Assumption 6 $\Delta' = E[\nabla_\theta r_0'(\theta_0)G_0']$ *has full rank* $p + q + 2$, *where* $\nabla_\theta r_0'(\theta) = \partial r_0'(\theta)/\partial\theta$.

Note that the above assumptions are not more restrictive than the usual assumptions for the asymptotic properties of GMM estimators in the literature. They are formulated for the general forms of the instrumental functions f_1 and f_2 (which are also on the diagonal of matrix G_t). For example, if f_1 and f_2 are taken to be the linear projections of the lagged Z_t, then Assumption 1 simply means the Z_t process has finite second and third moments. Similarly, Assumption 4 means Z_t has finite fourth and sixth moments. In particular, the identifiability Assumption 3 is based on the moment conditions (5)–(7) which is given in $r_t(\theta)$. Again, if f_1 and f_2 are taken to be the linear projections then this assumption follows directly from (5)–(7).

Proof of Theorem 1

To simplify notation in the following we will omit the subscript n in $\hat{\theta}_n$ and denote it as $\hat{\theta}$. First, since $\{X_t\}$ is strictly stationary and ergodic, and $\{\delta_t\}$ is iid and independent of $\{\eta_t\}$, $\{Z_t\}$ is strictly stationary and ergodic. It follows from Assumption 1 and White (1996, Th. A.2.2) that $E[G_t r_t(\theta)]$ is continuous on Θ and, furthermore, by the strong uniform law of large numbers (ULLN), as $n \to \infty$,

$$\sup_{\Theta} \left\| \frac{1}{n} \sum_{i=1}^{n} G_t r_t(\boldsymbol{\theta}) - E[G_0 r_0(\boldsymbol{\theta})] \right\| \overset{a.s.}{\to} 0. \tag{26}$$

The result (1) follows then from Assumption 2 and White (1996, Th. 3.4).

To prove the asymptotic normality, note that for sufficiently large n, the score

$$S_n(\hat{\boldsymbol{\theta}}, \Lambda_n) = \left[\sum_{t=1}^{n} \nabla_{\boldsymbol{\theta}} r_t'(\hat{\boldsymbol{\theta}}) G_t' \right] \Lambda_n \left[\sum_{t=1}^{n} G_t r_t(\hat{\boldsymbol{\theta}}) \right] = \boldsymbol{0}, \quad w.p.1, \tag{27}$$

where $\nabla_{\boldsymbol{\theta}} r_t'(\boldsymbol{\theta}) = \partial r_t'(\boldsymbol{\theta})/\partial \boldsymbol{\theta}$. Then using the mean-value theorem (Jennrich 1969), we have

$$\left[\sum_{t=1}^{n} \nabla_{\boldsymbol{\theta}} r_t'(\hat{\boldsymbol{\theta}}) G_t' \right] \Lambda_n \left[\sum_{t=1}^{n} G_t r_t(\boldsymbol{\theta}_0) \right] = - \left[\sum_{t=1}^{n} \nabla_{\boldsymbol{\theta}} r_t'(\hat{\boldsymbol{\theta}}) G_t' \right] \Lambda_n \left[\sum_{t=1}^{n} G_t \nabla_{\boldsymbol{\theta}} r_t(\tilde{\boldsymbol{\theta}}) \right] (\hat{\boldsymbol{\theta}} - \boldsymbol{\theta}_0),$$
$$\tag{28}$$

where $\left\| \tilde{\boldsymbol{\theta}} - \boldsymbol{\theta}_0 \right\| \leq \left\| \hat{\boldsymbol{\theta}} - \boldsymbol{\theta}_0 \right\|$. Again by the ULLN (White 1996, Th. A.2.2 and Cor. 3.8), we have, as $n \to \infty$,

$$\frac{1}{n} \sum_{t=1}^{n} \nabla_{\boldsymbol{\theta}} r_t'(\hat{\boldsymbol{\theta}}) G_t' \overset{a.s.}{\to} E\left[\nabla_{\boldsymbol{\theta}} r_0'(\boldsymbol{\theta}_0) G_0' \right] \tag{29}$$

which has full rank by Assumption 6. Further, by Assumption 3–5 and (White 1996, Th. A.3.2), we can use the so-called Cramer–Wold device (Rao 1973) to show that

$$\frac{1}{\sqrt{n}} \sum_{t=1}^{n} G_t r_t(\boldsymbol{\theta}_0) \overset{d}{\to} N(0, \boldsymbol{\Sigma}), \tag{30}$$

where $\boldsymbol{\Sigma} = E[G_t r_t(\boldsymbol{\theta}_0) r_t'(\boldsymbol{\theta}_0) G_t']$. Finally the result follows from (28)–(30) and Assumption 6.

Proof of Theorem 2

First, using the nonsingular factorization we can write

$$V_1 = \plim_{n \to \infty} V[n^{1/2} \boldsymbol{b}_{1n}(\boldsymbol{\gamma}_0)] = C_1 C_1'$$

and $V_{1n} = C_{1n} C_{1n}'$ such that $C_1 = \plim_{n \to \infty} C_{1n}$. Then by the mean-value theorem and Slutsky's theorem we have

$$\ell_1 = n^{1/2} C_{1n}' \boldsymbol{b}_{1n}(\hat{\boldsymbol{\gamma}}_1) = n^{1/2} M_1 C_1' \boldsymbol{b}_{1n}(\boldsymbol{\gamma}_0) + o_p(1), \tag{31}$$

where $M_1 = I_{k_1+k_2} - A_1(A_1'A_1)^{-1}A_1'$, $A_1 = C_1'D_1$, and $D_1' = E[\nabla_\gamma \tilde{r}_t'(\gamma_0)G_{1t}']$. Similarly, let $V_n = C_nC_n'$, where

$$C_n' = \begin{pmatrix} C_{1n}' & 0 \\ 0 & C_{2n}' \end{pmatrix} \begin{pmatrix} I_{k_1+k_2} & 0 \\ -H_n & I_{2p+q} \end{pmatrix},$$

$C_{2n}C_{2n}' = V^{-1}[n^{1/2}(b_{2n}(\gamma_0) - H_nb_{1n}(\gamma_0))]$, and

$$\operatorname*{plim}_{n\to\infty} H_n = E[b_{2n}(\gamma_0)b_{1n}(\gamma_0)']E^{-1}[b_{1n}(\gamma_0)b_{1n}(\gamma_0)'].$$

Then it is easy to show that $\operatorname{plim}_{n\to\infty} C_nC_n' = \lim_{n\to\infty} V^{-1}[n^{1/2}b_n(\gamma_0)]$, and similarly to (31), we have

$$\ell = n^{1/2}C_n'b_n(\hat{\gamma}) = n^{1/2}MC'b_n(\gamma_0) + o_p(1), \tag{32}$$

where $M = I_{k_1+k_2+2p+q} - A(A'A)^{-1}A'$, $C = \operatorname{plim}_{n\to\infty} C_n$, $A = C'D$, $D' = (D_1', D_2')$, and $D_2' = E[\nabla_\gamma \tilde{r}_t'(\gamma_0)G_{2t}']$. Further, denote

$$M_2 = \begin{pmatrix} M_1 & 0 \\ 0 & 0 \end{pmatrix}.$$

Then out test statistic is

$$SW = nb_n'(\gamma_0)C(M - M_2)C'b_n(\gamma_0) + o_p(1). \tag{33}$$

Finally, since clearly $(M - M_2)M_2 = 0$ and $n^{1/2}C'b_n(\gamma_0) \xrightarrow{d} N(0, I_{k_1+k_2+2p+q})$ under H_0, we have $SW \xrightarrow{d} \chi^2_{2p+q}$.

References

Alberini, A., & Filippini, M. (2011). Response of residential electricity demand to price: The effect of measurement error. *Energy Economics, 33*(5), 889–895.

Arellano, M. (2003). *Panel data econometrics*. Oxford: Oxford University Press.

Bollerslev, T. (1986). Generalized autoregressive conditional heteroskedasticity. *Journal of Econometrics, 31*(3), 307–327.

Buonaccorsi, J. P. (2010). *Measurement Error: Models, Methods, and Applications*. New York: CRC Press.

Buonaccorsi, J. P. (2013). Measurement error in dynamic models. In *ISS-2012 Proceedings Volume On Longitudinal Data Analysis Subject to Measurement Errors, Missing Values, and/or Outliers* (pp. 53–76). Berlin: Springer.

Caporale, G. M., Onorante, L., & Paesani, P. (2012). Inflation and inflation uncertainty in the Euro area. *Empirical Economics, 43*(2), 597–615.

Carroll, R. J., Ruppert, D., Crainiceanu, C. M., & Stefanski, L. A. (2006). *Measurement Error in Nonlinear Models: A Modern Perspective*. West Palm Beach: Chapman and Hall/CRC.

Chen, X., Hong, H., & Nekipelov, D. (2011). Nonlinear models of measurement errors. *Journal of Economic Literature, 49*(4), 901–937.

Engle, R. F. (1982). Autoregressive conditional heteroscedasticity with estimates of the variance of united kingdom inflation. *Econometrica, 50*(4), 987–1007.

Engle, R. F., Focardi, S. M., & Fabozzi, F. J. (2008). ARCH/GARCH models in applied financial econometrics. In *Handbook of Finance, 3*.

Fan, J., & Wang, Y. (2007). Multi-scale jump and volatility analysis for high-frequency financial data. *Journal of the American Statistical Association, 102*(480), 1349–1362.

Fang, W., & Miller, S. M. (2009). Modeling the volatility of real GDP growth: The case of Japan revisited. *Japan and the World Economy, 21*(3), 312–324.

Francq, C., & Zakoïan, J.-M. (2000). Estimating weak GARCH representations. *Econometric Theory, 16*(5), 692–728.

Francq, C., & Zakoian, J.-M. (2011). *GARCH Models: Structure, Statistical Inference and Financial Applications*. New York: Wiley.

Gourieroux, C., Monfort, A., & Renault, E. (1993). Indirect inference. *Journal of applied econometrics, 8*(S1), S85–S118.

Grier, K. B., & Perry, M. J. (2000). The effects of real and nominal uncertainty on inflation and output growth: some GARCH-M evidence. *Journal of Applied Econometrics, 15*(1), 45–58.

Handbury, J., Watanabe, T., & Weinstein, D. E. (2013). How much do official price indexes tell us about inflation? Technical report, National Bureau of Economic Research.

Harvey, A., Ruiz, E., & Sentana, E. (1992). Unobserved component time series models with arch disturbances. *Journal of Econometrics, 52*(1–2), 129–157.

Jennrich, R. I. (1969). Asymptotic properties of non-linear least squares estimators. *The Annals of Mathematical Statistics, 40*(2), 633–643.

Ramirez, O. A., & Fadiga, M. (2003). Forecasting agricultural commodity prices with asymmetric-error GARCH models. *Journal of Agricultural and Resource Economics, 28*(1), 71–85.

Rao, C. R. (1973). Linear Statistical Inference and Its Applications. New York: Wiley.

Reitz, S., & Westerhoff, F. (2007). Commodity price cycles and heterogeneous speculators: a STAR–GARCH model. *Empirical Economics, 33*(2), 231–244.

Roche, M. J., & McQuinn, K. (2003). Grain price volatility in a small open economy. *European Review of Agricultural Economics, 30*(1), 77–98.

Staudenmayer, J., & Buonaccorsi, J. P. (2005). Measurement error in linear autoregressive models. *Journal of the American Statistical Association, 100*(471), 841–852.

Teräsvirta, T. (2009). An introduction to univariate GARCH models. In *Handbook of Financial Time Series* (pp. 17–42). Berlin: Springer.

Wang, L., & Hsiao, C. (2011). Method of moments estimation and identifiability of semiparametric nonlinear errors-in-variables models. *Journal of Econometrics, 165*(1), 30–44.

Wansbeek, T. J., & Meijer, E. (2000). *Measurement Error and Latent Variables in Econometrics*, vol. 37. Amsterdam: Elsevier.

White, H. (1996). *Estimation, Inference and Specification Analysis*. Cambridge: Cambridge University Press.

White, H. (2001). Asymptotic Theory for Econometricians. New York: Academic Press.

Wooldridge, J. M. (1994). Estimation and inference for dependent processes. In Handbook of Econometrics, vol. 4, pp 2639-2738.

Yi, G. Y., Delaigle, A., & Gustafson, P. (2021). *Handbook of Measurement Error Models*. London: Chapman and Hall/CRC.

Modal Regression for Skewed, Truncated, or Contaminated Data with Outliers

Sijia Xiang and Weixin Yao

Abstract Built on the ideas of mean and quantile, mean regression and quantile regression are extensively investigated and popularly used to model the relationship between a dependent variable Y and covariates $\mathbf{x}$. However, the research about the regression model built on the mode is rather limited. In this article, we introduce a new regression tool, named modal regression, that aims to find the most probable conditional value (mode) of a dependent variable Y given covariates $\mathbf{x}$ rather than the mean that is used by the traditional mean regression. The modal regression can reveal new interesting data structure that is possibly missed by the conditional mean or quantiles. In addition, modal regression is resistant to outliers and heavy-tailed data and can provide shorter prediction intervals when the data are skewed. Furthermore, unlike traditional mean regression, the modal regression can be directly applied to the truncated data. Modal regression could be a potentially very useful regression tool that can complement the traditional mean and quantile regressions.

Keywords Modal regression · Mode · Skewed data

1 Introduction

When talking about location measurements of a data set or distribution, mean, quantile and mode are most commonly used. They have their own merits and complement each other. Up till now, mean and quantile regressions have been extensively studied and popularly used to model the relationship between a response Y and covariates $\mathbf{x}$. However, there is not much research about the regression built on

S. Xiang
School of Data Sciences, Zhejiang University of Finance and Economics, Hangzhou, China
e-mail: sjxiang@zufe.edu.cn

W. Yao (✉)
Department of Statistics, University of California at Riverside, Riverside, CA, USA
e-mail: weixin.yao@ucr.edu

© The Author(s), under exclusive license to Springer Nature Switzerland AG 2022
W. He et al. (eds.), *Advances and Innovations in Statistics and Data Science*, ICSA
Book Series in Statistics, https://doi.org/10.1007/978-3-031-08329-7_12

257

the mode (i.e., modal regression). Different from mean/quantile regression, modal regression is another important tool to study the relationship between a response Y given a set of predictors $\mathbf{x}$, which estimates the conditional modes of Y given $\mathbf{x}$. The developed new regression tool complements the mean and quantile regression and is especially useful for skewed and truncated data and has broad applicability throughout science, such as economics, sociology, behavior, medicine, and biology.

Indeed, the skewed data or truncated data can be commonly found in many applications. For example, Cardoso and Portugal (2005) stated that wages, prices, and expenditures are typical examples of skewed data. In sociology, Healy and Moody (2014) showed that "many of the distributions typically studied in sociology are extremely skewed," for example, church sizes in sociology of religion (Weber 1993), symptoms indices in sociology of mental health (Mirowsky 2013), and so on. Besides, truncated data can be commonly found in many applications such as econometrics (Amemiya 1973; Lewbel & Linton 2002; Park et al. 2008) when dependent variable is an economic index measured within some range. Some examples of truncated data are a sample of Americans whose income is above the poverty line, military height records with a minimum height requirement in many armies, a central bank intervenes to stop an exchange rate falling below or going above certain levels.

We use the following example (Yao & Li 2014) to demonstrate the difference between the modal regression and the mean regression.

Example 1 Let $(\mathbf{x}, Y)$ be coming from the model Use the standard equation environment to typeset your equations, e.g.,

$$Y = m(\mathbf{x}) + \sigma(\mathbf{x})\epsilon, \tag{1}$$

where ϵ has a density $q(\cdot)$, which is a skewed density with mean 0 and mode 1.

1. If $m(\mathbf{x}) = 0$ and $\sigma(\mathbf{x}) = \mathbf{x}^\top \alpha$, then

$$E(Y|\mathbf{x}) = 0 \quad \text{and} \quad Mode(Y|\mathbf{x}) = \mathbf{x}^\top \alpha.$$

That is to say, the conditional mean does not contain any information of the covariate, while the conditional mode does. As a result, various techniques based on modal regression could reveal more important covariates than conditional mean.

2. If $\sigma(\mathbf{x}) = \mathbf{x}^\top \alpha - m(\mathbf{x})$ and $m(x)$ is a nonlinear smooth function, then

$$E(Y|\mathbf{x}) = m(\mathbf{x}) \quad \text{and} \quad Mode(Y|\mathbf{x}) = \mathbf{x}^\top \alpha.$$

In this case, the conditional mode is linear in $\mathbf{x}$ while the conditional mean does not. Of course, the opposite situation could also happen.

In Fig. 1, we also use two plots to illustrate the difference between linear mean and linear mode regression.

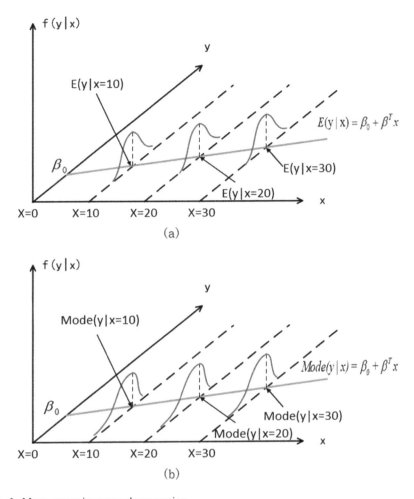

Fig. 1 Mean regression vs mode regression

Many authors have made efforts to identify the modes in the one sample problem. See, for example, Parzen (1962); Scott (1992); Friedman and Fisher (1999); Chauduri and Marron (1999); Hall et al. (2004); Ray and Lindsay (2005); Yao and Lindsay (2009); Henderson and Russell (2005); Henderson et al. (2008); Henderson and Parmeter (2015). Modal hunting has received much interest and wide applications in economy and econometrics too. For example, Henderson and Russell (2005) applied a nonparametric production frontier model to show that international polarization (shift from a uni-modal to a bimodal distribution) is brought primarily by technological catch-up. Cardoso and Portugal (2005) studied the impact of union bargaining power and the degrees of employer coordination on the wage distribution in Portugal wage computed by the mode of the contractual wage set by collective bargaining. Henderson et al. (2008) applied recent advances from statistics literature to test for unconditional multimodality of worldwide distributions of several (unweighted and population-weighted) measures of labor productivity, which is of great interest in economics. They also examined the movements of economies between modal clusters and relationships between certain key development factors and multimodality of the productivity distribution. Einbeck and Tutz (2006) used the value(s) maximizing the conditional kernel density estimate as estimator(s) for the conditional mode(s), and proposed a plug-in estimator using kernel density estimator.

Most of the above modal hunting methods require first nonparametrically estimating the joint density $f(\mathbf{x}, y)$ and $f(y \mid \mathbf{x})$, and then estimating the mode based on the estimated conditional density $f(y \mid \mathbf{x})$, which is practically challenging when the dimension of $\mathbf{x}$ is large due to the well-known "curse of dimensionality." Motivated by the result that the conditional mode from the truncated data provides consistent estimates of the conditional mean for the original non-truncated data, Lee (1989) proposed to model $\text{Mode}(y|\mathbf{x}) = \mathbf{x}^\top \boldsymbol{\beta}$ and derived the mode regression estimator. The identification of $\boldsymbol{\beta}$ and strong consistency of its estimator were derived. However, the objective function used by Lee (1989) is based on kernels with bounded support and thus is difficult to implement in practice. This might explain why modal regression has not drawn too much attention in the last century. In addition, the tuning parameter h used by Lee (1989) is fixed and does not depend on the sample size n. Therefore, it requires the error to be symmetric to get the consistent modal line. Note that in such cases the modal line is indeed the same as the mean regression line and thus their modal regression estimator is essentially a type of robust regression estimate under the assumption of symmetric error density. This limitation of requiring a symmetric error density also applies to the nonparametric modal regression proposed by Yao et al. (2012).

Kemp and Santos Silva (2012) and Yao and Li (2014) are among the first who proposed consistent linear modal regression estimates without requiring a symmetric error density. They established asymptotic properties of the proposed modal estimates, under very general conditions, allowing a skewed error density and a more general kernel function, by letting the bandwidth h go to zero. Since the work of Kemp and Santos Silva (2012) and Yao and Li (2014), modal regression has received much attention recently and been widely applied to various problems. Chen et al. (2016) considered a nonparametric modal regression and used it to build confidence sets based on a kernel density estimate of the joint distribution. Zhou and Huang (2016) considered estimating local modes of the food frequency questionnaire (FFQ) intake given one's long-term usual intake using dietary data. Noticing that the neuroimaging features and cognitive assessment are often heavy-tailed and skewed, Wang et al. (2017) argued that a traditional regression approach might fail to capture the relationship, and applied a regularized modal regression to predict for Alzheimer's disease. Yao and Li (2014) also applied the modal linear regression to a forest fire data, and the results showed that the modal regression gave shorter predictive intervals than traditional methodologies. In order to accurately forecast the energy that will be consumed in the evening, so as to optimize the capacity of storage and consequently to increase the batteries life, Chaouch et al. (2017) applied modal regression to analyze electricity consumption. Kemp et al. (2019) applied both mode- and mean-based autoregressive models to compare the estimates and forecasts of monthly US data on inflation and personal income growth. Please also see Krief (2017); Chen (2018); Li and Huang (2019); Ota et al. (2019); Feng et al. (2020) for some other extensions of the linear modal regression. Ullah et al. (2021) extended the modal regression to the panel data setting.

The rest of the article is organized as follows. In Sect. 2, we formally define the linear modal regression model and discuss its estimator. In Sect. 3, we introduce the nonparametric modal regression. The semiparametric modal regression, which combines the linear modal regression and nonparametric modal regression, is introduced in Sect. 4. A discussion section with some possible future works are presented in Sect. 5.

2 Linear Modal Regression

2.1 Introduction of Linear Modal Regression

Suppose $\{(\mathbf{x}_i, y_i), i = 1, \ldots, n\}$ is a random sample, where $\mathbf{x}_i$ is a p-dimensional column vector, and $f(y|\mathbf{x})$ is the conditional density function of Y given $\mathbf{x}$. In conventional regression models, the mean of $f(y|\mathbf{x})$ is used to investigate the relationship between Y and $\mathbf{x}$. However, when the conditional density of Y given $\mathbf{x}$ is skewed, truncated, or contaminated data with outliers, the conditional mean may not provide a good representation of the $\mathbf{x}$-Y relationship. In this scenario, it is well-known that the mode provides a more meaningful location estimator than the mean. Therefore, the modal regression model is more preferable in this scenario.

The traditional modal estimation is to first estimate the joint density $f(\mathbf{x}, y)$ based on kernel density estimation and then derive the conditional density $f(y|\mathbf{x})$ and its conditional mode. Such method works reasonably well when the dimension of $\mathbf{x}$ is low, however, it is practically infeasible when the dimension of $\mathbf{x}$ is large, due to the "curse of dimensionality".

Borrowing the idea from linear mean/quantile regression, Kemp and Santos Silva (2012) and Yao and Li (2014) proposed linear modal regression (LMR), which assumes that the mode of $f(y|\mathbf{x})$ is a linear function of $\mathbf{x}$. Suppose that the mode of $f(y|\mathbf{x})$ is unique, and denote it by

$$\text{Mode}(Y|\mathbf{x}) = \arg\max_y f(y|\mathbf{x}),$$

then, the LMR assumes that $\text{Mode}(Y|\mathbf{x})$ is a linear function of $\mathbf{x}$, that is,

$$\text{Mode}(Y|\mathbf{x}) = \mathbf{x}^\top \boldsymbol{\beta}, \tag{2}$$

where the first element of $\mathbf{x}$ is assumed to be 1 to represent the intercept. Denote the error term as $\epsilon = y - \mathbf{x}^\top \boldsymbol{\beta}$, and let $q(\epsilon|\mathbf{x})$ to be the conditional distribution of ϵ given $\mathbf{x}$, which is referred to as the error distribution. Note that we allow the error distribution to depend on $\mathbf{x}$. Based on the model assumption of (2), the error density $q(\epsilon|\mathbf{x})$' has the mode at 0.

Unlike one sample mode estimators, the proposed linear modal regression (Yao and Li 2014) puts some model assumptions on Mode($Y|\mathbf{x}$) to transform the original multivariate problems to a much simpler one-dimensional problem and thereby avoid directly estimating the conditional density $f(y|\mathbf{x})$. Note that if the error distribution $q(\epsilon|\mathbf{x})$ is symmetric, then $\boldsymbol{\beta}$ in (2) is nothing but the regression coefficient in traditional linear regression model. However, if $q(\epsilon|\mathbf{x})$ is skewed or heavy-tailed, then, (2) will be quite different from the conventional mean regression model.

Next we explain how we can use a kernel based objective function to estimate the modal regression parameter $\boldsymbol{\beta}$ in (2) consistently. Note that if $\boldsymbol{\beta} = \beta_0$ is a scalar, then β_0 is the mode of $f(y)$, i.e., 0 is the mode of $f(y - \beta_0)$. Therefore, β_0 can be estimated by the maximizer of

$$Q_h(\boldsymbol{\beta}_0) = \frac{1}{n} \sum_{i=1}^{n} \phi_h(y_i - \beta_0), \tag{3}$$

which is a kernel density estimate of $f(y)$, where $\phi_h(\cdot) = h^{-1}\phi(\cdot/h)$ with $\phi(\cdot)$ being a kernel density function symmetric about 0 and h being a tuning parameter. Such a modal estimator has been proposed by Parzen (1962). It has been proved that as $n \to \infty$ and $h \to 0$, the mode of kernel density function will converge to the mode of the distribution of Y.

If $\boldsymbol{\beta}$ does include predictors like in the model (2), by extending the objective function (3), we can then estimate $\boldsymbol{\beta}$ by maximizing

$$Q_h(\boldsymbol{\beta}) = \frac{1}{n} \sum_{i=1}^{n} \phi_h(y_i - \mathbf{x}_i^\top \boldsymbol{\beta}), \tag{4}$$

which can be also considered as the kernel density estimate of the residual $\epsilon_i = y_i - \mathbf{x}_i^\top \boldsymbol{\beta}$ at 0. Then, maximizing (4) with respect to $\boldsymbol{\beta}$ yields $\mathbf{x}^\top \hat{\boldsymbol{\beta}}$ so that the kernel density function of ϵ_i at 0 is maximized. It has been proved by Yao and Li (2014) that as $h \to 0$ as $n \to \infty$, the maximizer of (4), named the linear modal regression estimator (LMRE), is a consistent estimate of $\boldsymbol{\beta}$ in (2) for very general error density without requiring symmetry.

Note that if $\phi_h(t) = (2h)^{-1}I(|t| \le h)$, a uniform kernel, then maximizing (4) is equivalent to maximizing

$$\frac{1}{n} \sum_{i=1}^{n} I(|y_i - \mathbf{x}_i^\top \boldsymbol{\beta}| \le h) = \frac{1}{n} \sum_{i=1}^{n} I(\mathbf{x}_i^\top \boldsymbol{\beta} - h \le y_i \le \mathbf{x}_i^\top \boldsymbol{\beta} + h).$$

Therefore, the LMR tries to find the linear regression $\mathbf{x}^\top \hat{\boldsymbol{\beta}}$ such that the band $\mathbf{x}^\top \hat{\boldsymbol{\beta}} \pm h$ contains the largest proportion/number of response y_i. Therefore, modal regression provides more meaningful point predictions, i.e., larger coverage probability of prediction intervals with a fixed small window around the estimate, and shorter predication intervals than the mean and quantile regression for a fixed confidence limit.

2.2 Asymptotic Properties

In this section, the consistency, convergence rate and asymptotic distribution of the LMR estimator (Kemp & Santos Silva 2012; Yao & Li 2014) are discussed.

Theorem 1 *As $h \to 0$ and $nh^5 \to \infty$, and under the regularity conditions (A1)–(A3) given in the Appendix, there exists a consistent maximizer of (4) such that*

$$\left\| \hat{\boldsymbol{\beta}} - \boldsymbol{\beta}_0 \right\| = O_p\{h^2 + (nh^3)^{-1/2}\},$$

and the asymptotic distribution of the estimator is

$$\sqrt{nh^3} \left[\hat{\boldsymbol{\beta}} - \boldsymbol{\beta}_0 - \frac{h^2}{2} J^{-1} K \{1 + o_p(1)\} \right] \xrightarrow{D} N\{0, v_2 J^{-1} L J^{-1}\},$$

where $\boldsymbol{\beta}_0$ denotes the true coefficient of (4), $v_2 = \int t^2 \phi^2(t)dt$ with $\phi(\cdot)$ being the standard normal density and $q(\cdot)$ is the density of the error term.

$$J = E\{q''(0|\mathbf{x}_i)\mathbf{x}_i\mathbf{x}_i^\top\}, \quad K = E\{q'''(0|\mathbf{x}_i)\mathbf{x}_i\}, \quad L = E\{q(0|\mathbf{x}_i)\mathbf{x}_i\mathbf{x}_i^\top\}. \tag{5}$$

Readers are referred to Yao and Li (2014) for the proofs. One striking but reasonable finding is that the convergence rate of modal regression estimator is slower than the root-n convergence rate of traditional mean/median regression estimators. That is the cost we need to pay in order to estimate the conditional mode (Parzen 1962). Note that for the distribution of Y (without conditioning on $\mathbf{x}$), Parzen (1962) and Eddy (1980) have proven similar asymptotic results for kernel estimators of the mode. Therefore, the results of Parzen (1962) and Eddy (1980) can be considered as special cases of the above theorem with no predictor.

Based on the asymptotic bias and asymptotic variance of $\hat{\boldsymbol{\beta}}$, a theoretical optimal bandwidth h for estimating $\boldsymbol{\beta}$ is to minimize the asymptotic weighted mean squared errors

$$E\{(\hat{\boldsymbol{\beta}} - \boldsymbol{\beta}_0)^\top W(\hat{\boldsymbol{\beta}} - \boldsymbol{\beta}_0)\} \approx (4)^{-1} K^\top J^{-1} W J^{-1} K h^4 + (nh^3)^{-1} v_2 \mathrm{tr}(J^{-1} L J^{-1} W),$$

where $tr(\cdot)$ denotes the trace and W is a diagonal matrix, whose elements reflect the importance of the accuracy in estimating different coefficients. As a result, an asymptotic optimal bandwidth h can be calculated as

$$\hat{h}_{opt} = \left[\frac{3\nu_2 tr(J^{-1}LJ^{-1}W)}{K^\top J^{-1}WJ^{-1}K}\right]^{1/7} n^{-1/7},$$

where J, K, and L are listed in (5).

If W is set to be $W = (J^{-1}LJ^{-1})^{-1} = JL^{-1}J$, which is proportional to the inverse of the asymptotic variance of $\hat{\beta}$, then

$$\hat{h}_{opt} = \left[\frac{3\nu_2(p+1)}{K^\top L^{-1}K}\right]^{1/7} n^{-1/7}.$$

We can then use a plug-in method (Yao and Li 2014) to choose the bandwidth based on the above results.

Another computationally extensive way to choose the bandwidth is to use a cross validation criterion proposed by Zhou and Huang (2019) for modal regression. In addition, instead of just estimating the conditional mode for a chosen value of h, Kemp and Santos Silva (2012) proposed estimating the parameters of interest for a wide range of h, and obtain a more detailed picture of how the parameter estimators perform. The authors further argued that since the inference will not be based on a single value of h, the choice of the limits of h is not as critical as the choice of an optimal value of h.

2.3 Estimation Algorithm

Since there is no closed-form solution to maximize (4), a modal expectation-maximization (MEM) algorithm (Yao 2013) is extended to find the maximizer, which consists of an E-step and an M-step. Note that the choice of the kernel function is not crucial, and Yao and Li (2014) used the standard Gaussian kernel to simplify the computation in the M-step of a modal EM (MEM) algorithm.

Algorithm 2.1 *For $t = 0, 1, \ldots$, at the $(t+1)$-th iteration,*
E-step *For $i = 1, \ldots, n$, calculate the weight as*

$$p(i|\boldsymbol{\beta}^{(t)}) = \frac{\phi_h(y_i - \mathbf{x}_i^\top \boldsymbol{\beta}^{(t)})}{\sum_{j=1}^n \phi_h(y_j - \mathbf{x}_j^\top \boldsymbol{\beta}^{(t)})} \propto \phi_h(y_i - \mathbf{x}_i^\top \boldsymbol{\beta}^{(t)}).$$

M-step *Update the estimate $\boldsymbol{\beta}^{(t+1)}$ as*

$$\boldsymbol{\beta}^{(t+1)} = \arg\max_{\beta} \sum_{i=1}^{n} \{ p(i|\boldsymbol{\beta}^{(t)}) \log \phi_h(y_i - \mathbf{x}_i^\top \boldsymbol{\beta}) \}$$

$$= (\mathbf{X}^\top \mathbf{W}_t \mathbf{X})^{-1} \mathbf{X}^\top \mathbf{W}_t \mathbf{y}, \tag{6}$$

where $\mathbf{X} = (\mathbf{x}_1, \ldots, \mathbf{x}_n)^\top$, $\mathbf{W}_t$ *is an* $n \times n$ *diagonal matrix whose diagonal element is* $p(i|\boldsymbol{\beta}^{(t)})$ *and* $\mathbf{y} = (y_1, \ldots, y_n)^\top$.

Remark 2.1

1. From the above algorithm, we can see that the major difference between the mean regression estimated by the least squares (LSE) criterion and the modal regression lies in the weight $p(i|\boldsymbol{\beta}^{(t)})$. For LSE, each observation has equal weight $1/n$, while for modal regression, the weight $p(i|\boldsymbol{\beta}^{(t)})$ depends on how close y_i is to the modal regression curve. This weight scheme allows the modal regression to reduce the effect of observations far away from the regression curve, so as to achieve robustness.
2. Note that when a normal kernel is used in (4), the function optimized in the M-step is a weighted sum of log-likelihoods corresponding to weighted least squares estimator in the ordinary linear regression. In this case, we obtain a closed-form expression for the maximizer in (6). If other kernels are used, then some optimization algorithms are needed in the M-step.
3. It should be noted that the converged value of this MEM algorithm depends on the starting value. Therefore, it is prudent that we start from several different starting values and choose the best local optima.

2.4 Prediction Intervals Based on Modal Regression

As we explained after the objective function (4), the modal regression could provide more representative point predictions and shorter prediction intervals. In this section, we explain how to construct asymmetric prediction intervals for new observations based on the linear modal regression. The described methods can be also applied to other nonparametric or semiparametric modal regression models introduced in Sects. 3 and 4.

For the simplicity of explanation, we assume that the error distribution of ϵ is independent of $\mathbf{x}$. Let $\hat{\epsilon}_1, \ldots, \hat{\epsilon}_n$ be the residuals of the linear modal regression estimate, where $\hat{\epsilon}_i = y_i - \mathbf{x}_i^\top \hat{\boldsymbol{\beta}}$, and $\hat{\epsilon}_{[i]}$ be the ith smallest value of the residuals. The traditionally used prediction interval with confidence level $1 - \alpha$ for a new covariate $\mathbf{x}_{new}$ is $(\mathbf{x}_{new}^\top \hat{\boldsymbol{\beta}} + \hat{\epsilon}_{[n_1]}, \mathbf{x}_{new}^\top \hat{\boldsymbol{\beta}} + \hat{\epsilon}_{[n_2]})$, where $n_1 = \lfloor n\alpha/2 \rfloor$, and $n_2 = n - n_1$. This symmetric method works best if the error distribution is symmetric. Since the linear modal regression focuses on the highest conditional density region and does not assume a symmetric error density, Yao and Li (2014) proposed the following method for modal regression to use the information of the skewed error density to construct prediction intervals. Suppose $\hat{q}(\cdot)$ is a kernel density estimate of ϵ based on the residuals $\hat{\epsilon}_1, \ldots, \hat{\epsilon}_n$. We find the indexes $k_1 < k_2$ such that $k_2 - k_1 = \lceil n(1-\alpha) \rceil$ and $\hat{q}(\hat{\epsilon}_{[k_1]}) \approx \hat{q}(\hat{\epsilon}_{[k_2]})$. The proposed prediction interval by Yao and Li (2014) for a new covariate $\mathbf{x}_{new}$ is then $(\mathbf{x}_{new}^\top \hat{\beta} + \hat{\epsilon}_{[k_1]}, \mathbf{x}_{new}^\top \hat{\beta} + \hat{\epsilon}_{[k_2]})$.

To find indexes k_1 and k_2, we could use the following iterative algorithm.

Algorithm 2.2 *Starting from $k_1 = \lfloor n\alpha/2 \rfloor$ and $k_2 = n - n_1$,*

Step 1: *If $\hat{q}(\hat{\epsilon}_{[k_1]}) < \hat{q}(\hat{\epsilon}_{[k_2]})$ and $\hat{q}(\hat{\epsilon}_{[k_1+1]}) < \hat{q}(\hat{\epsilon}_{[k_2+1]})$, $k_1 = k_1 + 1$ and $k_2 = k_2 + 1$; if $\hat{q}(\hat{\epsilon}_{[k_1]}) > \hat{q}(\hat{\epsilon}_{[k_2]})$ and $\hat{q}(\hat{\epsilon}_{[k_1-1]}) > \hat{q}(\hat{\epsilon}_{[k_2-1]})$, $k_1 = k_1 - 1$ and $k_2 = k_2 - 1$.*

Step 2: *Iterate Step 1 until none of above two conditions is satisfied or $(k_1 - 1)(k_2 - n) = 0$.*

Based on Yao and Li (2014)'s numerical studies, the above proposed prediction intervals have superior performance to existing symmetric prediction intervals when the data is skewed.

3   Nonparametric Modal Regression

Similar to the traditional linear regression, linear modal regression requires a strong parametric assumption which might not hold in practice. To relax the parametric assumption, there are also nonparametric modal regression that is built based on kernel density estimation. Readers are referred to Chen (2018) for a detailed review of nonparametric modal regressions. For simplicity of explanation, in this section, the covariate X is assumed to be univariate with a compactly supported density function. The estimation procedure can be easily extended to multivariate case but practically difficult due to the "curse of dimensionality."

Let $f(z)$ denote the probability density function (pdf) of a random variable Z and be twice differentiable. Then, define the global mode and local modes of $f(z)$, respectively, as:

$$\mathrm{UniMode}(Z) = \arg\max_z f(z)$$

and

$$\mathrm{MultiMode}(Z) = \{z : f'(z) = 0, f''(z) < 0\}.$$

UniMode(Z), which focuses on the conditional global mode, is called the uni-modal regression, as studied by Lee (1989); Manski (1991). MultiMode(Z), on the other hand, studies the conditional local modes, and is sufficiently investigated by Chen et al. (2016).

The uni-modal regression searches for the function

$$m(x) = \text{UniMode}(Y|X = x) = \arg\max_y f(y|x)$$

and multi-modal regression targets at

$$M(x) = \text{MultiMode}(Y|X = x) = \left\{ y : \frac{\partial}{\partial y} f(y|x) = 0, \frac{\partial^2}{\partial y^2} f(y|x) < 0 \right\},$$

where $f(y|x) = f(x, y)/f(x)$ is the conditional density of Y given $X = x$. Note that, for a given x, the modes or local modes of $f(y|x)$ and $f(x, y)$ are the same. Therefore, the uni-modal and multi-modal regression can be also defined as

$$m(x) = \text{UniMode}(Y|X = x) = \arg\max_y f(x, y), \qquad (7)$$

and

$$M(x) = \left\{ y : \frac{\partial}{\partial y} f(x, y) = 0, \frac{\partial^2}{\partial y^2} f(x, y) < 0 \right\}, \qquad (8)$$

respectively.

3.1 Estimating Uni-Modal Regression

First, we estimate the joint density $f(x, y)$ by the kernel density estimator (KDE) as

$$\hat{f}_n(x, y) = \frac{1}{n h_1 h_2} \sum_{i=1}^{n} K_1 \left(\frac{x_i - x}{h_1} \right) K_2 \left(\frac{y_i - y}{h_2} \right), \qquad (9)$$

where K_1 and K_2 are kernel densities such as Gaussian functions and $h_1 > 0$ and $h_2 > 0$ are tuning parameters. Then, a nonparametric modal regression estimator of $m(x)$ in (7) is

$$\hat{m}_n(x) = \arg\max_y \hat{f}_n(x, y).$$

If K_2 is assumed to be a spherical kernel such as $K_2(z) = \frac{1}{2} I(|z| \leq 1)$, then it has been shown that the maximization operation is equivalent to the minimization operator on a flattened $0 - 1$ loss.

Yao and Xiang (2016) proposed a local polynomial modal regression (LPMR) estimation procedure to estimate the nonparametric modal regression, which maximizes

$$\ell(\boldsymbol{\theta}) = \frac{1}{n} \sum_{i=1}^{n} K_{h_1}(x_i - x_0)\phi_{h_2}\left(y_i - \sum_{j=1}^{p} \beta_j(x_i - x_0)^j\right) \qquad (10)$$

over $\boldsymbol{\theta} = (\beta_0, \ldots, \beta_p)$. Similar to Yao et al. (2012), the authors used an EM algorithm to maximize (10) since it has a mixture type form. The asymptotic properties were discussed and proved.

Feng et al. (2020) also studied nonparametric modal regression from a statistical learning viewpoint through the classical empirical risk minimization (ERM) scheme and investigated its theoretical properties.

3.2 Estimating Multi-Modal Regression

Similar to the estimation of uni-modal regression, Chen et al. (2016) proposed estimating the multi-modal regression by a plug-in estimate from the KDE, as follows:

$$\hat{M}_n(x) = \left\{ y : \frac{\partial}{\partial y} \hat{f}_n(x, y) = 0, \ \frac{\partial^2}{\partial y^2} \hat{f}_n(x, y) < 0 \right\},$$

where $\hat{f}_n(x, y)$ is from (9).

By assuming K_1 and K_2 to be Gaussian kernels, $\hat{M}_n(x)$ can be estimated through a mean-shift algorithm (Chen et al. 2016) which is actually equivalent to the mode hunting EM algorithm (Yao 2013, MEM). The results can be applied to other radially symmetric kernels as well. The partial mean-shift algorithm is summarized in Algorithm 3.1.

Algorithm 3.1 *Partial mean-shift*
Input: *Samples* $\mathcal{D} = \{(x_1, y_1), \ldots, (x_n, y_n)\}$, *bandwidths* h_1 *and* h_2.
1. Find a starting set $\mathcal{M} \in \mathbb{R}^2$, *such as* $\mathcal{D}$.
2. For each $(x, y) \in \mathcal{M}$, *fix x and update y by*
$$y \leftarrow \frac{\sum_{i=1}^{n} y_i K(|x-x_i|/h_1) K(|y-y_i|/h_2)}{\sum_{i=1}^{n} K(|x-x_i|/h_1) K(|y-y_i|/h_2)}$$
until convergence. Let y^∞ *be the converged value.*
Output: $\mathcal{M}^\infty$, *which contains the points* (x, y^∞).

Comparing between uni-modal and multi-modal regression, we can see that multi-modal regression is more preferred in situations where there are hidden heterogeneous relations in the data set. In addition, if the there are several modes in the original data, since the uni-modal regression can only detect the main component, the prediction regions tend to be wider than that of the multi-modal regression, as shown in Fig. 2. However, it is obvious that the uni-modal regression is easier to interpret, which is quite important in data applications.

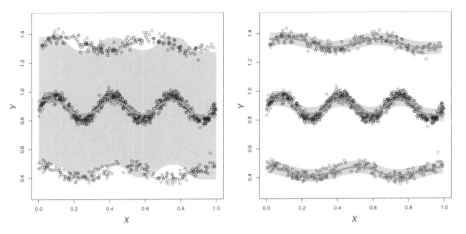

Fig. 2 Uni-modal vs multi-modal regression

4 Semiparametric Modal Regression

Many authors have extended the linear modal regression (Kemp & Santos Silva 2012; Yao & Li 2014) to semiparametric models. See, for example, Krief (2017), Ota et al. (2019), and Yao and Xiang (2016). In this section, we explain the idea of semiparametric modal regression using the varying coefficient modal regressions proposed by Yao and Xiang (2016).

To be more specific, given a random sample $\{(\mathbf{x}_i, u_i, y_i); 1 \leq i \leq n\}$, where y_i is the response variable and $(\mathbf{x}_i, u_i)$ are covariates, Yao and Xiang (2016) proposed a nonparametric varying coefficient modal regression, defined as

$$\text{Mode}(y|\mathbf{x}_i, u_i) = \max_y f(y|\mathbf{x}_i, u_i) = \sum_{j=1}^{p} g_j(u_i)x_{ij}, \qquad (11)$$

where $\mathbf{x}_i = (x_{i1}, \ldots, x_{ip})^\top$ and $\{g_1(u), \ldots, g_p(u)\}^\top$ are unknown smooth functions. If $g_j(u)$ is constant for all j, then the above model becomes the linear modal regression (2). In addition, the nonparametric uni-modal regression introduced in Sect. 3 is a special case of (11) when $p = 1$ and $x_i = 1$. Allowing $g_j(u)$ to depend on some index u, the varying coefficient modal regression can relax the constant coefficient assumption of the linear modal regression, and also better model how the modal regression coefficients dynamically change over the index u, which could be a time or location index. Compared to the fully nonparametric modal regression, the above model can easily adopt multivariate covariates by imposing some model assumption on the conditional mode. Therefore, the semiparametric modal regression can combine the benefits of both the parametric modal regression and the nonparametric modal regression.

Yao and Xiang (2016) proposed estimating the varying coefficient modal regression (11) by a local linear approximation of $g_j(u)$ in a neighborhood of u_0,

$$g_j(u) \approx g_j(u_0) + g_j'(u_0)(u - u_0) = b_j + c_j(u - u_0).$$

Let $\theta = (b_1, \ldots, b_p, h_1 c_1, \ldots, h_1 c_p)^\top$. Then θ is found by maximizing

$$\ell(\theta) = \sum_{i=1}^{n} K_{h_1}(u_i - u_0) \phi_{h_2} \left[y_i - \sum_{j=1}^{p} \{ b_j + c_j(u_i - u_0) \} x_{ij} \right], \tag{12}$$

over θ. Let $\hat{\theta} = (\hat{b}_1, \ldots, \hat{b}_p, h_1 \hat{c}_1, \ldots, h_1 \hat{c}_p)^\top$ be the maximizer of (12). Then $\hat{g}(u_0) = (\hat{b}_1, \ldots, \hat{b}_p)^\top$ is the estimate of $\{ g_1(u_0), \ldots, g_p(u_0) \}^\top$, and $\hat{g}'(u_0) = (\hat{c}_1, \ldots, \hat{c}_p)^\top$ is the estimate of $\{ g_1'(u_0), \ldots, g_p'(u_0) \}^\top$.

The algorithm proposed to maximize (12) is summarized as follows.

Algorithm 4.1 *Starting with $t = 0$:*

E-Step: *Update $\pi(j \mid \theta^{(t)})$*

$$\pi(j \mid \theta^{(t)}) = \frac{K_{h_1}(u_j - u_0) \phi_{h_2} \left[y_j - \sum_{l=1}^{p} \left\{ b_l^{(t)} + c_l^{(t)}(u_j - u_0) \right\} x_{jl} \right]}{\sum_{i=1}^{n} K_{h_1}(u_i - u_0) \phi_{h_2} \left[y_i - \sum_{l=1}^{p} \left\{ b_l^{(t)} + c_l^{(t)}(u_i - u_0) \right\} x_{il} \right]},$$

$$j = 1, \ldots, n.$$

M-Step: *Update $\theta^{(t+1)}$*

$$\theta^{(t+1)} = \arg\max_\theta \sum_{j=1}^{n} \pi(j \mid \theta^{(t)}) \log \phi_{h_2} \left[y_j - \sum_{l=1}^{p} \left\{ b_l^{(t)} + c_l^{(t)}(u_j - u_0) \right\} x_{jl} \right],$$

which has an explicit solution since $\phi(\cdot)$ is the Gaussian density.

Denote by $f_u(u)$ the marginal density of u, $q(\epsilon \mid \mathbf{x}, u)$ the conditional density of $\epsilon = y - \sum_{j=1}^{p} g_j(u) x_j$ given $\mathbf{x}$ and u, and $q^{(v)}(\epsilon \mid \mathbf{x}, u)$ the v-th derivative of $q(\epsilon \mid \mathbf{x}, u)$. Let

$$\alpha_j(u) = E\{ \mathbf{x} X_j q^{(2)}(0 \mid \mathbf{x}, u) \mid u \}, \quad \beta(u) = E\{ \mathbf{x} q^{(3)}(0 \mid \mathbf{x}, u) \mid u \}$$

$$\Delta(u) = E\{ \mathbf{x} \mathbf{x}^\top q^{(2)}(0 \mid \mathbf{x}, u) \mid u \}, \quad \tilde{\Delta}(u) = E\{ \mathbf{x} \mathbf{x}^\top q(0 \mid \mathbf{x}, u) \mid u \}.$$

Yao and Xiang (2016) provided the following asymptotic properties for the proposed varying coefficient modal regression estimator.

Theorem 2 *Under the regularity conditions (A4)|(A6) in the Appendix, if the bandwidths h_1 and h_2 go to 0 such that $nh_1^3 h_2^5 \to \infty$ and $h_1^2/h_2 \to 0$ the asymptotic bias of $\hat{\mathbf{g}}(u_0)$ is given by*

$$Bias\left\{\hat{\mathbf{g}}(u_0)\right\} = \frac{1}{2}\Delta^{-1}(u_0)\left\{\mu_2 h_1^2 \sum_{j=1}^{p} g_j''(u_0)\alpha_j(u_0) - h_2^2\beta(u_0)\right\}\left\{1 + o_p(1)\right\},$$

(13)

and the asymptotic covariance is

$$Cov\left\{\hat{\mathbf{g}}(u_0)\right\} = \frac{\tilde{\nu}\nu_0}{nh_1 h_2^3 f_u(u_0)}\Delta^{-1}(u_0)\tilde{\Delta}(u_0)\Delta^{-1}(u_0)\left\{1 + o_p(1)\right\},$$

(14)

where $\mu_j = \int t^j K(t)dt$, $\nu_j = \int t^j K^2(t)dt$, and $\tilde{\nu} = \int t^2\phi^2(t)dt$.

Theorem 3 *Under the same condition as in Theorem 2, if the bandwidths h_1 and h_2 go to 0 such that $nh_1 h_2^5 \to \infty$ and $h_1^2/h_2 \to 0$, the estimate $\mathbf{g}(u_0)$ has the following asymptotic distribution*

$$[Cov\{\hat{\mathbf{g}}(u_0)\}]^{-1/2}[\hat{\mathbf{g}}(u_0) - \mathbf{g}_0(u_0) - Bias\{\hat{\mathbf{g}}(u_0)\}] \xrightarrow{L} N(0, I),$$

where $Bias\{\hat{\mathbf{g}}(u_0)\}$ is defined in (13) and $Cov\{\hat{\mathbf{g}}(u_0)\}$ is defined in (14).

5 Discussion

In this article, we introduced modal regressions, which can be a good complement to mean/quantile regression, and are especially suitable for skewed, truncated, or contaminated data with outliers. Compared to traditional mean regression models, the modal regression models are more robust and have better prediction performance. Simulation studies and real data analysis are done to illustrate the numerical performance of the new methods. Due to the length of the article, the readers are referred to Yao and Li (2014) and Yao and Xiang (2016) for the details.

The development of modal regression is still in its early stage. Parallel to the traditional mean/quantile regression, the modal regression can be extended to a broad variety of parametric, nonparametric, and semiparametric modal regression models. For high dimensional models, it is interesting to investigate how to perform feature screening and variable selection for modal regression. In addition, it also requires more research to extend the modal regression to the longitudinal/panel data (Ullah et al. 2021), time series data, data with measurement errors, and missing data problems.

Appendix

The conditions used by the theorems are listed below. They are not the weakest possible conditions, but they are imposed to facilitate the proofs.

Technical Conditions:

(A1) $q^{(v)}(t \mid x)$, $v = 0, 1, 2, 3$ is continuous in a neighborhood of 0 , and $q'(0 \mid x) = 0$ for any x.

(A2) $n^{-1} \sum_{i=1}^{n} q''(0 \mid x_i) x_i x_i^T = J + o_p(1)$, $n^{-1} \sum_{i=1}^{n} q'''(0 \mid x_i) x_i = K + o_p(1)$ and $n^{-1} \sum_{i=1}^{n} q(0 \mid x_i) x_i x_i^T = L + o_p(1)$, where $J < 0$, that is, $-J$ is a positive definite matrix.

(A3) $n^{-1} \sum_{i=1}^{n} \|x_i\|^4 = O_p(1)$, and $q'(0 \mid x) = 0$ any x.

(A4) $g_j(x)$ has continuous 2nd derivative at the point x_0, $j = 1, ..., p$.

(A5) $q'(0 \mid \mathbf{x}, u) = 0$, $q''(0 \mid \mathbf{x}, u) < 0$, $q^{(v)}(t \mid \mathbf{x}, u)$ is bounded in a neighbor of $(\mathbf{x}_0, u_0)$ and has continuous first derivative at the point $(\mathbf{x}_0, u_0)$ as a function of $(\mathbf{x}, u)$, for $v = 0, \ldots, 4$.

(A6)   The $f_u(u)$ is bounded and has continuous first derivative at the point u_0 and $f(u_0) > 0$.

References

Amemiya, T. (1973). Regression analysis when the dependent variable is truncated normal. *Econometrica, 41,* 997–1016.

Cardoso, A. R., & Portugal, P. (2005). Contractual wages and the wage cushion under different bargaining settings. *Journal of Labor Economics, 23,* 875–902.

Chaouch, P., Laïb, N., & Louani, D. (2017). Rate of uniform consistency for a class of mode regression on functional stationary ergodic data. *Statistical Methods & Applications, 26*(1), 19–47.

Chauduri, P., & Marron, J. (1999). Sizer for exploration of structures in curves. *Journal of the American Statistical Association, 94,* 807–823.

Chen, Y. (2018). Modal regression using kernel density estimation: a review. *Advanced Review, 10,* 1–14.

Chen, Y. C., Genovese, C. R., Tibshirani, R. J., & Wasserman, L. (2016). Nonparametric modal regression. *The Annals of Statistics, 44,* 489–514.

Eddy, W. P. (1980). Optimum kernel estimators of the mode. *The Annals of Statistics, 8,* 870–882.

Einbeck, J., & Tutz, G. (2006). Modelling beyond regression functions: an application of multimodal regression to speed-flow data. *Applied Statistics, 55,* 461–475.

Feng, Y., Fan, J., & Suykens, J. A. (2020). A statistical learning approach to modal regression. *Journal of Machine Learning Research, 21*(2), 1–35.

Friedman, J. H., & Fisher, N. I. (1999). Bump hunting in high-dimensional data. *Statistics and Computing, 9,* 123–143.

Hall, P., Minnotte, M. C., & Zhang, C. (2004). Bump hunting with non-gaussian kernels. *The Annals of Statistics, 32,* 2124–2141.

Healy, K., & Moody, J. (2014). Data visualization in sociology. *Annual Review of Sociology, 40,* 105–128.

Henderson, D. J., & Parmeter, C. F. (2015). *Applied nonparametric econometrics.* Cambridge University Press.

Henderson, D. J., & Russell, R. R. (2005). Human capital and convergence: a production frontier approach. *International Economic Review, 46*, 1167–1205.

Henderson, D. J., Parmeter, C. F., & Russell, R. R. (2008). Modes, weighted modes, and calibrated modes: evidence of clustering using modality tests. *Journal of Applied Econometrics, 23*, 607–638.

Kemp, G. C. R., & Santos Silva, J. M. C. (2012). Regression towards the mode. *Journal of Economics, 170*, 92–101.

Kemp, G. C. R., Parente, P., & Santos Silva, J. M. C. (2019). Dynamic vector mode regression. *Journal of Business & Economic Statistics, 38*, 647–661.

Krief, J. M. (2017). Semi-linear mode regression. *The Econometrics Journal, 20*(2), 149–167.

Lee, M. J. (1989). Mode regression. *Journal of Econometrics, 42*, 337–349.

Lewbel, A., & Linton, O. (2002). Nonparametric censored and truncated regression. *Econometrica, 70*, 765–779.

Li, X., & Huang, X. (2019). Linear mode regression with covariate measurement error. *Canadian Journal of Statistics, 47*(2), 262–280.

Manski, C. (1991). Regression. *Journal of Economic Literature, 29*, 34–50.

Mirowsky, J. (2013). Analyzing associations between mental health and social circumstances. In *Handbook of the sociology of mental health* (pp. 143–165).

Ota, H., Kato, K., Hara, S., et al. (2019). Quantile regression approach to conditional mode estimation. *Electronic Journal of Statistics, 13*(2), 3120–3160.

Park, B. U., Simar, L., & Zelenyuk, V. (2008). Local likelihood estimation of truncated regression and its partial derivatives: Theory and application. *Journal of Econometrics, 146*, 185–198.

Parzen, E. (1962). On estimation of a probability density function and mode. *Journal of American Statistical Association, 33*, 1065–1076.

Ray, S., & Lindsay, B. G. (2005). The topography of multivariate normal mixtures. *The Annals of Statistics*, 2042–2065.

Scott, D. W. (1992). *Multivariate density estimation: Theory, practice and visualization*. New York: Wiley.

Ullah, A., Wang, T., & Yao, W. (2021). Modal regression for fixed effects panel data. *Empirical Economics, 60*(1), 261–308.

Wang, X., Chen, H., Shen, D., & Huang, H. (2017). Cognitive impairment prediction in Alzheimer's disease with regularized modal regression. *Advances in Neural Information Processing Systems*, 1447–1457.

Weber, M. (1993). *The sociology of religion*.

Yao, W. (2013). A note on EM algorithm for mixture models. *Statistics Probability Letters, 83*, 519–526.

Yao, W., & Li, L. (2014). A new regression model: modal linear regression. *Scandinavian Journal of Statistics, 41*, 656–671.

Yao, W., & Lindsay, B. G. (2009). Bayesian mixture labelling by highest posterior density. *Journal of American Statistical Association, 104*, 758–767.

Yao, W., & Xiang, S. (2016). Nonparametric and varying coefficient modal regression. arXiv:1602.06609.

Yao, W., Lindsay, B. G., & Li, R. (2012). Local modal regression. *Journal of Nonparametric Statistics, 24*, 647–663.

Zhou, H., & Huang, X. (2016). Nonparametric modal regression in the presence of measurement error. *Electronic Journal of Statistics, 10*(2), 3579–3620.

Zhou, H., & Huang, X. (2019). Bandwidth selection for nonparametric modal regression. *Communications in Statistics-Simulation and Computation, 48*(4), 968–984.

Spatial Multilevel Modelling in the Galveston Bay Recovery Study Survey

Mary E. Thompson, Gang Meng, Joseph Sedransk, Qixuan Chen, and Rebecca Anthopolos

Abstract The Galveston Bay Recovery Study conducted a longitudinal survey of residents of two counties in Texas in the aftermath of Hurricane Ike, which made landfall on September 13, 2008 and caused widespread damage. An important objective was to chart the extent of symptoms of Post-Traumatic Stress Disorder (PTSD) in the resident population over the following months. Wave 1 of the survey was conducted between November 17, 2008 and March 24, 2009. Waves 2 and 3 consisted of two month and one year follow-ups, respectively. With the use of a stratified, 3-stage sampling design, data were collected from 658 residents. The first stage of sampling within strata was the selection of clusters, or *area segments*. Our objective is to model the course of the repeated PTSD measures as a function of individual characteristics and area segment, and to examine the analytical and visual evidence for spatial correlation of the area segment effect. To incorporate design information, our multilevel analysis uses the composite likelihood approach of Rao et al. (*Survey Methodology, 39*, 263–282, 2013) and Yi et al. (*Statistica Sinica, 26*, 569–587, 2016). We compare this with a Bayesian multilevel analysis and discuss the estimability of the model when the cluster-level variation has spatial dependence.

M. E. Thompson (✉) · G. Meng
Department of Statistics and Actuarial Sciences, University of Waterloo, Waterloo, ON, Canada
e-mail: methomps@uwaterloo.ca; gmeng@uwaterloo.ca

J. Sedransk
University of Maryland, College Park, MD, USA
e-mail: jxs123@case.edu

Q. Chen
Department of Biostatistics, Columbia University, New York, NY, USA
e-mail: qc2138@cumc.columbia.edu

R. Anthopolos
New York University, New York, NY, USA
e-mail: Rebecca.Anthopolos@nyulangone.org

© The Author(s), under exclusive license to Springer Nature Switzerland AG 2022
W. He et al. (eds.), *Advances and Innovations in Statistics and Data Science*, ICSA
Book Series in Statistics, https://doi.org/10.1007/978-3-031-08329-7_13

Keywords Bayesian analysis · Complex survey design · Longitudinal data ·
Multilevel model · Pairwise composite likelihood

1 Introduction

The Galveston Bay Recovery Study (GBRS) survey was conducted to study the
impact of Hurricane Ike, which had made landfall at Galveston Bay on September
13, 2008. The survey took place in Chambers County and Galveston County in
Texas. Galveston County includes Galveston Island and the Bolivar Peninsula, with
Goat Island just to the north. The hurricane caused severe damage, particularly on
the Bolivar Peninsula and Goat Island, but also on Galveston Island and further into
the Bay.

With the intention of gathering data close to the time of the disaster, the
investigators were able to design a three-wave longitudinal survey of which Wave
1 went into the field about two months after Hurricane Ike. Wave 1 continued until
March 24, 2009. Wave 2 was a half-hour follow-up intended to be conducted two to
three months after the initial interview. Wave 3 was a full follow-up survey intended
to be conducted about a year after the first interview (University of Michigan
Survey Research Center/Institute for Social Research 2010). The sampling design
was a two-stage area sample of households from address-based frames, while
interviewing took place by telephone. The main goal was to characterize trajectories
and determinants of post-disaster mental health outcomes, such as Post-Traumatic
Stress Disorder (PTSD), as measured through a severity score computed from
responses to a 17-item scale (Pietrzak et al. 2013). Another aim (Gruebner et al.
2016a,b) was to use spatial analysis to identify patterns of mental health and
wellness, and their predictors, across the geographic area in the aftermath of the
disaster.

With a view to incorporating the complex features of the sampling design,
Anthopolos et al. (2020) have proposed a Bayesian growth mixture model, where
the three-wave trajectory of the log of the PTSD severity score is modelled within
latent classes. The modelling of latent class membership is multilevel because of
the clustering of the sample, and incorporates spatial dependence across adjacent
clusters. Sampling design variables such as household size and auxiliary information
on the frames are incorporated as covariates. Inference concerning the cluster-level
variance components of latent class membership is part of the purpose.

The aim of this paper is to implement a frequentist approach to incorporating
complex sampling design features in a more basic repeated measures analysis of the
same data, where inference concerning the cluster-level variance components for the
log PTSD severity score itself is envisaged. The complex sampling design features
are incorporated using pairwise likelihood using the approach of Rao et al. (2013)
and Yi et al. (2016).

Section 2 will describe the sampling design in detail. Sections 3 and 4 will
document the construction of survey weights and the derivation of the inclusion
probabilities required for the illustrative analyses. Section 5 specifies the spatial

multilevel model under consideration. Sections 6 and 7 present a standard Bayesian analysis and the proposed frequentist analysis, respectively. Section 8 discusses the advantages and disadvantages of the two approaches, with reference to the ways in which they use the information in the sampling design and the weights.

2 Sampling Design

The following description is taken from Valliant et al. (2009) and University of Michigan Survey Research Center/Institute for Social Research (2010).

There were two sampling frames. One frame was the Experian Gold list for Galveston and Chambers Counties, purchased from the credit reporting agency Experian. This list had demographic information that could be used in an attempt to identify households and persons with higher probability of experiencing PTSD in the short or long run, based on earlier studies. A score was then constructed by the SRC to classify most of the households as high risk or low risk (or with insufficient data to determine) for PTSD after a disaster. The other frame was an area probability frame created by field staff listing procedures. Its coverage was more comprehensive, for example, including growth since the 2000 Census.

For the GBRS survey, FEMA maps of the flooding in the Galveston area immediately after Hurricane Ike and Census 2000 data were used to divide the two-county area into five geographic strata:

Stratum 1: Galveston Island and the Bolivar Peninsula, which suffered storm surge damage
Stratum 2: Flooded areas of the mainland
Stratum 3: Non-flooded areas of the mainland which had relatively high rates of poverty in the 2000 Census
Stratum 4: Non-flooded, non-poverty areas east of Route 146 (and thus close to the Bay)
Stratum 5: Non-flooded, non-poverty areas west of Route 146 and the remainder of Chambers County (not flooded for the most part)

Within strata, the researchers constructed *area segments* composed of census blocks from the 2000 Census. Eighty (80) of these were to be selected. It was initially decided that the relative sampling rates in the strata would be 4, 4, 2, 2, and 1, so that Stratum 1 and Stratum 2 would be oversampled, while Stratum 5 would be undersampled. Implementing these rates resulted in an allocation of area segments to strata of 42, 4, 16, 4, and 14. Within strata, the area segments were selected with probability proportional to a size measure, namely the number of occupied housing units in the 2000 census.

Three of the selected segments in Stratum 1 were in an area (the Bolivar Peninsula) that received extensive damage and could not be field-listed. Thus the final numbers of segments represented in the strata samples are 39, 4, 16, 4 and 14; or 77 in all. Figure 1 shows the locations of the census tracts of the sampled area segments, coloured according to stratum, superimposed on a map of population

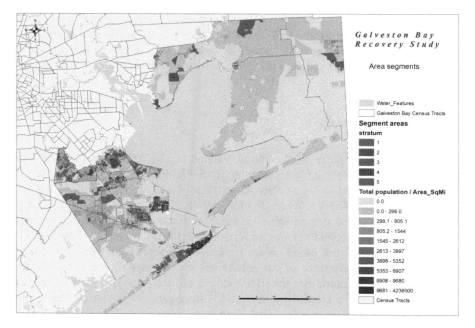

Fig. 1 Census blocks of the sampled area segments superimposed on a map of population density from the 2000 Census

density from the 2000 Census. From this map it is apparent that the sample is taken from areas of higher population density.

The area field listing included many housing units present in the area which did not appear on the Experian frame, and there were many cases where the same housing unit was recorded differently on the two frames. Within selected area segments, it was decided to use the Experian list as the primary sampling frame. Households therein were subdivided in each geographic stratum into *High Risk for PTSD* and *Other* (low risk or not determinable). The High Risk group was sampled at a rate 1.5 times that of the Other group. A separate sample was then taken from the subset of the area field frame listings which did not appear on the Experian frame. Whether this was the case could not always be determined perfectly: in some apartment buildings, there were cases that had a chance of selection on both frames. In the end, there were 124 Wave 1 interviews that came from the area frame (all coded as *other* for the risk variable) and 534 from the Experian frame.

In a *first phase* of sampling, selected households where it was possible to make contact were rostered, and in each, a member was selected at random from among those who were 18 years of age or older at the time of selection. *Respondent locating* was a major part of the effort, and this task was sent first to an outside vendor for internet locating of respondents, to be followed by in-person tracking.

In a *second phase* of sampling of households not responding in the first fieldwork period, cases from the first released sample, either in tracking or never contacted, were considered for further effort aimed at completing an interview. Of 489 eligible cases, 250 were selected.

Overall there were 2116 selected housing units, 420 of which were determined to be out of scope, and 658 of which resulted in a completed interview. Twenty (20) of the selected respondents were judged ineligible. Thus the Wave 1 response rate was approximately 40%. Weighted re-interview rates were 81.4% at Wave 2 and 73.3% at Wave 3.

3 Survey Weights

Survey weights were constructed for the GBRS survey data. Only the Wave 1 weights will be described here. The process is described in Valliant et al. (2009). The initial household weight was calculated as the reciprocal of the intended household inclusion probability, taking into account risk status (High Risk for PTSD or Other), the possibility of inclusion in both frames, and phase of sampling.

Consideration of phase of sampling leads to high variability of the initial household weight within strata.

The household weight was then adjusted for non-response, as follows. Contact, screening, and main interview completion were modelled in terms of housing unit characteristics: observed damage to the unit, observed destruction of the unit, stratum, Bolivar indicator, Experian indicator, High Damage Area indicator, Median Year Housing Units Built (an area segment variable), Ever a Refusal (15% of household refusals were converted), and Number of Calls.

Four adjustment strata were created, and weights were adjusted by the mean predicted contact, screening, and interview propensities in their adjustment strata. A few non-response adjustment factors were very large, and the corresponding weights were trimmed, with the reduction in weights being distributed across the other cases.

For each individual respondent, the person-level weight was the product of the non-response-adjusted household weight and the number of adults aged 18 or over in the household.

4 Inferring Inclusion Probabilities from the Weights

In the data file the household weights and person weights were provided, giving us the unconditional inclusion probability for each household and for each individual. For an illustrative design-based multilevel analysis, we needed to assign an estimated inclusion probability to each sampled area segment, and an estimated inclusion probability to each sampled individual, conditional on their area segment being sampled. The sampling of area segments was done using probability proportional to size sampling, where size was the 2000 census number of occupied housing units in the area segment. We were able to obtain an approximate value of the size of an area segment by summing the year 2000 occupied housing unit numbers of the census blocks of sampled households within the area segment, and adjusting the sum upward so that the totals over area segments in the strata would match known numbers. This produced an estimated size variable $\hat{N}_{hj}$ for each Stratum h and area segment j. It should be noted that the designers of the sampling plan would have had access to the true size values.

If we denote the initial household weight for household k in area segment j and Stratum h by w_{hjk}, we can write the reciprocal of w_{hjk} as

$$\pi_{k|hj}\pi_{j|h}, \tag{1}$$

where $\pi_{j|h}$ is the needed area segment inclusion probability and $\pi_{k|hj}$ is the design inclusion probability of household k within sampled area segment j in Stratum h. The value of $\pi_{k|hj}$ depends on the risk stratum (High Risk for PTSD vs Other) of the household.

The High Risk for PTSD vs Other variable is not included on the data set. However, within many area segments, the lower household weights follow a pattern: the lowest weights are about 2/3 of the next lowest weights. Thus it appears that the lowest weights may correspond to deliberate oversampling, and we have assumed that they belong to households that were sampled at a rate of 1.5 times the "usual" rate in the area segment. We have also noted that within strata, the inclusion probabilities for households from the area frame were a fixed multiple of the inclusion probability of lower risk households from the Experian frame. Using these facts, together with information about the inclusion probabilities for the second phase samples, and additional assumptions, we have assigned a value of the High Risk indicator to each household.

Except for some extreme values due to the second phase of sampling, the initial household weights are not highly variable within area segments, and we approximated household inclusion probabilities by assuming simple random sampling within risk indicator value to begin with. Let a_{hj} (to be estimated) be N_{hj} times the sampling rate for lower risk households in area segment j of stratum h, where N_{hj} is the number of census 2000 occupied housing units in the area segment (the "size" of the area segment), so that for household k, the probability of inclusion $\pi_{k|hj}$ is $1.5^{\delta_{hjk}}a_{hj}/N_{hj}$ where $\delta_{hjk} = 1$ if household k is of High Risk for PTSD, and 0 otherwise. Suppose the number of sampled households in the area segment is n_{hj}. Let the proportion of those households that appear (from their weights) to be High Risk for PTSD be $\hat{p}_{hj}$. Then a_{hj} can be estimated from the equation

$$n_{hj} = \hat{p}_{hj}(1.5\hat{a}_{hj}) + (1 - \hat{p}_{hj})\hat{a}_{hj}. \tag{2}$$

This gives a preliminary estimate of $N_{hj}\pi_{k|hj}$ for each household k in the sample in area segment j.

Taking this estimate and multiplying by initial household weight, i.e., the reciprocal of the expression in (1), we computed a household-specific preliminary estimate of $\pi_{j|h}/N_{hj}$. We averaged these over the households with non-extreme weights in area segment j to estimate $\pi_{j|h}/N_{hj}$. We multiplied by $\hat{N}_{hj}$ and took the minimum of the result and 1 to obtain an approximate value of $\pi_{j|h}$ for each area segment j.

We then estimated the post-nonresponse inclusion probability for a household, given inclusion of its area segment, as the reciprocal of (the non-response adjusted household weight times the approximate value of the area segment inclusion probability). If we set aside three area segments with unusually high inclusion probabilities in Stratum 1, the average estimated area segment inclusion probabilities in the five strata are, respectively, 0.516, 0.689, 0.239, 0.260, and 0.113. The relative values of these are not very different from those of the initial target sampling rates, which were to be proportional to 4, 4, 2, 2, and 1.

These calculations allowed us to construct, for illustrative purposes, approximate decompositions of the person-level inclusion probabilities as follows:

$$\pi_{hjki} = \pi_{j|h}\pi_{k|hj}\pi_{i|hjk},$$

where $\pi_{i|hjk}$ is the reciprocal of the number of people aged 18 or over in household k. In what follows it will be convenient most of the time so suppress the stratum index h and combine the selection of household and person, writing the inclusion probability of person i of area segment j as

$$\pi_{ji} = \pi_j\pi_{i|j}. \tag{3}$$

5   Spatial Multilevel Model

Let the outcome variable y_{jit} be the logarithm of self-reported Post-Traumatic Stress Disorder (PTSD) severity score for resident i living in sampling cluster j at Wave t, $t = 1, 2, 3$. The sampling clusters are taken to be the area segments. We suppress notation for the sampling stratum h and the household k for simplicity. The PTSD severity scores were calculated as the sum of responses to 17 symptoms of PTSD, such as "repeated, disturbing memories of Hurricane Ike," using the Checklist-Specific version (PCL-S) (Blanchard et al. 1996) with each symptom rated from 1 (not at all) to 5 (extremely). Questions were asked in reference to the period since the hurricane at Wave 1, and the period since the previous interview at Waves 2 and 3. Let $\mathbf{x}_{ji}$ be the row vector of p covariates of interest for resident i in cluster j, potentially including age, gender, ethnicity, highest education completed, pre-disaster trauma exposure, pre-disaster PTSD, pre-disaster depression, hurricane-related trauma and stressors, peri-event reactions, and community-level social assets (Gruebner et al. 2016a). The model for the outcome variable could also depend on the sampling design through the sampling stratum, and through determinants of w_{ij}, such as a smooth function of the logarithm of the size variable (the number of occupied housing units in the sampled census blocks of the area segment); the risk indicator for the household; the number of adult members of the household; and a function of the household non-response adjustment (Anthopolos et al. 2020). We have used all of these except the function of the size variable, this being omitted to keep the covariate space relatively simple.

The goal of this modelling approach is to examine risk factors, analytically and visually, associated with post-disaster scores of PTSD after accounting for longitudinal dependence, spatial correlation and the complex survey design. We propose a three-level model, where the three levels are the spatial cluster (the area segment), the individual within a cluster, and the survey wave within an individual. By an extension of notation j is the identifier of the *adjusted census tract* (CT) containing cluster j. Adjusted CTs were defined as follows: if two or more area segments (clusters) were in one official CT, the CT was split based on the number of area segments within it so that each area segment is in just one adjusted CT; if a CT has no area segment within it, that CT is combined with the nearest adjusted CT; thus after adjustment, the whole study area has the same number of adjusted CTs as the number of area segments.

The model for the outcome variable can be written as follows:

$$y_{jit} | \mu_{jit} \sim N(\mu_{jit}, \sigma_c^2)$$

$$\mu_{jit} = \alpha_{0ji} + \gamma_{02} I(t = 2) + \gamma_{03} I(t = 3)$$

$$\alpha_{0ji} = \beta_{0j} + \mathbf{x}_{ji}\beta + v_{0ji}$$

$$v_{0ji} \sim N(0, \sigma_{v0}^2)$$

$$\beta_{0j} = \gamma_{00} + w_{0j} + u_{0j}$$

$$w_{0j} \sim N(0, \sigma_{w0}^2),$$

where μ_{jit} is the expected value for individual i in area segment j at Wave t, and σ_c^2 is the within person variance component; the individual level intercept α_{0ji} depends on the covariates, and has an individual level variance component σ_{v0}^2; its area segment level intercept β_{0j} has the sum of two error terms, a spatially correlated term u_{0j} and an i.i.d. error term w_{0j} with variance component equal to σ_{w0}^2.

For the spatially correlated error term of the area segment level intercept a relatively simple choice is the intrinsic conditional autoregressive (ICAR) prior (Besag et al. 1991):

$$u_{0j}|u_{0j'}, j' \in \text{ne}(j) \sim N\left(\bar{u}_{0j}, \frac{\sigma_{u0}^2}{n_j}\right), \tag{4}$$

where $\text{ne}(j)$ is the set of adjusted CTs which are neighbours of Area j, n_j is the number of such neighbours, and $\bar{u}_{0j}$ is the mean of the neighbouring spatial random effects.

In this spatial multilevel model, we model the spatial dependence of clusters by the neighbourhood structure. Adjusted CTs are considered to be *neighbours* if they have a boundary edge or a corner in common.

A Note on Identifiability

An important reason for application of a multilevel spatial model is to try to estimate the response variable cluster means and to map them. Separating the cluster random effects into spatially correlated and independent parts can also be of interest, and that means not only estimating the variance components σ_c^2, σ_{v0}^2, σ_{w0}^2, and σ_{u0}^2 but also estimating (in a Bayesian analysis) or predicting (in a frequentist analysis) w_{0j} and u_{0j}. With the model of this section and the kind of data available from the Galveston Bay Recovery Study, the variance components are identifiable in a frequentist likelihood analysis, or in the composite likelihood approach of Sect. 7. The quantities β_{0j} and γ_{00} are also estimable if the β_{0j} are constrained to have mean value 0. However, the separation of the random effect $w_{0j} + u_{0j}$ into its two components is not identifiable in these contexts. (The Bayesian analysis of Sect. 6 would allow such a separation because of the prior assumption on the variance components.) See Eberly and Carlin (2000) and Best et al. (2005) for discussions of this non-identifiability of spatial and random effects.

Leroux et al. (1999) and MacNab (2003) proposed a different model for $b_{0j} = w_{0j} + u_{0j}$ under which this total cluster random effect can be estimated, as well as a parameter λ that expresses the extent of spatial dependence of the cluster means. In this model, the covariance of b_{0j} and $b_{0j'}$ is the jj'-th element of the matrix $[\sigma_{w0}^2 + \sigma_{u0}^2][\lambda(D-A) + (1-\lambda)I]^{-1}$ where D is the diagonal matrix with j-th entry equal to n_j, the number of neighbours of area segment j; A is the adjacency matrix for the area segment clusters; and I is the identity matrix. Our method in this paper could be adapted to working with this parameterization.

6 A Bayesian Analysis

If a Bayesian approach is taken, for example, using WINBUGS, the following prior distributions for the parameters may be adopted:

$$\gamma_{02} \sim N(0, 1000); \quad \gamma_{03} \sim N(0, 1000); \quad \beta \sim MVN(0, 1000 * I),$$

where I is the identity matrix with the same number of rows as the dimension of $\mathbf{x}_{ij}$ and the component standard deviations σ_c, σ_{u0}, σ_{v0} and σ_{w0} have a $Cauchy(25)$ distribution, where $Cauchy(h)$ signifies a half-Cauchy distribution with scale parameter h. The parameter γ_{00} is given an improper uniform prior. All parameters are *a priori* independent. In all analyses in this paper, we assume dropout is not informative.

The results of the Bayesian analysis are displayed in Table 1. The level of PTSD is seen to decrease after Wave 1, and to rise a little between Wave 2 and Wave 3. The level of PTSD tends to be higher among females, and to increase with age; it is higher for minorities; higher for people with PTSD prior to Hurricane Ike; higher for people with Ike-related trauma; higher for people with peri-event

Table 1 Results of the Bayesian analysis

Beta values		Mean	SD	2.50%	97.50%
Intercept		3.1500	0.1695	2.8230	3.4890
Survey waves	Wave 2	−0.1107	0.0131	−0.1367	−0.0850
	Wave 3	−0.0835	0.0135	−0.1096	−0.0570
Sex	Male	−0.0408	0.0224	−0.0842	0.0032
Age groups	35–54	0.0215	0.0303	−0.0379	0.0799
	55 and over	0.1180	0.0335	0.0511	0.1832
Race	Black non-hisp	0.1226	0.0356	0.0529	0.1932
	Hispanic	0.0929	0.0317	0.0312	0.1557
	Other non-hisp	0.0328	0.0497	−0.0644	0.1314
Education	= high school	−0.1006	0.0353	−0.1690	−0.0313
	> high school	−0.1379	0.0327	−0.2017	−0.0741
# traumatic events prior to Ike	2–3	0.0179	0.0264	−0.0337	0.0701
	4+	0.0471	0.0295	−0.0103	0.1049
Depression prior to Ike	Yes	0.0359	0.0287	−0.0204	0.0929
PTSD prior to Ike	Yes	0.2017	0.0355	0.1328	0.2720
Ike-related trauma	Yes	0.1058	0.0342	0.0390	0.1734
Ike-related stress	Yes	0.0028	0.0499	−0.0951	0.0996
Peri-event emotional reactions	Medium	0.1608	0.0272	0.1087	0.2149
	High	0.3801	0.0285	0.3234	0.4359
Non-response adjustment		−0.0262	0.0625	−0.1503	0.0945
# adult household members	2–3	0.0371	0.0242	−0.0104	0.0851
	4+	0.0585	0.0629	−0.0657	0.1826
High PTSD risk indicator	Yes	0.0090	0.0232	−0.0361	0.0557
Average social support		0.0670	0.0541	−0.0397	0.1727
Average collective efficacy		−0.0635	0.0384	−0.1372	0.0132
Within person variance	σ_c^2	0.0474	0.0026	0.0427	0.0529
Within cluster variance	σ_{v0}^2	0.0456	0.0041	0.0381	0.0539
Between cluster variance (indep)	σ_{w0}^2	0.0033	0.0025	0.0001	0.0090
Between cluster variance (ICAR)	σ_{u0}^2	0.0064	0.0051	0.0007	0.0197

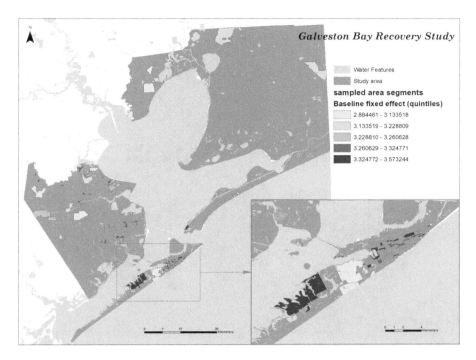

Fig. 2 Estimated cluster-level mean fixed effects of PTSD severity score

emotional reactions. The components of variance σ_c^2 and σ_{v0}^2 are estimated at 0.047 and 0.046, respectively, while the estimates of σ_{u0}^2 and σ_{w0}^2 are much smaller, and the posterior 2.50% quantiles of these last two variance components are very close to 0, suggesting that the variability within and between individuals dominates the area segment level variability.

Figures 2 and 3 display, respectively, the estimated cluster-level mean fixed effects and the estimated cluster-level random effects $u_0 + w_0$. (See Fig. 1 for comparison of the areas of high and low predicted PTSD severity with the stratum definitions.) The cluster-level mean fixed effects are the average, taken over sample members of the cluster at baseline, of the regression function with the coefficients replaced by their posterior mean values.

The estimated mean fixed effects have higher variability about their overall mean than do the estimated random effects. For the mean fixed effects, the values are mainly as expected given the characteristics of their strata. For example, higher values for the average predicted PTSD severity score are found in Stratum 1, in the eastern part of Galveston Island and Bolivar Island, and in some areas of Stratum 3, while lower values appear in parts of Stratum 5. The random effects also appear higher in Stratum 1.

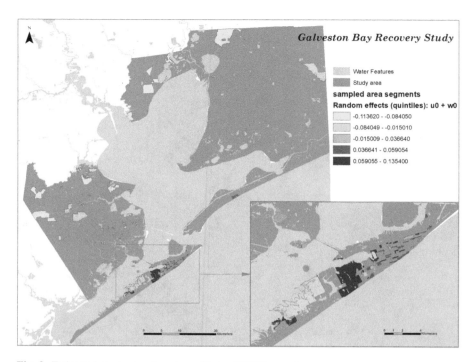

Fig. 3 Estimated cluster-level random effects of PTSD severity score

7 Frequentist Composite Likelihood Analysis

For a frequentist analysis, we consider adapting the weighted pairwise composite likelihood approach of Rao et al. (2013) and Yi et al. (2016). The idea in outline is as follows.

- Find (approximately) unbiased census estimating function terms for individual y values (for mean function parameters) and pairs of y values (for variance parameters).
- Combine them appropriately so that the combinations become maximum pairwise composite likelihood equations under the Gaussian model of Sect. 5.
- Estimate the census estimating functions by weighted sample estimating functions, and find their roots for point estimation.

7.1 Estimating Function System for Mean Parameters

For the mean parameters, the estimating function system could be a survey weighted GEE system:

$$\sum_j \sum_i w_{ji} X_{ji} (\Sigma_r)^{-1} (y_{ji.} - M_{ji.}),\qquad(5)$$

where $M_{jit} = \gamma_{00} + \mathbf{x}_{ji}\beta + \gamma_{02} I(t = 2) + \gamma_{03} I(t = 3)$ is the marginal mean of y_{jit}, and $y_{ji.} - M_{ji.}$ is the vector of observed y_{jit} minus the corresponding M_{jit}; X_{ji} is a $(p+3) \times 3$ matrix with columns equal to the transposes of $(\mathbf{x}_{ji}, 1, 1, 1)$, $(\mathbf{x}_{ji}, 0, 1, 0)$ and $(\mathbf{x}_{ji}, 0, 0, 1)$; and Σ_r is an exchangeable working correlation matrix, with 1's on the diagonal and with off-diagonal entries equal to a single correlation parameter ρ. The residuals are $\hat{z}_{jit} = y_{jit} - \hat{M}_{jit}$.

We note that the corresponding census estimating equation system is sub-optimal because the working covariance structure assumes independence of individuals, rather than the two-level model. Fitting this model using SUDAAN allows the stratification and two-stage design to be taken into account in estimation and testing hypotheses for the mean function parameters. This use of SUDAAN requires that the working correlation matrix be either exchangeable or independent.

7.2   Decomposition of the Error Term

The variance of

$$z_{jit} = y_{jit} - M_{jit} = e_{jit} + v_{0ij} + w_{0j} + u_{0j}$$

is

$$\sigma_c^2 + \sigma_{v0}^2 + \sigma_{w0}^2 + \sigma_{uj}^2,$$

where σ_{uj}^2 is the (unconditional) variance of u_{0j} under the ICAR model.

The covariance of z_{jit} and $z_{j'i't'}$ is the (unconditional) covariance of u_{0j}, $u_{0j'}$ under the ICAR model. This is expressible as $C_{ujj'}$, the jj'-th element of the matrix $\sigma_{u0}^2 (D - A)^{-1}$ (generalized inverse) where D is the diagonal matrix with j-th entry equal to n_j, the number of neighbours of area segment j; and A is the adjacency matrix for the area segment clusters.

7.3   Estimating Equation System for Variance Components

If $z_{jit} = y_{jit} - M_{jit}$, and s_j denotes the sample of respondents in cluster j, the estimating equation system for the variance components can be written as:

$$\sum_j w_j \sum_{i \in s(j)} w_{i|j} \sum_{t=1}^{3} (z_{jit}^2 - v_{1j}) = 0, \tag{6}$$

$$\sum_j w_j \sum_{i \in s(j)} w_{i|j} \sum_{t=1}^{3} \sum_{t' < t} (z_{jit} z_{jit'} - v_{2j}) = 0, \tag{7}$$

$$\sum_j w_j \sum_{i' < i \, \in s(j)} w_{ii'|j} \sum_{t=1}^{3} \sum_{t'=1}^{3} (z_{jit} z_{ji't'} - v_{3j}) = 0, \tag{8}$$

and

$$\sum_h \sum_{j' < j \in S_h} w_{jj'} \sum_{i' \in s(j')} \sum_{i \in s(j)} w_{i'|j'} w_{i|j} \sum_{t=1}^{3} \sum_{t'=1}^{3} (z_{jit} z_{j'i't'} - C_{jj'}) = 0. \tag{9}$$

In Eqs. (6)–(8), the notation $\sum_j$ signifies $\sum_h \sum_{j \in S_h}$, where S_h denotes Stratum h. In the system of equations (6)–(9)

$$v_{1j} = \sigma_{uj}^2 + \sigma_{w0}^2 + \sigma_{v0}^2 + \sigma_c^2$$

$$v_{2j} = \sigma_{uj}^2 + \sigma_{w0}^2 + \sigma_{v0}^2$$

$$v_{3j} = \sigma_{uj}^2 + \sigma_{w0}^2$$

$$C_{ujj'} = c_{jj'} \sigma_{u0}^2$$

and $c_{jj'}$ is a known constant.
The solutions to (5) and to (6)–(9) have closed forms:

$$\hat{\sigma}_{u0}^2 = \frac{\sum_h \sum_{j' < j \in S_h} w_{jj'} \sum_{i' \in s(j')} \sum_{i \in s(j)} w_{i'|j'} w_{i|j} \sum_{t=1}^{3} \sum_{t'=1}^{3} I_{it} I_{i't'} z_{jit} z_{j'i't'}}{\sum_h \sum_{j' < j \in S_h} w_{jj'} \sum_{i' \in s(j')} \sum_{i \in s(j)} w_{i'|j'} w_{i|j} \ell_i \ell_{i'} c_{jj'}} \tag{10}$$

$$\hat{\sigma}_{w0}^2 = \frac{\sum_j w_j \sum_{i \in s(j)} \sum_{i' < i \in s(j)} w_{ii'|j} \sum_{t=1}^{3} \sum_{t'=1}^{3} I_{it} I_{i't'} (z_{jit} z_{ji't'} - a_j \hat{\sigma}_{u0}^2)}{\sum_j w_j \sum_{i \in s(j)} \sum_{i' < i \in s(j)} w_{ii'|j} \ell_i \ell_{i'}} \tag{11}$$

$$\hat{\sigma}_{v0}^2 = \frac{\sum_j w_j \sum_{i \in s(j)} w_{i|j} \sum_{t=1}^3 \sum_{t'<t} I_{it} I_{it'} (z_{jit} z_{jit'} - a_j \hat{\sigma}_{u0}^2)}{\sum_j w_j \sum_{i \in s(j)} w_{i|j} \ell_i (\ell_i - 1)/2} - \hat{\sigma}_{w0}^2 \qquad (12)$$

$$\hat{\sigma}_c^2 = \frac{\sum_j w_j \sum_{i \in s(j)} w_{i|j} \sum_{t=1}^3 I_{it} (z_{jit}^2 - a_j \hat{\sigma}_{u0}^2)}{\sum_j w_j \sum_{i \in s(j)} w_{i|j} \ell_i} - \hat{\sigma}_{w0}^2 - \hat{\sigma}_{v0}^2. \qquad (13)$$

where I_{it} is the indicator function for i having an interview at t, and ℓ_i is the number of interviews of i.

7.4 Point Estimation

In a design-based analysis taking the weights to be the reciprocals of the corresponding inclusion probabilities, inclusion probabilities are needed for area segments j and for individuals within area segments $i \mid j$. Joint inclusion probabilities are needed for area segments jj' and for individuals within area segments $ii' \mid j$.

To illustrate the method with the GBRS data, having reconstructed inclusion probabilities from partial information on the data file as described in Section 4, we have used a Hájek approximation (Hájek et al. 1964) for the joint inclusion probabilities:

$$\pi_{ab} \simeq \pi_a \pi_b \left[1 - \frac{(1 - \pi_a)(1 - \pi_b)}{\sum_{a \in sample} (1 - \pi_a)} \right].$$

The paper by Haziza et al. (2008) gives an account of this and other joint inclusion approximations that can be used in variance estimation, including the one by Hartley and Rao (1962).

The residuals $z_{jit} = y_{jit} - M_{jit}$ were estimated using SUDAAN; the results of the SUDAAN analysis are displayed in Table 2:

In (5), the design weight for $y_{ji.}$ minus its marginal mean is the design weight for individual i in cluster j. This was taken to be the reciprocal of $\pi_{i|j}\pi_j$ as approximated in Sect. 4. These design weights were also applied in (13) and (12).

In (11), the design weight for $z_{ji't'}z_{jit}$ minus its marginal mean was taken to be the reciprocal of $\pi_j \pi_{ii'|j}$, where the second factor is the joint inclusion probability of i and i', given that cluster j is included. The second factor was taken to be the product of the reciprocals of the numbers of adults in their households, times the joint inclusion probabilities of their households, given that cluster j is included. This last factor was calculated by a Hájek approximation from the individual conditional inclusion probabilities. Finally, in (10), the weight $w_{jj'}$ was taken to be the reciprocal of the Hájek approximation to the joint cluster inclusion probability $\pi_{jj'}$.

Table 2 Results of the GEE analysis

Beta values		Point est	SE	2.50%	97.50%
Intercept		3.0554	0.1995	2.6656	3.4452
Survey waves	Wave 2	−0.1165	0.0162	−0.1489	−0.0842
	Wave 3	−0.0785	0.0241	−0.1265	−0.0304
Sex	Male	0.0005	0.0262	−0.0518	0.0527
Age groups	35–54	0.0440	0.0283	−0.0123	0.1004
	55 and over	0.1277	0.0282	0.0715	0.1840
Race	Black non-hisp	0.2176	0.0326	0.1525	0.2827
	Hispanic	0.1324	0.0407	0.0513	0.2136
	Other non-hisp	0.0634	0.0457	−0.0277	0.1544
Education	= high school	−0.0097	0.0449	−0.0991	0.0797
	> high school	−0.0480	0.0443	−0.1363	0.0403
# traumatic events prior to Ike	2–3	−0.0353	0.0305	−0.0961	0.0254
	4+	−0.0065	0.0275	−0.0613	0.0484
Depression prior to Ike	Yes	0.0165	0.0295	−0.0424	0.0754
PTSD prior to Ike	Yes	0.1975	0.0311	0.1354	0.2595
Ike-related trauma	Yes	0.2115	0.0653	0.0814	0.3416
Ike-related stress	Yes	−0.0106	0.0470	−0.1043	0.0830
Peri-event emotional reactions	Medium	0.1458	0.0284	0.0891	0.2024
	High	0.3354	0.0372	0.2613	0.4095
Non-response adjustment		−0.0033	0.0597	−0.1223	0.1157
# adult household members	2–3	0.0449	0.0317	−0.0183	0.1082
	4+	0.0522	0.0620	−0.0715	0.1758
High PTSD risk indicator	Yes	0.0245	0.0270	−0.0293	0.0784
Average social support		0.1401	0.0355	0.0694	0.2108
Average collective efficacy		−0.1200	0.0436	−0.2069	−0.0332
Within person correlation	ρ	0.2903			

The point estimates of the first two variance components from the Galveston Bay data are $\hat{\sigma}_c^2 = 0.0381$ and $\hat{\sigma}_{v0}^2 = 0.0314$. The sum of $\hat{\sigma}_{u0}^2$ and $\hat{\sigma}_{w0}^2$, the total cluster-level variance component, is estimated at 0.0023, indicating that in this data set, the within cluster (between person) and within person variances dominate. We note that the sample has not been designed to facilitate a spatial analysis with the multilevel model of Sect. 5, and that the model itself may be too simple to apply well to the whole area.

The point estimates of variance components are somewhat smaller than those arising from the Bayesian analysis, but despite the high variability of the survey weights, the relative values from the frequentist analysis are similar.

There is good agreement between the estimates in Tables 1 and 2. Considering exclusion of zero from a nominal 95% interval as evidence of a non-zero effect, there are only four variables (average social support, average collective efficacy and the two education variables) where the inferences are different. It should be noted that, although the GEE point estimation is sub-optimal, the standard errors from the GEE analysis do take into account the clustering and (through the design weights) the unequal probability sampling in the sampling design, and not surprisingly the SEs for the GEE analysis tend to be a little larger than the SDs of the Bayesian analysis.

7.5   *Uncertainty Estimation*

There are several methods that can be contemplated for the estimation of uncertainty in the point estimates arising from the system (5) and (6)–(8) or the system (5) and (10)–(13).

Applying a classical design-based approach would require the use of third and fourth order approximate inclusion probabilities. More appealing would be a model-based estimator of the mean-squared error of the design-based point estimators, using a *sandwich estimation* technique, described next in a simpler case.

Suppose $\hat{\theta}$ is the solution of the estimating equation

$$\sum_{i \in s} w_i \phi_i (y_i, \theta),$$

where under the model for the observations y_i, the terms $\phi_i (y_i, \theta)$ are correlated, with a correlation structure having parameters ρ. Then consider the Taylor series expression for the estimation error:

$$\hat{\theta} - \theta \simeq \left(\sum_{i \in s} w_i \frac{\partial \phi_i}{\partial \theta} \right)^{-1} \sum_{i \in s} w_i \phi_i.$$

The square of the left-hand side can be expressed as

$$(\hat{\theta} - \theta)^2 = \left(\sum_{i \in s} w_i \frac{\partial \phi_i}{\partial \theta} \right)^{-1} \sum_i \sum_{i'} w_i w_{i'} \phi_i \phi_{i'} \left(\sum_{i \in s} w_i \frac{\partial \phi_i}{\partial \theta} \right)^{-1}.$$

The factor in the middle can be replaced by its expectation in terms of the ρ parameters. The estimator of the variance of $\hat{\theta}$ could be the same expression evaluated at $\hat{\theta}$ and $\hat{\rho}$.

Another possible approach would be to treat the expressions in the left-hand sides for the sample-based maximum pairwise composite likelihood equations as analogous to the score function in a corresponding Gaussian model for the generation of the observations, as developed in the case of a simpler random effects model by Thompson et al. (2022). In that case, applying an adjustment to the curvature of the corresponding log likelihood along the lines of that proposed by

Ribatet et al. (2012) would make the pairwise log likelihood equations information unbiased and bring the inference based on them closer to that of a Bayesian analysis.

8 Discussion and Conclusions

We have outlined a frequentist design-based approach to estimation of the parameters of a multilevel repeated measures model with a continuous outcome, using data from a complex stratified three stage sampling design. The method uses the sample data to estimate population pairwise composite likelihood estimating functions. We have applied it to complex survey data from the Galveston Bay Recovery Study. In this application, the point estimates are broadly similar to those obtained from a Bayesian analysis of the same model.

Besides availability in software, important advantages of the Bayesian approach are the capacity to estimate the parameters of complex models and the principled expression of uncertainty through posterior distributions and credible intervals. From the frequentist perspective, a disadvantage of some Bayesian approaches is a requirement for knowledge of the variables influencing the sampling design, and the form of that influence. Incorporating this knowledge in the model accounts for the way in which the sampling design may distort the population relationships of interest. Other Bayesian approaches, such as the one used by Anthopolos et al. (2020), and used in Sect. 6, summarize the design features by including in the model the sample weights as covariates. When we include the survey design variables in the model, the interpretation of covariates of interest is altered, and may be changed in ways that do not align with scientific investigation.

The design-based frequentist approach attempts to address directly and compensate for this distortion. An advantage of this approach is that it can be applied in a straightforward manner to simple analytic uses of complex survey data with the use of a single set of survey weights supplied with the data. With this approach, there is also a natural extension to account for missing data by multiplying the baseline weight of someone who has responded at Wave t by the reciprocal of the probability of remaining in the sample up to that wave. Disadvantages are that the method as applied in this paper requires linear or quadratic estimating functions and that the variance components at the cluster-level tend to be weakly estimable.

We recommend the use of both methods for comparison in simple analytic uses of the data.

Acknowledgments The authors are grateful to Dr. Sandro Galea, Robert A. Knox Professor and Dean at the Boston University of Public Health, and to the National Center for Disaster Mental Health Research, for permission to use the data from the Galveston Bay Recovery Study. The work has been supported by a Discovery Grant to M. E. Thompson (RGPIN-2016-03688) from the Natural Sciences and Engineering Research Council of Canada.

References

Anthopolos, R., Chen, Q., Sedransk, J., Thompson, M. E., Meng, G., & Galea, S. (2020). A Bayesian growth mixture model for complex survey data: clustering post-disaster PTSD trajectories (21 p.).

Besag, J., York, J., & Mollié, A. (1991). Bayesian image restoration with two applications in spatial statistics. *Annals of the Institute of Statistical Mathematics, 43,* 1–59.

Best, N., Richardson, S., & Thomson, A. (2005). A comparison of Bayesian spatial models for disease mapping. *Statistical Methods in Medical Research, 14,* 35–39.

Blanchard, E. B., Jones-Alexander, J., Buckley, T.C., et al. (1996). Psychometric properties of the PTSD Checklist (PCL). *Behavioral Research Therapy, 34,* 669–673.

Eberly, L. E., & Carlin, B. P. (2000). Identifiability and convergence issues for Markov chain Monte Carlo fitting of spatial models. *Statistics in Medicine, 19,* 2279–2294.

Gruebner, O., Lowe, S. R., Tracy, M., Joshi, S., Cerdá, M., Norris, F. H., Subramanian, S. V., & Galea, S. (2016a). Mapping concentrations of posttraumatic stress and depression trajectories following Hurricane Ike. *Scientific Reports, 20166,* 32242.

Gruebner, O., Lowe, S. R., Tracy, M., Cerdá, M., Joshi, S., Norris, F. H., & Galea, S. (2016b). The geography of mental health and general wellness in Galveston Bay after Hurricane Ike: a spatial epidemiologic study with longitudinal data. *Disaster Medicine and Public Health Preparedness, 10,* 261–273.

Hájek, J. (1964). Asymptotic theory of rejective sampling with varying probabilities from a finite population. *Annals of Mathematical Statistics, 35,* 1491–1523.

Hartley, H. O., & Rao, J. N. K. (1962). Sampling with unequal probabilities and without replacement. *Annals of Mathematical Statistics, 33,* 350–374.

Haziza, D., Mecatti, F., & Rao, J. N. K. (2008). Evaluation of some approximate variance estimators under the Rao-Sampford unequal probability sampling design. *Metron - International Journal of Statistics, 66,* 91–108.

Leroux, B. G., Lei, X., & Breslow, N. (1999). Estimation of disease rates in small areas: a new mixed model for spatial dependence. In M. E. Halloran, & D. Berry (Eds.), *Statistical models in epidemiology, the environment and clinical trials* (pp. 135–178). New York: Springer Verlag.

MacNab, Y. C. (2003). Hierarchical Bayes spatial modeling of small-area rates of non-rare disease. *Statistics in Medicine, 22,* 1761–1773.

Pietrzak, R. H., Van Ness, P. H., Fried, T. R., Galea, S., & Norris, F. H. (2013). Trajectories of posttraumatic stress symptomatology in older persons affected by a large-magnitude disaster. *Journal of Psychiatric Research, 47,* 520–526.

Rao, J. N. K., Verret, F., & Hidiroglou, M. A. (2013). A weighted composite likelihood approach to inference for two-level models from survey data. *Survey Methodology, 39,* 263–282.

Ribatet, M., Cooley, D., & Davison, A. C. (2012). Bayesian inference from composite likelihoods, with an application to spatial extremes. *Statistica Sinica, 22,* 813–845.

Thompson, M. E., Sedransk, J., Fang, J., & Yi, G. Y. (2022). Bayesian inference for a variance component model using pairwise composite likelihood with survey data. *Survey Methodology, 48,* 73–93.

University of Michigan Survey Research Center/Institute for Social Research. (2010). *The Galveston Bay Recovery Study: Report on Survey Procedure and Approach.*

Valliant, R., Adams, T., & Wagner, J. (2009). Sample design documentation Galveston Bay recovery survey 2008–2009. *Survey Research Operations, Production Sampling Group, University of Michigan Survey Research Center,* 1–18.

Yi, G. Y., Rao, J. N. K., & Li, H. (2016). A weighted composite likelihood approach for analysis of survey data under two-level models. *Statistica Sinica, 26,* 569–587.

Efficient Experimental Design for Lasso Regression

Peter Chien, Xinwei Deng, and Chunfang Devon Lin

Abstract Lasso regression has attracted great attention in statistical learning and data science. However, there is sporadic work on constructing efficient data collection for regularized regression. In this work, we propose an experimental design approach, using nearly orthogonal Latin hypercube designs, to enhance the variable selection accuracy of Lasso regression. Systematic methods for constructing such designs are presented. The effectiveness of the proposed method is illustrated with several examples.

Keywords Design of experiments · Latin hypercube design · Nearly orthogonal design · Regularization · Variable selection

1 Introduction

In statistical learning and data sciences, regularized regression has attracted great attention across multiple disciplines (Fan et al. 2005; Hesterberg et al. 2008; Huang & Breheny 2012; Heinze et al. 2018). Among various regularized regression, the Lasso regression is one of the most well-known techniques on the L_1 regularization to achieve accurate prediction with variable selection (Tibshirani 1996). Statistical properties and various extensions of this method have been actively studied in recent years (Tibshirani & Taylor 2011; Zhao & Yu 2006; Zhao et al. 2009; Zou & Hastie 2005; Zou 2016). However, there is sporadic work on constructing efficient data

P. Chien
Department of Statistics, University of Wisconsin-Madison, Madison, WI, USA
e-mail: peter.chien@wisc.edu

X. Deng
Department of Statistics, Virginia Tech, Blacksburg, VA, USA
e-mail: xdeng@vt.edu

C. Devon Lin (✉)
Department of Mathematics and Statistics, Queen's University, Kingston, ON, Canada
e-mail: devon.lin@queensu.ca

collection for regularized regression (De Castro 2014; Ravi et al. 2016; Huang & Kong 2020). In this article, we study the data collection for the regularized regression from an experimental design perspective.

First, we give a brief description of the Lasso procedure. Consider a linear model

$$y = \mathbf{x}^T \boldsymbol{\beta} + \epsilon, \tag{1}$$

where $\mathbf{x} = (x_1, \ldots, x_p)^T$ is the vector of p continuous predictor variables, y is the response value, $\boldsymbol{\beta} = (\beta_1, \ldots, \beta_p)^T$ are the vector of regression parameters, and the error term ϵ is normally distributed with mean zero and variance σ^2. Throughout, assume data are centered so that the model in (1) has no intercept. Suppose this model has a *sparse* structure for which only p_0 predictor variables are *active* with non-zero regression coefficients, where $p_0 < p$. Let $\mathcal{A}(\boldsymbol{\beta}) = \{j : \beta_j \neq 0, j = 1, \ldots, p\}$ be the set of the indices of the active variables. Then the cardinality of the set $\mathcal{A}(\boldsymbol{\beta})$ is p_0.

For a given $n \times p$ regression matrix $\mathbf{X} = (\mathbf{x}_1, \ldots, \mathbf{x}_n)^T$, and a given response vector $\mathbf{y} = (y_1, \ldots, y_n)^T$, the Lasso solution is

$$\hat{\boldsymbol{\beta}} = \arg \min_{\boldsymbol{\beta}} [(\mathbf{y} - \mathbf{X}\boldsymbol{\beta})^T (\mathbf{y} - \mathbf{X}\boldsymbol{\beta}) + \lambda \|\boldsymbol{\beta}\|_{l_1}], \tag{2}$$

where $\|\boldsymbol{\beta}\|_{l_1} = \sum_{i=1}^{p} |\beta_i|$ and λ is a tuning parameter. Because the l_1 norm $\| \cdot \|_{l_1}$ is singular at the origin, a desirable property of the Lasso is that some components of $\hat{\boldsymbol{\beta}}$ are exactly zero. Then $\mathcal{A}(\boldsymbol{\beta})$ can be estimated by $\mathcal{A}(\hat{\boldsymbol{\beta}}) = \{j : \hat{\beta}_j \neq 0, j = 1, \ldots, p\}$. The number of false selections of the Lasso is

$$\gamma = \#\{j : j \in \mathcal{A}(\hat{\boldsymbol{\beta}}) \text{ but } j \notin \mathcal{A}(\boldsymbol{\beta})\} + \#\{j : j \notin \mathcal{A}(\hat{\boldsymbol{\beta}}) \text{ but } j \in \mathcal{A}(\boldsymbol{\beta})\}, \tag{3}$$

where # denotes the set cardinality, the first term counts the number of false positives and the second term counts the number of false negatives.

The scope of this work is in developing experimental design techniques to construct the regression matrix $\mathbf{X}$ in (2) in order to minimize the value of γ in (3), the number of false selection. Based on the probability properties of regularized regression, it often requires large randomness in the regression matrix (Jung et al. 2019). Thus, a straightforward way is to take $\mathbf{X}$ to be an independently and identically distributed (i.i.d.) sample. However, from an experimental design perspective, the points of an i.i.d. sample is not well stratified in the design space (Box et al. 2005; Wu & Hamada 2009). To improve upon this scheme, we propose to take $\mathbf{X}$ to be a nearly orthogonal Latin hypercube design (NOLHD) that is a Latin hypercube design with nearly orthogonal columns. A Latin hypercube design is a space-filling design that achieves maximum uniformity when the points are projected onto any one dimensional space (McKay et al. 1979). An NOLHD simultaneously possesses two desirable properties: low-dimensional stratification and nearly orthogonality. Owen (1992) stated the advantage of using Latin hypercube designs for learning additive models. It was discussed in Section 3 of Owen (1992) that the least-squares estimates of the regression coefficients of an additive regression with a Latin hypercube design can have significant smaller variability than their counterparts under an i.i.d. sample. Since the model in (1) is additive, $\hat{\boldsymbol{\beta}}$ in (2) associated with a Latin hypercube design is expected to be superior to that with an i.i.d. sample. Both random Latin hypercube designs and NOLHDs are popular in computer experiments (Lin 2015). It is advantageous to use NOLHDs instead of random Latin hypercube designs for the Lasso problem because the former have guaranteed small columnwise correlations. When the regression matrix $\mathbf{X}$ is taken to be an NOLHD, its small columnwise correlations allow the active variables less correlated with the inactive variables, thus improving the selection accuracy of the Lasso.

There is some consistency between the concept of NOLHDs and the sparsity concept in variable selection. The sparsity assumption we have made earlier for the model in (1) states that only p_0 variables in the model are active and does not specify which p_0 variables are active. If the regression matrix $\mathbf{X}$ for this model is an NOLHD of n runs for p input variables, when the points of this design are projected onto any p_0 dimensions, the resulting design still retains the NOLHD structure for the p_0 factors. Note that an NOLHD has more than two levels and spreads the points evenly in the design space, not restricted to the boundaries only. Since the number of false selections γ in (3) has a nonlinear relation with the regression matrix $\mathbf{X}$, the use of an NOLHD for the Lasso problem is more appropriate than a two-level design to exploit this complicated relation between γ and $\mathbf{X}$.

The remainder of the article is organized as follows. Section 2 introduces a new criterion to measure NOLHDs and presents two systematic methods for constructing such designs for the Lasso problem. Section 3 provides numerical examples to bear out the effectiveness of the proposed method. The numerical examples in Sect. 3 clearly indicate the superiority of NOLHDs over two-level designs for the Lasso problem. We provide a brief discussion in Sect. 4.

2   Methodology

In this section we discuss the construction of NOLHDs and how to use them for the Lasso problem. We prefer NOLHDs over random Latin hypercube designs because the latter are not guaranteed to have small columnwise correlations. An illustration, let $n = 64$ and $p = 192$ and compute γ in (3) for two different choices of $\mathbf{X}$ in (2). Assume the model in (1) has $\sigma = 8$ and $\boldsymbol{\beta} = (0.05, 0.2, \ldots, 3.0, 0 \ldots, 0)^T$, where only the first 20 coefficients are nonzeros, and the predictor variables take values on the hypercube $[-(64 - 1)/2, (64 - 1)/2]^p$. The first method takes the design matrix $\mathbf{X}$ to be a random Latin hypercube design constructed by (7). Figure 1 depicts the histogram of the columnwise sample correlations of one random Latin hypercube design, where 21% of the columnwise correlations of the matrix are larger than 0.1 in absolute values. This method gives $\gamma = 36$ in one realization of the model. The second method takes the design matrix to be a 64×192 NOLHD from Sect. 2.1,

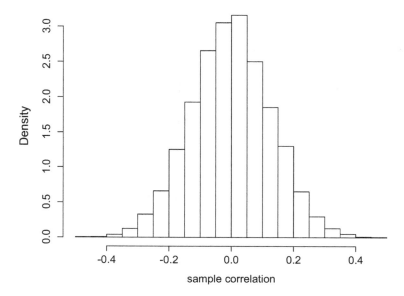

Fig. 1 Histogram of the sample correlations of a 64×192 random Latin hypercube design

where the columnwise correlations of the matrix are very small. The second method gives $\gamma = 20$ in one realization of the model. The difference of γ values of the two methods indicates that the Lasso solution with an NOLHD can be far more superior.

Here are some useful notation and definitions for constructing NOLHDs. The Kronecker product of an $n \times p$ matrix $\mathbf{A} = (a_{ij})$ and an $m \times q$ matrix $\mathbf{B} = (b_{ij})$ is

$$
\mathbf{A} \otimes \mathbf{B} =
\begin{bmatrix}
a_{11}\mathbf{B} & a_{12}\mathbf{B} & \dots & a_{1p}\mathbf{B} \\
a_{21}\mathbf{B} & a_{22}\mathbf{B} & \dots & a_{2p}\mathbf{B} \\
\vdots & \vdots & \ddots & \vdots \\
a_{n1}\mathbf{B} & a_{n2}\mathbf{B} & \dots & a_{np}\mathbf{B}
\end{bmatrix},
$$

where $a_{ij}\mathbf{B}$ is an $m \times q$ matrix whose (k, l) entry is $a_{ij}b_{kl}$. The correlation matrix of an $n \times p$ matrix $\mathbf{X} = (x_{ij})$ is

$$
\rho =
\begin{pmatrix}
\rho_{11} & \rho_{12} & \dots & \rho_{1p} \\
\rho_{21} & \rho_{22} & \dots & \rho_{2p} \\
\vdots & \vdots & \ddots & \vdots \\
\rho_{p1} & \rho_{p2} & \dots & \rho_{pp}
\end{pmatrix},
\tag{4}
$$

where

$$\rho_{ij} = \frac{\sum_{k=1}^{n}(x_{ki} - \bar{x}_i)(x_{kj} - \bar{x}_j)}{\sqrt{\sum(x_{ki} - \bar{x}_i)^2 \sum(x_{kj} - \bar{x}_j)^2}}, \tag{5}$$

represents the correlation between the ith and jth columns of $\mathbf{X}$, $\bar{x}_i = n^{-1}\sum_{k=1}^{n}x_{ki}$ and $\bar{x}_j = n^{-1}\sum_{k=1}^{n}x_{kj}$. The matrix $\mathbf{X}$ is orthogonal if ρ in (4) is an identity matrix.

Let $\mathbf{D} = (d_{ij})$ be an $n \times p$ random Latin hypercube in which each column is a random permutation of $1, \ldots, n$, and all columns are generated independently. Using $\mathbf{D}$, a random Latin hypercube design $\mathbf{Z} = (z_{ij})$ on $[0, 1]^p$ is generated through

$$z_{ij} = \frac{d_{ij} - u_{ij}}{n}, i = 1, \ldots, n; j = 1, \ldots, p, \tag{6}$$

where the u_{ij}'s are independent uniform random variables on $[0,1)$, and the d_{ij}'s and the u_{ij}'s are mutually independent. If $\mathbf{Z}$ needs to be defined on $[a, b]^p$ for general $a < b$, rescale z_{ij} in (6) as

$$z_{ij} \leftarrow (b - a)z_{ij} + a. \tag{7}$$

We use NOLHD(n, p) to denote an $n \times p$ NOLHD. For a pre-specified vector $\mathbf{t} = (t_1, \ldots, t_q)$ with $0 \leq t_q \leq \cdots \leq t_1 \leq 1$, the orthogonality of an NOLHD $\mathbf{X}$ can be assessed by using the *proportion correlation vector* given by

$$\delta_{\mathbf{t}}(\mathbf{X}) = (\delta_{t_1}(\mathbf{X}), \ldots, \delta_{t_q}(\mathbf{X})), \tag{8}$$

where $\delta_{t_k}(\mathbf{X}) = \{p(p - 1)\}^{-1}\sum_{i=1}^{p}\sum_{j \neq i}I(|\rho_{ij}| \leq t_k), k = 1, \ldots, q$, and $I(\cdot)$ is an indicator function. For $k = 1, \ldots, q$, this criterion computes the proportion of the $|\rho_{ij}|$'s not exceeding t_k. For two designs $\mathbf{X}_1$ and $\mathbf{X}_2$, $\mathbf{X}_1$ is preferred over $\mathbf{X}_2$ if $\delta_{t_k}(\mathbf{X}_1) > \delta_{t_k}(\mathbf{X}_2)$ for $t_1, \ldots, t_q$. For the Lasso problem, this new criterion has more discriminating power than the *maximum correlation* ρ_m and *root average squared correlation* ρ_{ave} criteria proposed in Bingham et al. (2009), where $\rho_m(\mathbf{X}) = \max_{i,j}|\rho_{ij}|$ and and $\rho_{ave}(\mathbf{X}) = \{\sum_{i<j}\rho_{ij}^2/[p(p - 1)/2]\}^{1/2}$. Designs with similar values of ρ_m and ρ_{ave} may have different values of $\delta_{\mathbf{t}}$. For illustration, compare a randomly generated 64×192 i.i.d. sample with an NOLHD(64, 192) from Sect. 2.1. The former has $\rho_{ave} = 0.124$ and $\rho_m = 0.493$ and the latter has $\rho_{ave} = 0.112$ and $\rho_m = 0.786$. The two designs are indistinguishable in terms of ρ_{ave}. But for $\mathbf{t} = (0.1, 0.05, 0.01, 0.005)$, $\delta_{\mathbf{t}} = (0.562, 0.305, 0.064, 0.033)$ for the i.i.d. sample and $\delta_{\mathbf{t}} = (0.906, 0.894, 0.883, 0.883)$ for the NOLHD, clearly indicating the superiority of the latter.

Sections 2.1 and 2.2 present two systematic methods for constructing NOLHDs. The first method was proposed by Lin et al. (2009) and the second method is a generalization of the method in Lin et al. (2010). To assist readers in machine learning who may not be familiar with NOLHDs, we describe these two methods in a self-contained fashion. These two methods are easy to implement. Other construction methods for (nearly) orthogonal Latin hypercube designs include Owen (1994), Tang (1998), Ye (1998), Steinberg and Lin (2006), Pang et al. (2009), and Sun et al. (2009, 2010), among others. However, they have run-size constraints and thus we do not consider here. In the two constructions we will present, an NOLHD with n runs is obtained from a Latin hypercube in which the n levels in each column are $\{-(n-1)/2, \ldots, 0, \ldots, (n-1)/2\}$ if n is odd and $\{-(n-1)/2, \ldots, -1/2, 1/2, \ldots, (n-1)/2\}$ if n is even.

2.1 A Construction Method Using Orthogonal Arrays

Lin et al. (2009) proposed a method for constructing nearly orthogonal Latin hypercubes using orthogonal arrays. Recall that an orthogonal array $OA(n, p, s)$ of strength two is an $n \times p$ matrix with levels $1, \ldots, s$ such that, for any two columns, all level combinations appear equally often (Hedayat et al. 1999). Let $\mathbf{A}$ be an $OA(s^2, 2f, s)$ and let $\mathbf{B} = (b_{ij})$ be an $s \times p$ Latin hypercube. This method works as follows.

Step 1. For $j = 1, \ldots, p$, obtain an $s^2 \times (2f)$ matrix $\mathbf{A}_j$ from $\mathbf{A}$ by replacing the symbols $1, \ldots, s$ in the latter by $b_{1j}, \ldots, b_{sj}$, respectively, and partition $\mathbf{A}_j$ to $\mathbf{A}_{j1}, \ldots, \mathbf{A}_{jf}$, each of two columns.
Step 2. Let

$$\mathbf{V} = \begin{bmatrix} 1 & -s \\ s & 1 \end{bmatrix}.$$

For $j = 1, \ldots, p$, obtain an $s^2 \times (2f)$ matrix

$$\mathbf{M}_j = [\mathbf{A}_{j1}\mathbf{V}, \ldots, \mathbf{A}_{jf}\mathbf{V}].$$

Step 3. For $n = s^2$ and $q = 2pf$, define an $n \times q$ matrix $\mathbf{M} = [\mathbf{M}_1, \ldots, \mathbf{M}_p]$.

Lemma 1 from Lin et al. (2009) captures the structure of $\mathbf{M}$.

Lemma 1

(a) *The matrix $\mathbf{M}$ constructed above is an $s^2 \times (2pf)$ Latin hypercube.*
(b) *The correlation matrix of $\mathbf{M}$ is $\rho(\mathbf{M}) = \rho(\mathbf{B}) \otimes \mathbf{I}_{2f}$, where $\mathbf{I}_{2f}$ is the identity matrix of order $2f$.*

Observe that the proportion correlation δ_{t_k} in (8) of $\mathbf{M}$ is

$$\delta_{t_k}(\mathbf{M}) = [p(2f-1) + (p-1)\delta_{t_k}(\mathbf{B})]/(2pf-1), \text{ for } k = 1, \ldots, q. \tag{9}$$

Example 1 Let $\mathbf{A}$ be an $OA(49, 8, 7)$ from Hedayat et al. (1999) and let $\mathbf{B}$ be an NOLHD(7, 12) given by

$$
\begin{pmatrix}
-3 & 0 & -1 & 0 & 3 & 3 & 0 & -2 & 1 & -3 & -1 & -3 \\
-2 & -1 & 1 & -3 & -1 & -3 & 1 & -3 & -2 & -1 & 1 & 3 \\
-1 & 3 & 0 & 3 & 0 & -2 & 2 & 0 & -1 & 3 & -3 & -1 \\
0 & -2 & 3 & 2 & -2 & 2 & -2 & 1 & -3 & 1 & 2 & -2 \\
1 & 1 & -3 & -1 & -3 & 1 & -3 & -1 & 3 & 2 & 0 & 1 \\
2 & -3 & -2 & 1 & 1 & -1 & 3 & 2 & 2 & 0 & 3 & 0 \\
3 & 2 & 2 & -2 & 2 & 0 & -1 & 3 & 0 & -2 & -2 & 2
\end{pmatrix},
$$

where $\rho_{ave}(\mathbf{B}) = 0.3038$, $\rho_m(\mathbf{B}) = 0.9643$, and $\delta_{\mathbf{t}}(\mathbf{B}) = (\delta_{0.1}, \delta_{0.05}, \delta_{0.01}, \delta_{0.005}) = (0.500, 0.364, 0.136, 0.136)$. Here, the matrix $\mathbf{M}$ from Lemma 1 is an NOLHD$(49, 96)$ with $\rho_{ave}(\mathbf{M}) = 0.1034$ and $\rho_m(\mathbf{M}) = 0.9643$. From (9), $\delta_{\mathbf{t}}(\mathbf{M}) = (\delta_{0.1}, \delta_{0.05}, \delta_{0.01}, \delta_{0.005}) = (0.942, 0.926, 0.9, 0.9)$. In general, if $\mathbf{B}$ is an NOLHD$(7, p)$, Lemma 1 gives an NOLHD$(49, 8p)$.

2.2 A Construction Method Using the Kronecker Product

We now propose a generalization of the method in Lin et al. (2010) for constructing NOLHDs. This generalization provides designs with better low-dimensional projection properties than those obtained in Lin et al. (2010).

For $j = 1, \ldots, m_2$, let $\mathbf{C}_j = (c_{ik}^j)$ be an $n_1 \times m_1$ Latin hypercube and let $\mathbf{A}_j = (a_{ik}^j)$ be an $n_1 \times m_1$ matrix with entries ± 1. Let $\mathbf{B} = (b_{ij})_{n_2 \times m_2}$ be an $n_2 \times m_2$ Latin hypercube, let $\mathbf{D} = (d_{ij})_{n_2 \times m_2}$ be a matrix with entries ± 1, and let r be a real number. Our proposed method constructs

$$
\mathbf{M} = \begin{bmatrix}
b_{11}\mathbf{A}_1 + rd_{11}\mathbf{C}_1 & b_{12}\mathbf{A}_2 + rd_{12}\mathbf{C}_2 & \ldots & b_{1m_2}\mathbf{A}_{m_2} + rd_{1m_2}\mathbf{C}_{m_2} \\
b_{21}\mathbf{A}_1 + rd_{21}\mathbf{C}_1 & b_{22}\mathbf{A}_2 + rd_{22}\mathbf{C}_2 & \ldots & b_{2m_2}\mathbf{A}_{m_2} + rd_{2m_2}\mathbf{C}_{m_2} \\
\vdots & \vdots & \ddots & \vdots \\
b_{n_21}\mathbf{A}_1 + rd_{n_21}\mathbf{C}_1 & b_{n_22}\mathbf{A}_2 + rd_{n_22}\mathbf{C}_2 & \ldots & b_{n_2m_2}\mathbf{A}_{m_2} + rd_{n_2m_2}\mathbf{C}_{m_2}
\end{bmatrix}. \tag{10}
$$

In contrast, the method in Lin et al. (2010) constructs

$$
\mathbf{L} = \mathbf{A} \otimes \mathbf{B} + r\mathbf{C} \otimes \mathbf{D}, \tag{11}
$$

where $\mathbf{A} = (a_{ij})_{n_1 \times m_1}$ is a matrix with entries ± 1, $\mathbf{C} = (c_{ij})_{n_1 \times m_1}$ is an $n_1 \times m_1$ Latin hypercube, and $\mathbf{B}$, $\mathbf{D}$ and r are as in (10). Lin et al. (2010) provided the conditions for $\mathbf{L}$ to be a nearly orthogonal Latin hypercube. When projected onto some pairs of predictor variables, points in the design in (11) lie on straight lines, which may not be desirable for the Lasso problem. Such projection patterns are due to the use of the same $\mathbf{A}$ and the same $\mathbf{C}$ for each entry of $\mathbf{B}$ and $\mathbf{D}$ in (11). The generalization in (10) uses different $\mathbf{A}_j$'s and $\mathbf{C}_j$'s to eliminate this undesirable projection pattern. Proposition 1 establishes conditions for $\mathbf{M}$ in (10) to be a Latin hypercube.

Proposition 1 *Let $r = n_2$. Then the design $\mathbf{M}$ in (10) is a Latin hypercube if one of the following two conditions holds:*

(a) *For $j = 1, \ldots, m_2$, the $\mathbf{A}_j$ and $\mathbf{C}_j$ satisfy that for $i = 1, \ldots, m_1$, $c^j_{pi} = -c^j_{p'i}$ and $a^j_{pi} = a^j_{p'i}$ hold simultaneously.*
(b) *For $k = 1, \ldots, m_2$, the entries of $\mathbf{B}$ and $\mathbf{D}$ satisfy the condition that $b_{qk} = -b_{q'k}$ and $d_{qk} = d_{q'k}$ hold simultaneously.*

Proposition 1 can be verified by using an argument similar to the proof of Lemma 1 in Lin et al. (2010) and thus is omitted. Proposition 2 studies the orthogonality of $\mathbf{M}$ in terms of $\mathbf{A}_j$'s, $\mathbf{B}$, $\mathbf{C}_j$'s and $\mathbf{D}$.

Proposition 2 *Suppose $\mathbf{A}_j$'s, $\mathbf{B}$, $\mathbf{C}_j$'s, $\mathbf{D}$ and r in (10) satisfy condition (a) or (b) in Proposition 1 and $\mathbf{M}$ in (10) is a Latin hypercube. In addition, assume that $\mathbf{A}_j$s, $\mathbf{B}$, and $\mathbf{D}$ are orthogonal and that $\mathbf{B}^T \mathbf{D} = 0$ or $\mathbf{A}_j^T \mathbf{C}_j = 0$ holds for all js. Then we have that*

(a) $\rho_m(\mathbf{M}) = Max\{w_1 \rho_m(\mathbf{C}_j), j = 1, \ldots, m_2\}$, *where* $w_1 = n_2^2(n_1^2 - 1)/(n_1^2 n_2^2 - 1)$.
(b) $\rho_{ave}(\mathbf{M}) = \sqrt{w_2 \sum_{j=1}^{m_2} \rho_{ave}^2(\mathbf{C}_j)/m_2}$, *where* $w_2 = (m_1 - 1)w_1^2/(m_1 m_2 - 1)]$.
(c) $\delta_{t_k}(\mathbf{M}) \geq \sum_{j=1}^{m_2} \delta_{t_k}(\mathbf{C}_j)/m_2$ *for* $k = 1, \ldots, q$.
(d) *The matrix $\mathbf{M}$ is orthogonal if and only if $\mathbf{C}_1, \ldots, \mathbf{C}_{m_2}$ are all orthogonal.*

Proof Let $\mathbf{M}_{jk}$ and $\mathbf{M}_{j'k'}$ be the $[(j-1)m_2 + k]$th and $[(j'-1)m_2 + k']$th columns of $\mathbf{M}$ in (10), respectively. Take $n = n_1 n_2$. Let $\rho(\mathbf{M}_{jk}, \mathbf{M}_{j'k'})$ be the correlation between $\mathbf{M}_{jk}$ and $\mathbf{M}_{j'k'}$ defined in (5). Express $12^{-1}n(n^2 - 1)\rho(\mathbf{M}_{jk}, \mathbf{M}_{j'k'})$ as

$$\sum_{i_1=1}^{n_2} \sum_{i_2=1}^{n_1} (b_{i_1 j} a^j_{i_2 k} + n_2 d_{i_1 j} c^j_{i_2 k})(b_{i_1 j'} a^{j'}_{i_2 k'} + n_2 d_{i_1 j'} c^{j'}_{i_2 k'}),$$

which equals

$$\sum_{i_1=1}^{n_2} b_{i_1 j} b_{i_1 j'} \sum_{i_2=1}^{n_1} a^j_{i_2 k} a^{j'}_{i_2 k'} + n_2 \sum_{i_1=1}^{n_2} d_{i_1 j} b_{i_1 j'} \sum_{i_2=1}^{n_1} c^j_{i_2 k} a^{j'}_{i_2 k'}$$

$$+ n_2 \sum_{i_1=1}^{n_2} b_{i_1 j} d_{i_1 j'} \sum_{i_2=1}^{n_1} a^j_{i_2 k} c^{j'}_{i_2 k'} + n_2^2 \sum_{i_1=1}^{n_2} d_{i_1 j} d_{i_1 j'} \sum_{i_2=1}^{n_1} c^j_{i_2 k} c^{j'}_{i_2 k'}$$

$$= \sum_{i_1=1}^{n_2} b_{i_1 j} b_{i_1 j'} \sum_{i_2=1}^{n_1} a^j_{i_2 k} a^{j'}_{i_2 k'} + n_2^2 \sum_{i_1=1}^{n_2} d_{i_1 j} d_{i_1 j'} \sum_{i_2=1}^{n_1} c^j_{i_2 k} c^{j'}_{i_2 k'}.$$

Thus, $\rho(\mathbf{M}_{jk}, \mathbf{M}_{j'k'})$ is zero for $j \neq j'$ and is $n_2^2(n_1^2 - 1)\rho_{kk'}(\mathbf{C}_j)/(n^2 - 1)$ for $j = j'$ and $k \neq k'$. By the definitions of ρ_m and ρ_{ave}, the results in (a) and (b) hold.

Note that for $k = 1, \ldots, q$,

$$\delta_{t_k}(\mathbf{M}) = \{m_2(m_2 - 1)m_1^2 + m_1(m_1 - 1)\sum_{j=1}^{m_2} \delta_{t_k}(\mathbf{C}_j)\}/\{m_1 m_2(m_1 m_2 - 1)\}$$

$$= \sum_{j=1}^{m_2} \delta_{t_k}(\mathbf{C}_j)/m_2 + [(m_2 - 1)m_1\{1 - \sum_{j=1}^{m_2} \delta_{t_k}(\mathbf{C}_j)/m_2\}]/(m_1 m_2 - 1).$$

The result in (c) now follows because $\sum_{j=1}^{m_2} \delta_{t_k}(\mathbf{C}_j)/m_2 \leq 1$. By (a), (b), and (c), (d) is evident. This completes the proof. $\qquad\square$

Proposition 2 expresses the near orthogonality of $\mathbf{M}$ in (10) in terms of that of $\mathbf{C}_j$'s and establishes conditions for $\mathbf{A}_j$, $\mathbf{B}$, and $\mathbf{D}$ in order for $\mathbf{M}$ to be an orthogonal Latin hypercube. The required matrices in Proposition 2 can be chosen as follows. First, orthogonal matrices $\mathbf{A}_j$'s and $\mathbf{D}$ are readily available from Hadamard matrices when n_1 and n_2 are multiples of four. Second, orthogonal Latin hypercubes $\mathbf{B}$ are available from Pang et al. (2009), Lin et al. (2009), Lin et al. (2010), among others. If $\mathbf{A}_j$, $\mathbf{B}$, and $\mathbf{D}$ are orthogonal, and either $\mathbf{B}^T\mathbf{D} = 0$ or $\mathbf{A}_j^T\mathbf{C}_j = 0$, then $\mathbf{M}$ is orthogonal when $\mathbf{C}_j$'s are orthogonal Latin hypercubes. If $\mathbf{C}_j$'s are NOLHDs like those from Lin et al. (2009) and Lin et al. (2010), then $\mathbf{M}$ is nearly orthogonal. If $\mathbf{C}_1$ is an NOLHD, $\mathbf{C}_2, \ldots, \mathbf{C}_{m_2}$ can be obtained by permuting the rows of $\mathbf{C}_1$.

Example 2 Let

$$\mathbf{B} = \frac{1}{2}\begin{pmatrix} 1 & -3 & 7 & 5 \\ 3 & 1 & 5 & -7 \\ 5 & -7 & -3 & -1 \\ 7 & 5 & -1 & 3 \\ -1 & 3 & -7 & -5 \\ -3 & -1 & -5 & 7 \\ -5 & 7 & 3 & 1 \\ -7 & -5 & 1 & -3 \end{pmatrix}, \mathbf{D} = \begin{pmatrix} 1 & 1 & 1 & 1 \\ 1 & 1 & -1 & -1 \\ 1 & -1 & 1 & -1 \\ 1 & -1 & -1 & 1 \\ -1 & 1 & 1 & 1 \\ -1 & 1 & -1 & -1 \\ -1 & -1 & 1 & -1 \\ -1 & -1 & -1 & 1 \end{pmatrix},$$

$$\mathbf{A}_1 = \begin{pmatrix} 1 & 1 & 1 & 1 & 1 & 1 \\ 1 & -1 & 1 & 1 & 1 & -1 \\ -1 & 1 & -1 & 1 & 1 & 1 \\ -1 & -1 & 1 & -1 & 1 & 1 \\ 1 & -1 & -1 & 1 & -1 & 1 \\ -1 & 1 & -1 & -1 & 1 & -1 \\ -1 & -1 & 1 & -1 & -1 & 1 \\ -1 & -1 & -1 & 1 & -1 & -1 \\ 1 & -1 & -1 & -1 & 1 & -1 \\ 1 & 1 & -1 & -1 & -1 & 1 \\ 1 & 1 & 1 & -1 & -1 & -1 \\ -1 & 1 & 1 & 1 & -1 & -1 \end{pmatrix}, \text{ and } \mathbf{C}_1 = \frac{1}{2}\begin{pmatrix} -11 & -9 & 9 & 11 & 5 & 1 \\ -9 & 5 & -1 & -5 & -9 & 11 \\ -7 & 11 & -3 & 3 & 1 & -7 \\ -5 & -1 & -9 & -9 & -1 & -9 \\ -3 & -7 & 5 & -11 & 7 & -1 \\ -1 & 9 & -7 & 5 & 9 & 5 \\ 1 & -3 & 7 & -7 & -7 & 3 \\ 3 & -11 & -11 & 9 & -11 & -3 \\ 5 & 7 & 11 & 7 & -5 & -5 \\ 7 & -5 & -5 & 1 & 11 & 7 \\ 9 & 1 & 3 & -3 & 3 & -11 \\ 11 & 3 & 1 & -1 & -3 & 9 \end{pmatrix}.$$

For $j = 2, 3, 4$, obtain $\mathbf{A}_j$ and $\mathbf{C}_j$ by permuting the rows of $\mathbf{A}_1$ and $\mathbf{C}_1$, respectively. Using the above matrices, $\mathbf{M}$ in (10) is a 96×24 orthogonal Latin hypercube.

Example 3 Let $\mathbf{C}_1$ be an NOLHD(25, 24) constructed by Lemma 1 using an OA(25, 6, 5) from Hedayat et al. (1999) and an NOLHD(5, 4). Permute the rows of $\mathbf{C}_1$ to get an NOLHD $\mathbf{C}_2$. Generate two 25×24 nearly orthogonal matrices, $\mathbf{A}_1$ and $\mathbf{A}_2$, by using the Gendex DOE software associated with Nguyen (1996). Using

$$\mathbf{B} = \begin{pmatrix} \frac{1}{2} & -\frac{1}{2} \\ -\frac{1}{2} & \frac{1}{2} \end{pmatrix} \text{ and } \mathbf{D} = \begin{pmatrix} 1 & 1 \\ 1 & 1 \end{pmatrix},$$

$\mathbf{M}$ in (10) is an NOLHD(50, 48).

3 Numerical Illustration

In this section we provide numerical examples to compare the number of false selections γ in (3) with four different types of design matrices. Method I uses an NOLHD from Sect. 2. Method II uses a two-level design at levels $\pm(n - 1)/2$. If $p > n - 1$, a two-level design is often called a supersaturated design (Lin 1993; Wu 1993). Method III uses a random Latin hypercube design (RLHD) constructed in (7). Method IV uses an i.i.d. sample. Denote by γ_{NOLHD}, γ_{FD}, γ_{RLHD}, and γ_{IID} the γ values of these methods, respectively. Since the focus here is to compare the effect of the regression matrix $\mathbf{X}$ on the accuracy of the Lasso solution, the response vector $\mathbf{y}$ from the model in (1) is generated with the same $\boldsymbol{\epsilon} = (\epsilon_1, \ldots, \epsilon_n)^T$ for the four methods. The tuning parameter λ in (2) is selected by the five-fold cross-validation. The package *lars* (Efron et al. 2003) in R (R, 2010) is used to compute the Lasso solution $\hat{\boldsymbol{\beta}}$ in (2). Examples below have different p/n ratios.

Example 4 For the model in (1), let $p = 48$, $\sigma = 8$, and $\boldsymbol{\beta} = (0.8, 1.0, \ldots, 3, 0, \ldots, 0)^T$ with the last 36 coefficients being zero. Take $n = 50$ with $n \approx p$. Method I takes the NOLHD(50, 48) in Example 3. Method II uses a 50×48 nearly orthogonal two-level design from the Gendex software based on the algorithm in Nguyen (1996). Table 1 compares three quartiles of the γ_{NOLHD}, γ_{FD}, γ_{RLHD} and γ_{IID} values over 50 replications. Figure 2 depicts the boxplots of γ values of these methods. Table 1 and Fig. 2 clearly indicate that γ_{NOLHD} is smaller than γ_{FD}, γ_{RLHD}, and γ_{IID}.

Table 1 Three quartiles of the γ_{NOLHD}, γ_{FD}, γ_{RLHD}, and γ_{IID} values over 50 replications for Example 4

	NOLHD	FD	RLHD	IID
Median	13.00	18.00	18.00	20.00
1st quartile	12.00	14.00	15.00	16.00
3rd quartile	15.00	21.00	23.00	23.00

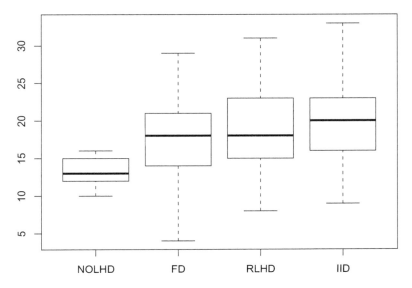

Fig. 2 Boxplots of the γ_{NOLHD}, γ_{FD}, γ_{RLHD}, and γ_{IID} values over the 50 replications for Example 4

Table 2 Three quartiles of the γ_{NOLHD}, γ_{FD}, γ_{RLHD} and γ_{IID} values over 50 replications for Example 5

	NOLHD	FD	RLHD	IID
Median	17.50	27.00	25.00	27.00
1st quartile	15.00	24.00	22.25	23.25
3rd quartile	22.75	30.00	28.00	29.00

Example 5 For the model in (1), let $p = 96$, $\sigma = 8$ and $\boldsymbol{\beta} = (0.2, 0.4, \ldots, 3, 0, \ldots, 0)^T$ with the last 81 coefficients being zero. Take $n = 49$ with $p > n$. Method I uses the NOLHD$(49, 96)$ in Example 1. Method II uses an $E(s^2)$-optimal supersaturated design from the Gendex software associated with Nguyen (1996). Table 2 compares three quartiles of the γ_{NOLHD}, γ_{FD}, γ_{RLHD} and γ_{IID} values over 50 replications. Figure 3 depicts the boxplots of γ values of these methods. Table 2 and Fig. 3 show that γ_{NOLHD}, once more, significantly outperforms γ_{FD}, γ_{RLHD}, and γ_{IID}.

Example 6 For the model in (1), let $p = 192$, $\sigma = 8$ and $\boldsymbol{\beta} = (0.05, 0.2, \ldots, 3, 0, \ldots, 0)^T$ with the last 172 coefficients being zero. Take $n = 64$ with $p > n$. Method I uses an NOLHD$(64, 192)$ from Lemma 1 in Sect. 2.1. Method II uses an $E(s^2)$-optimal supersaturated design from the Gendex software associated with Nguyen (1996). Table 3 compares three quartiles of the γ_{NOLHD}, γ_{FD}, γ_{RLHD}, and γ_{IID} values over 50 replications. Figure 4 depicts the boxplots of γ values for these methods, where γ_{NOLHD} is much smaller than γ_{FD}, γ_{RLHD}, and γ_{IID}. This example clearly demonstrates that the use of an NOLHD leads to significant improvement of the Lasso solution.

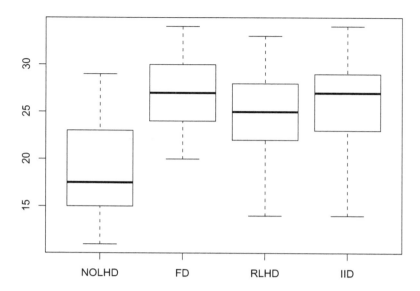

Fig. 3 Boxplots of the γ_{NOLHD}, γ_{FD}, γ_{RLHD} and γ_{IID} values over the 50 replications for Example 5

Table 3 Three quartiles of the γ_{NOLHD}, γ_{FD}, γ_{RLHD} and γ_{IID} values over 50 replications in Example 6

	NOLHD	FD	RLHD	IID
Median	27.00	42.50	43.00	41.00
1st quartile	23.00	40.00	34.25	34.00
3rd quartile	33.00	46.00	45.00	45.00

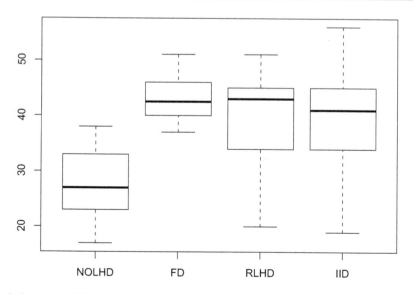

Fig. 4 Boxplots of the γ_{NOLHD}, γ_{FD}, γ_{RLHD} and γ_{IID} values over the 50 replications for Example 6

These examples suggest that the Lasso solution with an NOLHD is more accurate than those of the competing designs. Comparison of Figs. 2, 3, 4 indicates that the advantage of using NOLHDs in the Lasso problem grows as the ratio p/n increases.

4 Discussion

In this work, we proposed a method using NOLHDs from computer experiments to significantly enhance the variable selection accuracy of the Lasso procedure. The effectiveness of this method has been successfully illustrated by several examples. Design construction for sparse regressions is a new research direction in design of experiments, which can be applied in many areas, such compressed sensing (Song et al. 2016; Jung et al. 2019), and actuator placement (Du et al. 2019).

As an alternative to the proposed method, one may develop a model-based optimal design approach by extending the ideas of Meyer et al. (1996) and Bingham and Chipman (2007). Because the Lasso solution in (2) does not have an analytic form, a potential difficulty in developing such an approach is to introduce a sensible and computationally efficient design criterion for the Lasso problem. Another possible direction is to consider the Bayesian optimal design with proper priors for the sparsity on the regression parameters. It will be of interest as a future research project to study the proposed design strategy for various sparse regression under linear and generalized linear models.

Acknowledgments Chien is supported by U. S. National Science Foundation Grant 0969616 and an IBM Faculty Award. Deng is supported by the National Science Foundation CISE Expedition (Division of Computing and Communication Foundations) Grant CCF-1918770. Lin is supported by grants from the Natural Sciences and Engineering Research Council of Canada.

References

Bingham, D., & Chipman, H. A. (2007). Incorporating prior information in optimal design for model selection. *Technometrics*, *49*, 155–163.

Bingham, D., Sitter, R. R., & Tang, B. (2009). Orthogonal and nearly orthogonal designs for computer experiments. *Biometrika*, *96*, 51–65.

Box, G. E. P., Hunter, W. G., & Hunter, J. S. (2005). *Statistics for experimenters: design, innovation, and discovery, 2nd edition*. New York: John Wiley & Sons.

De Castro, Y. (2014). Optimal designs for Lasso and Dantzig selector using expander codes. *IEEE Transactions on Information Theory*, *60*, 7293–7299. Vancouver

Du, J., Yue, X., Hunt, J. H., & Shi, J. (2019). Optimal placement of actuators via sparse learning for composite fuselage shape control. *Journal of Manufacturing Science and Engineering*, *141*(10), 101004.

Efron, B., Hastie, T., Johnstone, I., & Tibshirani R. (2003). Least angle regression. *Annals of Statistics*, *32*, 407–499.

Fan, J., Li. G., & Li. R. (2005). An overview on variable selection for survival analysis. In *Contemporary multivariate analysis and design of experiments: In celebration of Professor Kai-Tai Fang's 65th birthday* (pp. 315–336).

Hedayat, A. S., Sloane, N. J. A., & Stufken, J. (1999). *Orthogonal arrays: theory and applications.* New York: Springer-Verlag.

Heinze, G., Wallisch, C., & Dunkler, D. (2018). Variable selection - A review and recommendations for the practicing statistician. *Biometrical Journal, 60,* 431–449.

Hesterberg, T., Choi, N. H., Meier, L., & Fraley, C. (2008). Least angle and l_1 penalized regression: a review. *Statistics Surveys, 2,* 61–93.

Huang, J., Breheny, P., & Ma, S. (2012). A selective review of group selection in high-dimensional models. *Statistical Science, 27.*

Huang, Y., Kong, X., & Ai, M. (2020). Optimal designs in sparse linear models. *Metrika, 83,* 255–273.

Jung, P., Kueng, R., & Mixon, D. G. (2019). Derandomizing compressed sensing with combinatorial design. *Frontiers in Applied Mathematics and Statistics, 5,* 26.

Lin, D. K. J. (1993). A new class of supersaturated designs. *Technometrics, 35,* 28–31.

Lin, C. D., & Tang, B. (2015). Latin Hypercubes and Space-filling Designs. In Bingham, D., Dean, A., Morris, M., & Stufken, J. (Ed.), *Handbook of design and analysis of experiments,* (pp. 593–626). CRC Press.

Lin, C. D., Mukerjee, R., & Tang, B. (2009). Construction of orthogonal and nearly orthogonal latin hypercubes. *Biometrika, 96,* 243–247.

Lin, C. D., Bingham, D., Sitter, R. R., & Tang, B. (2010). A new and flexible method for constructing designs for computer experiments. *Annals of Statistics, 38,* 1460–1477.

McKay, M. D., Beckman, R. J., & Conover, W. J. (1979). A comparison of three methods for selecting values of input variables in the analysis of output from a computer code. *Technometrics, 21,* 239–245.

Meyer, R. D., Steinberg, D. M., & Box, G. E. P. (1996). Follow-up designs to resolve confounding in multifactor experiments. *Technometrics, 38,* 303–313.

Nguyen, N. (1996). A note on constructing near-orthogonal arrays with economic run size. *Technometrics, 38,* 279–283.

Owen, A. B. (1992). A central limit theorem for latin hypercube sampling. *Journal of the Royal Statistical Society, Series B, 54,* 541–551.

Owen, A. B. (1994). Controlling correlations in latin hypercube samples. *Journal of the American Statistical Association, 89,* 1517–1522.

Pang, F., Liu, M. Q., & Lin, D. K. J. (2009). A construction method for orthogonal latin hypercube designs with prime power levels. *Statistica Sinica, 19,* 1721–1728.

R (2010). The R project for statistical computing.

Ravi, S. N., Ithapu, V., Johnson, S., & Singh, V. (2016). Experimental design on a budget for sparse linear models and applications. In *International conference on machine learning* (pp. 583–592).

Song, P., Mota, J. F., Deligiannis, N., & Rodrigues, M. R. D. (2016). Measurement matrix design for compressive sensing with side information at the encoder. In *2016 IEEE statistical signal processing workshop (SSP).* DOI:10.1109/SSP.2016.7551810.

Steinberg, D. M., & Lin, D. K. J. (2006). A construction method for orthogonal latin hypercube designs. *Biometrika, 93,* 279–288.

Sun, F., Liu, M. Q., & Lin, D. K. J. (2009). Construction of orthogonal latin hypercube designs. *Biometrika, 96,* 971–974.

Sun, F., Liu, M. Q., & Lin, D. K. J. (2010). Construction of orthogonal latin hypercube designs with flexible run sizes. *Journal of Statistical Planning and Inference, 140,* 3236–3242.

Tang, B. (1998). Selecting latin hypercubes using correlation criteria. *Statistica Sinica, 8,* 965–977.

Tibshirani, R. (1996). Regression shrinkage and selection via the lasso. *Journal of the Royal Statistical Society, Series B, 58,* 267–288.

Tibshirani, R. J., & Taylor, J. (2011). The solution path of the generalized lasso. *The Annals of Statistics, 39*(3), 1335–1371.

Wu, C. F. J. (1993). Construction of supersaturated designs through partially aliased interactions. *Biometrika*, *80*, 661–669.

Wu, C. F. J., & Hamada, M. (2009). *Experiments: planning, analysis, and parameter design optimization, 2nd edition*. New York: John Wiley & Sons.

Ye, K. Q. (1998). Orthogonal column latin hypercubes and their application in computer experiments. *Journal of the American Statistical Association*, *93*, 1430–1439.

Zhao, P., & Yu, B. (2006). On model selection consistency of the lasso. *Journal of Machine Learning Research*, *7*, 2541–2567.

Zhao, P., Rocha, G., & Yu, B. (2009). Grouped and hierarchical model selection through composite absolute penalties. *Annals of Statistics*, *37*(6A), 3468–3497.

Zou, H., & Hastie, T. (2005). Regularization and variable selection via the elastic net. *Journal of the Royal Statistical Society: Series B (statistical methodology)*, *67*(2), 301–320.

Zou, H. (2006). The adaptive lasso and its oracle properties. *Journal of the American Statistical Association*, *101*, 1418–1429.

Zou, H. (2016). Discussion of "Estimating structured high-dimensional covariance and precision matrices: Optimal rates and adaptive estimation". *Electronic Journal of Statistics*, *10*(1), 60–66.

A Selective Overview of Statistical Methods for Identification of the Treatment-Sensitive Subsets of Patients

Xinyi Ge, Yingwei Peng, and Dongsheng Tu

Abstract Identification of a subset of patients who may benefit from or be sensitive to a specific type of treatment has become a very important research topic in clinical trials and other types of clinical research. Statistical methods are essential in helping clinical researchers to identify the subset. In this article, we provide a selective overview of statistical methods developed in recent years in this research areas. Specifically, we consider first the cases where the outcome of the clinical studies is time-to-event or survival time and the subset is defined by one continuous covariate, such as the expression level of a gene, or by multiple covariates which can be continuous or categorical, such as mutation statuses of multiple genes. The cases where the outcomes of the clinical studies are longitudinal or repeated measurements, such as patient reported quality of life scores before, during, and after a treatment, are considered next. Gaps between the needs in clinical research and the methods available in statistical literature are identified and future research topics to bridge these gaps are discussed based on this overview.

Keywords Censored survival times · Clinical trials · Interaction · Longitudinal data · Predictive function

1 Introduction

For many diseases, such as cancer, it is often difficult to find a treatment that benefits all patents. There is an interest to identify a subset of patients, defined by individual characteristics, such as age, gender, blood test results, or gene expression levels,

X. Ge
Department of Mathematics and Statistics, Queen's University, Kingston, ON, Canada
e-mail: xinyi.ge@queensu.ca

Y. Peng · D. Tu (✉)
Departments of Public Health Sciences and Mathematics and Statistics, Queen's University, Kingston, ON, Canada
e-mail: yingwei.peng@queensu.ca; dtu@ctg.queensu.ca

© The Author(s), under exclusive license to Springer Nature Switzerland AG 2022
W. He et al. (eds.), *Advances and Innovations in Statistics and Data Science*, ICSA
Book Series in Statistics, https://doi.org/10.1007/978-3-031-08329-7_15

who may be more sensitive to a specific treatment and have a larger treatment effect in comparison with a standard treatment. Conversely, if a treatment is costly or has potential negative side effects, there is also an interest to look for subsets of patients for which the treatment has less side effects. Therefore, identification of treatment-sensitive subsets of patients for a specific treatment has become a very important topic in clinical research. For example, in a recent secondary analysis of data from CO.17 and CO.20 trials conducted by the Canadian Cancer Trials Group (CCTG), the investigators were interested to know whether older patients with advanced colorectal cancer treated by, respectively, cetuximab alone or cetuximab plus brivanib had a less benefit, in comparison with younger patients, in terms of various outcomes including overall survival and quality of life (Wells et al. 2008).

Subset analysis, which includes (1) identification of the subsets, (2) estimation of treatment effects in the subsets, and (3) tests for the significance of the differences in the treatment effects in these subsets, is a main statistical tool to assess the heterogeneity in treatment effects in subsets defined by certain characteristics of patients. For example, in the analyses of CO.17 and CO.20 data mentioned above, patients were divided into two age subsets based on whether their age was 70 years or older and differential treatment effects in these two age subsets were assessed through a test of interaction between the subset and treatment. However, it is unclear whether 70 years is an optimal cutpoint to define the age subsets when assessing the heterogeneity of treatment effects by age. This issue arises in many studies where the variable to define subsets is continuous but a pre-specified cutpoint is not available from previous studies or clinical experience, and a statistical approach is often needed to determine the optimal cutpoints based on data.

When the outcomes for the subgroup analyses are times to an event or survival times, such as progression-free or overall survivals, several approaches have been proposed for the determination of cutpoints in the definition of subsets. For example, Jiang et al. (2007) proposed a biomarker-adaptive threshold design, which combines a test for overall treatment effect in all patients with the determination and validation of a cutpoint for a biomarker which is used to define a sensitive subset. Chen et al. (2014) developed a hierarchical Bayesian procedure to estimate simultaneously the interaction parameter and cutpoint in a threshold Cox proportional hazards model. He et al. (2018) proposed a single-index threshold Cox proportional hazard model, which includes a smoothly clipped absolute deviation (SCAD) penalty function, to select and linearly combine multiple biomarkers in identification of treatment-sensitive subsets. Su et al. (2008) developed an interaction tree procedure, which recursively partitions the patients into two subsets based on the greatest interaction between the subset and treatment, to obtain treatment-sensitive subsets.

When the outcomes are longitudinal measurements, Moineddin et al. (2008) used multilevel models including patient-specific random effects to identify subsets of patients with differential treatment effects of gabapentin versus placebo on longitudinal measurements of hot flashes based on the baseline measurements in a double-blind randomized controlled trial for treatment of hot flashes in women who enter menopause naturally but a median was used as the cutpoint in defining subsets. Andrews et al. (2017) considered a random effects linear model for longitudinal outcomes to determine whether a patient had a positive response to the treatment and supervised learning algorithms were proposed to estimate a predictive function for the positive response but 0.5 was used as an ad hoc cutpoint for the predictive function to assign patients into subsets. Recently, Ge et al. (2020) introduced a threshold linear mixed model for the identification of treatment-sensitive subsets of patients based on longitudinal outcomes.

The objectives of this article are to provide a detailed review of the methods mentioned above and, based on this review, to discuss some future directions in this interesting and important area of research.

The remainder of this article is organized as follows. Sections 2 and 3 present a detailed review of statistical methods developed when, respectively, survival times and longitudinal measurements are the outcomes of the clinical research. Discussions on the future research directions are presented in the last section.

2 Statistical Methods for Treatment-Sensitive Subset Identification with Survival Times

Time to an event, which is denoted as F in this article and usually called as the survival time with overall survival or progression-free survival as examples, is usually a primary endpoint in a cancer clinical trial. Before we give detailed descriptions on the approaches proposed to identify treatment-sensitive subsets of patients based on survival times, some conventional notations, and a commonly used statistical model for the survival times are introduced below.

Denote F_i and C_i as, respectively, the potential survival and censoring times of a patient i ($i = 1, 2, \cdots, n$). The observed survival times T_i and survival status indicator δ_i are defined, respectively, as

$$
\begin{cases}
T_i & = \min(F_i, C_i), \\
\delta_i & = I_{(F_i < C_i)}.
\end{cases}
\tag{1}
$$

Let $h(t|\mathbf{W_i})$ be the hazard function of survival time F_i for a patient with a vector of covariates $\mathbf{W_i}$, which may include treatment indicators $\mathbf{X_i}$ and biomarkers of interest $\mathbf{Z_i}$. In the survival analysis, Cox's proportional hazards model (Cox 1972, 1975) is usually used to model the relationship between $h(t|\mathbf{W_i})$ and $\mathbf{W_i}$ as follows:

$$
h(t|\mathbf{W_i}) = h_0(t)g(\mathbf{W_i}, \boldsymbol{\beta}),
$$

where $g(\cdot)$ is a given link function, $h_0(t)$ is an unknown baseline hazard function, and $\boldsymbol{\beta}$ is an unknown vector of regression coefficients. A non-informative censoring is assumed, which implies that, given the covariates W_i, F_i, and C_i are independent.

2.1 An Approach Based on a Biomarker-Adaptive Threshold Design

We first review an approach based on a biomarker-adaptive threshold design proposed by Jiang et al. (2007), which tests first for an overall treatment effect in all patients and, if the overall treatment effect is not significant, proceeds to the next step to determine a cutpoint for a biomarker to identify a potential treatment-sensitive subset of patients.

Specifically, consider the following threshold Cox's proportional hazards model:

$$\log\{h(t|\mathbf{W_i})\} = \log h_0(t) + \beta_1 X_{1i} + \beta_2 I_{(Z_{1i}>c)} + \beta_3 X_{1i} I_{(Z_{1i}>c)}, \qquad (2)$$

where, for $i = 1, 2, \cdots, n$, $\mathbf{W_i} = (X_{1i}, Z_{1i})$ with X_{1i} an treatment indicator equal to 1 if patient i is assigned into a treatment group or 0 if into a control group and Z_{1i} the value of a continuous biomarker which is used to define the treatment-sensitive subset, c is an unknown threshold parameter for the definition of the sensitive subset, β_1 is the main treatment effect, β_2 is the main biomarker effect, and β_3 is the treatment by biomarker interaction effect. Without loss of generality, c and Z_{1i} are assumed to take values in the interval $(0, 1)$.

In the first step of their procedure, the effect of treatment over all patients is assessed, which can be achieved by taking $\beta_2 = \beta_3 = 0$ in model (2) and testing the null hypothesis that $\beta_1 = 0$ in the reduced model

$$\log h(t|\mathbf{W_i}) = \log h_0(t) + \beta_1 X_{1i}$$

by a likelihood ratio test. If the test rejects the null hypothesis of no treatment effect over all patients, the procedure stops and one can conclude that the treatment will benefit all patients. Otherwise, the procedure will continue to assess whether there is a subset of patients defined by a biomarker who may benefit from the treatment by testing the null hypothesis that $\beta_3 = 0$ in the full model (2).

Since the threshold parameter c is unknown, the following procedure is proposed to test the null hypothesis that $\beta_3 = 0$ under the assumption that $\beta_1 = 0$: For each candidate biomarker threshold in the range $(0, 1)$, a reduced model (2) with $\beta_1 = 0$ is fitted on the subset of patients with biomarker values over c to obtain a log-likelihood ratio statistic $S(c)$ for testing the null hypothesis $\beta_3 = 0$ under the given c. Maximizing $S(c)$ over a range of possible cutpoint values would give a test statistic for testing null hypothesis $\beta_3 = 0$ with c unspecified. In order to obtain a reasonable power, a test statistic T is defined as $\max((S(0)+R), \max_{0<c<1} S(c))$, where R is a positive constant which was suggested to be 2.2 by Jiang et al. (2007). The p-value of this test statistic can be calculated from a resampling-based approach by randomly permutating treatment labels. If the test rejects the null hypothesis $\beta_3 = 0$, the optimal threshold c_0 can be estimated as

$$\hat{c}_0 = \arg\max_{c_0} l(c_0),$$

where $l(c_0)$ is the partial log-likelihood function based on model (2):

$$l(c_0) = \max_{\beta_1, \beta_2, \beta_3} l(\beta_1, \beta_2, \beta_3, c_0).$$

Therefore, the treatment-sensitive subset of patients can be defined by $\{i : I(Z_{1i} > \hat{c}_0)\}$, that is, a patient will be sensitive to the treatment if the observed value of the biomarker from this patients is over $\hat{c}_0$.

2.2 A Hierarchical Bayesian Method

Chen et al. (2014) proposed a hierarchical Bayesian method to estimate all unknown parameters, including the threshold c, in model (2) simultaneously without assumption $\beta_1 = 0$.

For simplicity of presentation, denote $[X_{1i}, I(Z_{1i} > c), X_{1i}I(Z_{1i} > c)]'$ as $\mathbf{W_i}(c)$ and $[\beta_1, \beta_2, \beta_3]'$ as $\boldsymbol{\beta}$. With these notations, model (2) can be rewritten as

$$h(t|\mathbf{W_i}(c)) = h_0(t) \exp\{\mathbf{W_i'}(c)\boldsymbol{\beta}\}. \tag{3}$$

Chen et al. (2014) assumed that the threshold parameter c has a prior Beta distribution Beta(2,q) for a given hyper-parameter $q > 1$, which can be written as

$$p_1(c|q) \propto q(q+1)c(1-c)^{q-1}.$$

This prior is flexible enough to accommodate any prior distribution in a family with its mode taking any specific value in the interval $(0, 1)$. In order to assign a specific prior distribution of c, instead of taking an arbitrary value for q, it is considered that q has a hyper-prior distribution with the following density function form

$$p_2(q) \propto \frac{q-1}{q(q+1)}, \quad q > 1.$$

At the same time, $\boldsymbol{\beta}$ is assumed to has a uniform improper prior distribution $p(\boldsymbol{\beta}) \propto 1$. For every given $0 < c < 1$, the corresponding partial likelihood function of $\boldsymbol{\beta}$ in model (3) is given by

$$p_3(\boldsymbol{\beta}|c) = \prod_{i=1}^{n} \left[\frac{\exp\{\mathbf{W_i'}(c)\boldsymbol{\beta}\}}{\sum_{j \in R(T_i)} \exp\{\mathbf{W_j'}(c)\boldsymbol{\beta}\}} \right]^{\delta_i},$$

where the risk set $R(t)$ is the index set of patients who are at risk of experiencing an event at time t. Consequently, given the observed data, the joint posterior distribution of β, c, q can be written as

$$p(\beta, c, q | data) \propto p_1(c|q) p_2(q) p_3(\beta|c)$$

$$= \prod_{i=1}^{n} \left[\frac{\exp\{\mathbf{W}_i'(c)\beta\}}{\sum_{j \in R(T_i)} \exp\{\mathbf{W}_j'(c)\beta\}} \right]^{\delta_i} c(1-c)^{q-1}(q-1).$$

Therefore, the marginal posterior distributions of β and c can be calculated, respectively, as

$$p(\beta) = \int_{c,q} p(\beta, c, q | data) dc dq$$

$$p(c) = \int_{\beta,q} p(\beta, c, q | data) d\beta dq.$$

Statistical inferences, such as point estimation, confidence interval and hypothesis testing, on the threshold parameter c and the regression coefficient β can be obtained based on these marginal distributions. After obtaining the estimation of the threshold c, the treatment-sensitive subset of patients consequently can be defined if β_3 is significantly different from 0.

2.3 A Procedure Based on a Single-index Threshold Cox Model

In some clinical trials, it may be difficult to identify a treatment-sensitive subset of patients based on a single biomarker, but a combination of multiple biomarkers may have a potential to identify a treatment-sensitive subset. For example, in a randomized control trial PA.3 conducted by NCIC Clinical Trials Group, 35 key proteins were selected from a global genetic analysis of pancreatic cancers with the purpose of identifying a subset of patients with locally advanced or metastatic pancreatic cancer who will be sensitive to the treatment of erlotinib in addition to gemcitabine (Shultz et al. 2016). However, no significant interaction was found between the treatment and any of these biomarkers, which implies that it is impossible to identify a treatment-sensitive subset according to a single biomarker. He et al. (2018) found that a combination of some of these biomarkers (CA 19-9 and Axl) had the potential to define a treatment-sensitive subset of patients with pancreatic cancer. It is more complicated to identify a treatment-sensitive subset based on multiple biomarkers, compared to the cases where there is only a single biomarker.

Several approaches have been proposed in subgroup analysis based on multiple biomarkers. He et al. (2018) proposed a single-index threshold Cox's proportional hazards model to identify treatment-sensitive subsets for each treatment using multiple biomarkers based on a linear combination of the multiple biomarkers. Let $\mathbf{X_i} = (x_{i1}, x_{i2}, \cdots, x_{id})'$ be a d-dimensional vector of exposure variables, such as treatment group indicators, for a patient i and $\mathbf{Z_i} = (z_{i1}, z_{i2}, \cdots, z_{ip})'$ be a p-dimensional vector which are the observed values of p biomarkers from the i-th patient ($i = 1, 2, \cdots, n$). Define an indicator function $I_{(\mathbf{Z_i'}\boldsymbol{\gamma_j} > c_j)}$ to be used to define the treatment-sensitive subset of patients for the j-th treatment, where $\boldsymbol{\gamma_j}$ is a p-dimensional vector used to combine biomarkers linearly and c_j is the threshold parameter. Denote $\mathbf{W_i} = (\mathbf{X_i'}, \mathbf{Z_i'})$. The proposed model can be written as

$$h(t|\mathbf{W_i}) = h_0(t) \exp\left\{ \boldsymbol{\beta}'X_i + \sum_{j=1}^{d} \eta_j I_{(\mathbf{Z_i'}\boldsymbol{\gamma_j} > c_j)} + \sum_{j=1}^{d} \alpha_j x_j I_{(\mathbf{Z_i'}\boldsymbol{\gamma_j} > c_j)} \right\}, \qquad (4)$$

where $h(t)$, $h_0(t)$, and $\boldsymbol{\beta}$ are the same defined in last section. The parameters $\boldsymbol{\eta} = (\eta_1, \eta_2, \cdots, \eta_d)'$ and $\boldsymbol{\alpha} = (\alpha_1, \alpha_2, \cdots, \alpha_d)'$ model the main effect of biomarker and the treatment-biomarker interaction, respectively. A significant treatment-biomarker interaction implies the treatment effect varies across subsets defined by $I_{(\mathbf{Z_i'}\boldsymbol{\gamma_j} > c_j)}$ and, consequently, the treatment-sensitive subsets for each treatment can be determined.

To obtain estimators of the parameters in the model, a maximum penalized smoothed partial likelihood method has been proposed. First, assume that data are available from n independent patients, where $i = 1, 2, \cdots, n$. Denote $\boldsymbol{\Gamma} = (\gamma_1, \gamma_2, \cdots, \gamma_d)'$, $\mathbf{c} = (c_1, c_2, \cdots, c_d)'$, and $\boldsymbol{\theta} = (\boldsymbol{\beta}', \boldsymbol{\eta}', \boldsymbol{\alpha}', \mathbf{c}', \boldsymbol{\Gamma}')'$. Then the partial likelihood of the parameters in model (4) can be written as

$$L(\boldsymbol{\theta})$$

$$= \prod_{i=1}^{n} \left[\frac{\exp\left\{ \boldsymbol{\beta}'X_i + \sum_{j=1}^{d} \eta_j I_{(\mathbf{Z_i'}\boldsymbol{\gamma_j} > c_j)} + \sum_{j=1}^{d} \alpha_j x_{ij} I_{(\mathbf{Z_i'}\boldsymbol{\gamma_j} > c_j)} \right\}}{\sum_{k \in R(T_i)} \exp\left\{ \boldsymbol{\beta}'X_k + \sum_{j=1}^{d} \eta_j I_{(\mathbf{Z_k'}\boldsymbol{\gamma_j} > c_j)} + \sum_{j=1}^{d} \alpha_j x_{kj} I_{(\mathbf{Z_k'}\boldsymbol{\gamma_j} > c_j)} \right\}} \right]^{\delta_i}.$$

$$(5)$$

Since the partial likelihood function is not continuous at some parameters, the estimator of $\boldsymbol{\theta}$ cannot be obtained by maximizing the partial likelihood function (5). He et al. (2018) proposed a local distribution function $\Phi((\mathbf{Z_i'}\boldsymbol{\gamma}_j - c_j)/h)$ as a smooth approximation to the indicator function $I(\mathbf{Z_i'}\boldsymbol{\gamma_j} > c_j)$, where Φ is the distribution function of the standard normal variable and the bandwidth h converges to zero as the sample size increases. With this approximation, the smoothed partial likelihood (SPL) function can be defined as

$$S(\boldsymbol{\theta}) =$$

$$\prod_{i=1}^{n} \left[\frac{\exp\{\boldsymbol{\beta}'X_i + \sum_{j=1}^{d} \eta_j \Phi((Z_i'\boldsymbol{\gamma}_j - c_j)/h) + \sum_{j=1}^{d} \alpha_j x_{ij} \Phi((Z_i'\boldsymbol{\gamma}_j - c_j)/h)\}}{\sum_{k \in R(T_i)} \exp\{\boldsymbol{\beta}'X_k + \sum_{j=1}^{d} \eta_j \Phi((Z_k'\boldsymbol{\gamma}_j - c_j)/h) + \sum_{j=1}^{d} \alpha_j x_{kj} \Phi((Z_k'\boldsymbol{\gamma}_j - c_j)/h)\}} \right]^{\delta_i} . \tag{6}$$

Because a large number of covariates may be available but only a few of them may be relevant in the definition of treatment-sensitive subsets, He et al. (2018) added a penalty function to the SPL function for efficiently selecting relevant biomarkers from large amount of biomarkers in practice. In their procedure, the smoothly clipped absolute deviation (SCAD) penalty function was used and the penalized smoothed partial likelihood (PSPL) function was defined as

$$L_n(\boldsymbol{\theta}) = \log\{S(\boldsymbol{\theta})\} - n \sum_{j=1}^{d} \sum_{k=1}^{p} P_\lambda(|\lambda_{jk}|), \tag{7}$$

where λ_{jk} is the component k of $\boldsymbol{\gamma}_j$ and $P_\lambda(\cdot)$ is the SCAD penalty function with a regularization parameter λ. By maximizing PSPL function (7), the estimations of $\boldsymbol{\theta}$ can be obtained. Therefore, when at least one of the α_j is significantly different from 0, corresponding treatment-sensitive subset of patients for the treatment j can be determined by the estimate $\hat{c}_j$ of c_j as $\{i : I_{(Z_i'\boldsymbol{\gamma}_j > \hat{c}_j)}\}$.

2.4 An Interaction Tree Approach

Su et al. (2008) proposed a procedure to construct an interaction tree $\mathscr{T}$ based on survival outcomes which can be used to identify treatment-sensitive subsets of patients. There are three steps in the construction of an interaction tree which are introduced in details below.

The first step is to grow a large initial tree. Let s be a single binary split of patients in the tree construction based on a biomarker z measured on patients. If z is continuous, then the split s is induced by whether or not $z \leq c$, where the threshold c can be any constant. However, in practice the threshold c is chosen as one of the observed values of z. If z is ordinal, the split s can be induced by the similar procedure. If z is a categorical variable with categories $C = \{c_1, \cdots, c_r\}$, then the split can be induced by the form of $z \in A$ with $A \subset C$. In order to reduce the computational burden, the treatment effect within each category is often estimated first and then the categories of z are reordered according to the treatment effect.

Splitting on z can then be induced by treating z as an ordinal variable. Next we need to select the best split from all possible splits, which has the greatest difference in the treatment effect between its two child nodes. The splitting selection approach in Su et al. (2008) is to choose the split to maximize a statistic for test $H_0 : \beta_3 = 0$ in the following Cox model:

$$h(t|\mathbf{W_i}) = h_0(t) \exp\{\beta_1 X_i + \beta_2 I^{(s)} + \beta_3 X_i I^{(s)}\}, \tag{8}$$

where X_i is a treatment indicator, $I^{(s)} = I_{(z \in A)}$ or $I^{(s)} = I_{(z \leq c)}$, and $W_i = (X_i, I^{(s)})$. In their method, they chose to use the following partial likelihood ratio test (PLRT) statistic as the test statistic for $H_0 : \beta_3 = 0$:

$$G(s) = -2(l_2 - l_1), \tag{9}$$

where l_2 is the maximized partial likelihood (Cox 1975) of model (8) and l_1 is the maximized partial likelihood of the reduced model under H_0:

$$h(t|\mathbf{W_i}) = h_0(t) \exp\{\beta_1 X_i + \beta_2 I^{(s)}\}. \tag{10}$$

The best split s^* can be determined by $G(s^*) = \max_s G(s)$. After choosing the best split, the patients can be divided into two subsets and therefore the tree grows two child nodes. The same procedure is then implemented to split both child nodes based on different variables such as the values of other biomarkers. A large initial tree $\mathscr{T}_0$ can be obtained by repeating the above process recursively.

Since the initial tree is large, it needs to be pruned until it has an appropriate size. Su et al. (2008) introduced the following penalty function for a node h of the initial tree:

$$g(h) = \frac{G(\mathscr{T}_h)}{|\mathscr{T}_h - \tilde{\mathscr{T}}_h|},$$

where $\mathscr{T}_h$ is the branch of tree with h as its root, $\tilde{\mathscr{T}}_h$ represents the set of all terminal nodes of $\mathscr{T}_h$, and $|\mathscr{T}_h - \tilde{\mathscr{T}}_h|$ denotes the number of all internal nodes of $\mathscr{T}_h$. By minimizing $g(h)$ over all the internal nodes of $\mathscr{T}_0$, the weakest link (or the most ineffective split) h^* can be determined. Denote $\mathscr{T}_1$ as the subtree after pruning off the branch $\mathscr{T}_{h^*}$ from $\mathscr{T}_0$ and apply the same pruning procedure to the subtree $\mathscr{T}_1$. After the above process is repeated recursively, a nested sequence of subtrees can be defined as $\mathscr{T}_M \prec \cdots \prec \mathscr{T}_m \prec \mathscr{T}_{m-1} \cdots \prec \mathscr{T}_1 \prec \mathscr{T}_0$, where $\mathscr{T}_M$ is a tree only having the root node and $\prec$ means "a subtree of."

After the pruning procedure is finished, the last step of the proposed procedure is to select the best size of the tree. For this purpose, following the split-complexity pruning algorithm for survival tree (LeBlanc & Crowley 1993), the following interaction-complexity measure is introduced to evaluate the overall goodness-of-interaction of a given tree $\mathcal{T}$:

$$G_\lambda(\mathcal{T}) = G(\mathcal{T}) - \lambda \cdot |\mathcal{T} - \tilde{\mathcal{T}}|, \tag{11}$$

where $\tilde{\mathcal{T}}$ denotes a set of all terminal nodes of $\mathcal{T}$ and $|\mathcal{T} - \tilde{\mathcal{T}}|$ the number of all internal nodes of $\mathcal{T}$, $G(\mathcal{T}) = \sum_{h \in \mathcal{T} - \tilde{\mathcal{T}}} G(h)$, which is the sum of $G(h)$, the splitting statistic defined in (9), over node h (including its split to its child nodes), and $\lambda (\geqslant 0)$ is a penalty parameter for each added node. With this measure, an optimally sized tree $\mathcal{T}^*$ can be determined by maximizing $G_\lambda(\mathcal{T})$ as following:

$$G_\lambda(\mathcal{T}^*) = \max_{m=0,\cdots,M} \{G(\mathcal{T}_m) - \lambda \cdot |\mathcal{T}_m - \tilde{\mathcal{T}}_m|\},$$

where the penalty parameter λ can be pre-specified within the range $2 \leqslant \lambda \leqslant 4$ (LeBlanc & Crowley 1993). After the optimally sized tree is determined, the treatment-sensitive subsets of patients can be defined based on the terminal nodes of the tree $\mathcal{T}^*$.

3 Statistical Methods for Treatment-Sensitive Subset Identification Based on Longitudinal Measurements

Longitudinal measurements, which are repeated observations measured on the same patients at different points in time, are often collected in clinical trials or other medical studies. For example, although the treatment effect in cancer clinical trials are traditionally evaluated by relatively objective endpoints such as tumor response, relapse-free survival, or overall survival, it is argued that these endpoints may not provide adequate information in understanding of the treatment effect. Recently, evaluations of more subjective endpoints, such as patient reported quality of life (QoL), have become increasingly recognized in cancer clinical trials, since these endpoints can help patients to make the treatment decisions by providing detailed information on side effects of the treatment (Blazeby et al. 2001). Also these endpoints can help future patients understand the consequences of their illness and treatment (Bezjak et al. 2006). These patient reported outcomes are usually assessed at several timepoints before, during, and after patients have received the treatment.

Multilevel or hierarchical models are often used for the analysis of longitudinal data, as these models incorporate the variation at different levels of the hierarchy into analysis. This class of models includes multilevel models, linear mixed models, random effects ANOVA models, generalized estimating equations (GEE), etc. In this section, some statistical methods proposed for identifying treatment-sensitive subsets of patients based on these models when the outcomes of clinical trials are longitudinal or repeated measures are reviewed.

3.1   A Procedure Based on Multilevel Models

To establish notations, let y_{ij} be the longitudinal measurement at j-th observation time t_{ij} ($j = 1, 2, \cdots, n_i$) from patient i ($i = 1, 2, \cdots, N$). The observation times are usually called as level-1 units in a multilevel model, while patients are called as the level-2 units. Also denote X_i as the treatment indicator with $X_i = 1$ if the patient is assigned into the treatment group and $X_i = 0$ if the patient is assigned into the control group. Consider the following two-level linear regression model proposed in Moineddin et al. (2008) for these longitudinal measurements: the first level of the model assumes that the measurement y_{ij} is a linear function of observation time t_{ij}, which can be written as

$$y_{ij} = \beta_{0i} + \beta_{1i} t_{ij} + e_{ij}, \tag{12}$$

where e_{ij} is the random error term assumed to follow a normal distribution with mean zero and a constant variance σ_e^2 and β_{0i} and β_{1i} are, respectively, a random intercept and slope associated with the ith patient. It is assumed further that β_{0i} and β_{1i} can be explained by a linear function of X_i in the following second level of the model:

$$\beta_{0i} = \gamma_{00} + \gamma_{01} X_i + u_{0i},$$

$$\beta_{1i} = \gamma_{10} + \gamma_{11} X_i + u_{1i},$$

where γ_{rs} ($r = 0, 1$ and $s = 0, 1$) are population average fixed effect parameters and u_{0i} and u_{1i} are random errors which follow a bivariate normal distribution with mean zero and variance-covariance $var(u_{0i}) = \sigma_0^2$, $var(u_{1i}) = \sigma_1^2$ and $cov(u_{0i}, u_{1i}) = \sigma_{01}^2$. From the definition of X_i as a treatment indicator, it can be seen that the fixed effects γ_{00} and γ_{10} are, respectively, the population average of the measurement y_{ij} at baseline (intercept) and the population average of change over time (slope) for patients in the control group, while the parameters γ_{01} and γ_{11} can be interpreted as the differences in, respectively, the population averages of the measurement y_{ij} at baseline (intercepts) and the population average of changes over time (slopes) between the treatment and the control groups. Parameter σ_0^2 is the residual variance of the measurement y_{ij} at baseline (intercept) , σ_1^2 is the residual variance of the change rate (slope), and σ_{01}^2 is the residual covariance between the baseline the measurement and rate of change.

It is known that u_{1i} represents the residuals of the regression slopes across the patients. When the variance of u_{1i} is significant at a two-sided 0.05 level, Moineddin et al. (2008) suggested that treatment-sensitive subsets of patients can be identified based on a baseline factor (age, gender, biomarker, etc.) of patients by correlating u_{1i} with this factor using a t-test or analysis of variance if the factor is categorical and the Pearson or Spearman correlations if the factor is continuous. When the association is significant at two-sided 0.05 level, treatment-sensitive subsets of patients can be defined by the natural grouping generated by the categories of the baseline factor when it is categorical (for example, female and male subsets if the gender is the baseline factor). When the factor is continuous such as the age or value of a biomarker, however, a cutpoint is required. Only an ad hoc approach using the median of the factor as a cutpoint was suggested and there was no formal procedure proposed to estimate the cutpoint.

3.2 A Prediction Model Approach

Andrews et al. (2017) proposed a complete procedure which can be used for both identification of the treatment-sensitive subsets of patients and validation of the subsets identified based on longitudinal measurements. First step in the proposed procedure is to use a linear mixed model which includes a random effect term to evaluate the individual treatment effect and a fixed effect term to evaluate the population average treatment effect. Based on the estimates of individual treatment effect, various classifying methods can then be used to build prediction models which can be used to identify treatment-sensitive subsets of patients based on the characteristics of patients. A validation step is then followed to select the best prediction model under a marginal regression framework.

Specifically, consider the following random intercept-slope linear mixed model:

$$y_{ij} = \beta_0 + \alpha_{0i} + (\beta_1 + \alpha_{1i})X_i t_{ij} + \beta_2 t_{ij} + e_{ij}, \tag{13}$$

where X_i, t_{ij}, y_{ij} and random error term e_{ij} are the same as defined in the last subsection, β_0 and β_1 represent, respectively, the population average of the initial status and the treatment effect over time, α_{0i} and α_{1i} are, respectively, the random intercept and slope for patient i, and β_2 is the fixed effect of time. The interaction effect $\beta_1 + \alpha_{1i}$ between the treatment and time in this model describes the trend of individual treatment effect over time.

To simplify the presentation of the procedure, model (13) can be rewritten in matrix form as

$$Y = X\beta + D\alpha + e, \tag{14}$$

where Y is a n-dimensional vector of the responses with $n = \sum_{i=1}^{N} n_i$, X and D are an $n \times 3$ and $n \times 2N$ matrices of covariates corresponding to the fixed effects $\beta = (\beta_0, \beta_1, \beta_2)'$ and random effects $\alpha = (\alpha_{01}, \cdots, \alpha_{0N}, \alpha_{11}, \cdots, \alpha_{1N})$, respectively, and e is a m-dimensional vector of the random errors. It is assumed that $E(\alpha) = 0$ and $E(e) = 0$. In addition, it is assumed that α and e are independent and distributed as multivariate normal as

$$\begin{bmatrix} \alpha \\ e \end{bmatrix} \sim N \left(\begin{bmatrix} 0 \\ 0 \end{bmatrix}, \begin{bmatrix} \mathbf{G} & \mathbf{0} \\ \mathbf{0} & \mathbf{R} \end{bmatrix} \right).$$

By using the conventional maximum likelihood method for the linear mixed model, the parameter estimates for the fixed and random effects can be obtained as following:

$$\hat{\beta} = (X'\hat{\Sigma}^{-1}X)^{-1}X'\hat{\Sigma}^{-1}Y,$$

$$\hat{\alpha} = \hat{G}D'\hat{\Sigma}^{-1}(Y - X\hat{\beta}),$$

where $\Sigma = DGD' + R$ and $\hat{G}$ and $\hat{R}$ are obtained by maximizing the following likelihood function:

$$l(R, G|Y, X) = -\frac{1}{2}(Y - X(X'\Sigma^{-1}X)^{-1}X'\Sigma^{-1}Y)'\Sigma^{-1}$$

$$(Y - X(X'\Sigma^{-1}X)^{-1}X'\Sigma^{-1}Y) - \frac{1}{2}\log|\Sigma| - \frac{n}{2}\log(2\pi),$$

where $|\Sigma|$ is the determinant of the variance-covariance matrix Σ. The asymptotic consistency and efficiency of these estimates were proved by Hartley and Rao (1967). Furthermore, if the variance estimation is biased, the restricted maximum likelihood would be a viable alternative method (Verbeke & Molenberghs 2009).

Since the random slope $\beta_1 + \alpha_{1i}$ describes the treatment effect over time, patients can be divided into two subsets based on whether its estimate $\hat{\beta}_1 + \hat{\alpha}_{1i}$ is positive. Define C_i as the subset indicator based on this definition. That is,

$$C_i = \begin{cases} 1 & \hat{\beta}_1 + \hat{\alpha}_{1i} > 0 \\ -1 & \hat{\beta}_1 + \hat{\alpha}_{1i} \leq 0. \end{cases}$$

Since some baseline characteristics or covariates $\mathbf{W}_i$ of patients, such as age, gender, blood pressure, and gene expression, might influence the treatment effect, a prediction model

$$f(\mathbf{W}_i) = P(C_i = 1|\mathbf{W}_i)$$

based on the subset indicator C_i and these baseline characteristics or covariates $\mathbf{W}_i$ may be used to classify patients into two subsets which have differential treatment effects. In general, the relationship between C_i and $\mathbf{W}_i$ is unknown, which could be linear or nonlinear, so the predictive function $f(\cdot)$ in the above prediction model needs to be estimated. Andrews et al. (2017) suggested various linear or nonlinear supervised learning algorithms, such as logistic regression, support vector machine (SVM) with linear kernel, linear discriminant analysis (LDA), decision tree, random forest, etc., may be used to estimate $f(\cdot)$. Once the estimated prediction function

$\hat{f}(\mathbf{W}_i)$ is obtained from the data, it was proposed that patient i can be classified in the subset of patients who may benefit from the treatment if $\hat{f}(\mathbf{W}_i) > 0.5$.

Andrews et al. (2017) also developed a validation procedure to assess the effectiveness of the method proposed above for the treatment-sensitive subset identification but the choice of 0.5 as the cutpoint for estimated predictive function to define the subsets is ad hoc, which may have large impact on the performance of the proposed method.

3.3   A Procedure Based on a Threshold Linear Mixed Model

Ge et al. (2020) introduced a threshold linear mixed model which can be used simultaneously to determine the cutpoint of a continuous covariate, such as age or the expression level of a biomarker, in the definition of treatment-sensitive subsets of patients and to assess the interaction effect between the treatment and subset indicator based on longitudinal measurements. The standard likelihood method is difficult to apply to the inference of the parameters in the model because the likelihood function is not continuous for some parameters. They therefore proposed a smoothing likelihood function to approximate the original likelihood function and developed an inference procedure for the parameters in the model based on this new likelihood function. Finally, they used the Broyden–Fletcher–Goldfarb–Shanno (BFGS) algorithm (Broyden 1970; Fletcher 1970; Goldfarb 1970; Shanno 1970), which belongs to quasi-Newton methods and is included in R package "maxLik" (Henningsen & Toomet 2011), to implement the proposed procedure.

Specifically, denote a column vector $\mathbf{Y}_i = (y_{i1}, y_{i2}, \cdots, y_{in_i})$ for the longitudinal measurements observed from the i-th patient. For each patient, denote also $\mathbf{X}_i = (\mathbf{x}_{i1}, \mathbf{x}_{i2}, \cdots, \mathbf{x}_{in_i})'$ as an $(n_i \times p)$ designed matrix of covariates for fixed effect $\boldsymbol{\beta}$ and $\mathbf{Z}_i = (\mathbf{z}_{i1}, \mathbf{z}_{i2}, \cdots, \mathbf{z}_{in_i})'$ as an $(n_i \times q)$ designed matrix of covariates for random effect $\boldsymbol{\alpha}_i$. Assume b_i is an indicator of the treatment received by patient i with either $b_i = 1$ if the patient receiving a new therapy or $b_i = 0$ if not. Denote w_i as a continuous covariate at baseline for patient i and assume two subsets of patients can be defined based on whether w_i exceeds an unknown cutpoint c. The following threshold linear mixed model was proposed to assess the potential differential treatment effects between these two subsets:

$$\mathbf{Y}_i = \mathbf{X}_i\boldsymbol{\beta} + \mathbf{Z}_i\boldsymbol{\alpha}_i + \eta_1 I(w_i > c)\mathbf{1} + \eta_2 b_i I(w_i > c)\mathbf{1} + \boldsymbol{\varepsilon}_i, \tag{15}$$

where $\boldsymbol{\varepsilon}_i = (\varepsilon_{i1}, \varepsilon_{i2}, \cdots, \varepsilon_{in_i})'$ is a vector of random errors and $\mathbf{1}$ is a n_i-dimensional vector with its all elements as 1. In model (15), the response y_{ij} of patient i measured at the time t_{ij} is modeled by three components: the fixed effects of all covariates $\mathbf{x}'_{ij}\boldsymbol{\beta} + \eta_1 I(w_i > c) + \eta_2 b_i I(w_i > c)$, the patient effect $\mathbf{z}'_{ij}\boldsymbol{\alpha}_i$, and the random error ε_{ij}. The columns of $\mathbf{X}_i$ may include intercept, time or its function, treatment, and other confounding variables, and the columns of $\mathbf{Z}_i$ are assumed to be a subset of the columns of $\mathbf{X_i}$. In order to simplify the presentation, model (15) can be rewritten in the matrix form as:

$$\mathbf{Y} = \mathbf{X}\boldsymbol{\beta} + \mathbf{W}\boldsymbol{\eta} + \mathbf{Z}\boldsymbol{\alpha} + \boldsymbol{\varepsilon}, \tag{16}$$

where $\mathbf{Y} = [\mathbf{Y}_1', \mathbf{Y}_2', \cdots, \mathbf{Y}_N']'$, $\mathbf{X} = [\mathbf{X}_1', \mathbf{X}_2', \cdots, \mathbf{X}_N']'$, $\boldsymbol{\alpha} = (\boldsymbol{\alpha}_1', \boldsymbol{\alpha}_2', \cdots, \boldsymbol{\alpha}_N')'$, $\boldsymbol{\varepsilon} = (\boldsymbol{\varepsilon}_1', \boldsymbol{\varepsilon}_2', \cdots, \boldsymbol{\varepsilon}_N')'$ and $\mathbf{W} = [\mathbf{W}_1', \mathbf{W}_2', \cdots, \mathbf{W}_N']'$, and

$$\mathbf{Z} = \begin{pmatrix} \mathbf{Z}_1 & 0 & 0 & \cdots & 0 \\ 0 & \mathbf{Z}_2 & 0 & \cdots & 0 \\ \vdots & \vdots & \vdots & \ddots & \\ 0 & 0 & 0 & & \mathbf{Z_N} \end{pmatrix} \quad, \quad W_i = \begin{pmatrix} I(w_i > c) & b_i \times I(w_i > c) \\ I(w_i > c) & b_i \times I(w_i > c) \\ \vdots & \vdots \\ I(w_i > c) & b_i \times I(w_i > c) \end{pmatrix}_{n_i \times 2}.$$

For the vector of random effects $\boldsymbol{\alpha}$ and vector of random errors $\boldsymbol{\varepsilon}$ in the model, it is assumed that $E(\boldsymbol{\alpha}) = \mathbf{0}$ and $E(\boldsymbol{\varepsilon}) = \mathbf{0}$. In addition, it is assumed that $\boldsymbol{\alpha}$ and $\boldsymbol{\varepsilon}$ are independent and distributed as multivariate normal, that is,

$$\begin{bmatrix} \boldsymbol{\alpha} \\ \boldsymbol{\varepsilon} \end{bmatrix} \sim N \left(\begin{bmatrix} \mathbf{0} \\ \mathbf{0} \end{bmatrix}, \begin{bmatrix} \mathbf{G} & \mathbf{0} \\ \mathbf{0} & \mathbf{R} \end{bmatrix} \right).$$

In the proposed model, they assumed that $\mathbf{R} = \sigma^2 \mathbf{I}$ (σ is an unknown parameter) and $\mathbf{G} = \sigma^2 \rho^2 \mathbf{I}$ (ρ is also an unknown parameter). Following Patterson and Thompson (1971), the covariance-variance matrix of the observation $\mathbf{Y}$ can be written as

$$Var(\mathbf{Y}) = \sigma^2(\rho^2 \mathbf{Z}\mathbf{Z}' + \mathbf{I}) = \sigma^2 \mathbf{H},$$

where $\mathbf{H} = \rho^2 \mathbf{Z}\mathbf{Z}' + \mathbf{I}$.

Under the assumptions and notations mentioned above, $\mathbf{Y}$ follows a multivariate normal distribution as $N(\mathbf{X}\boldsymbol{\beta} + \mathbf{W}\boldsymbol{\eta}, \sigma^2 \mathbf{H})$. Denote $n = \sum_{i=1}^{N} n_i$ as the total number of observations, The log-likelihood for the unknown parameters $\boldsymbol{\theta} = (\boldsymbol{\beta}, \boldsymbol{\eta}, c, \rho^2, \sigma^2)$ in model (16) based on longitudinal outcomes $\mathbf{Y}$ can be written as

$$l(\boldsymbol{\theta}|\mathbf{Y}, \mathbf{X}, \mathbf{Z}) = -\frac{1}{2} \Big\{ \log(2\pi) + n \log \sigma^2 +$$

$$\log |\mathbf{H}| + \frac{(\mathbf{Y} - \mathbf{X}\boldsymbol{\beta} - \mathbf{W}\boldsymbol{\eta})' \mathbf{H}^{-1} (\mathbf{Y} - \mathbf{X}\boldsymbol{\beta} - \mathbf{W}\boldsymbol{\eta})}{\sigma^2} \Big\}. \tag{17}$$

However, due to the presence of the indicator functions $I(w_i > c)$, the log-likelihood function is not continuous with respect to c, which makes the conventional maximum likelihood theory and algorithm difficult to apply. Following a smoothing procedure used by Brown and Wang (2007), they proposed to use a kernel smooth function

$$\Phi\left(\frac{w_i - c}{h}\right) \tag{18}$$

as a smooth approximation to the indicator function $I(w_i > c)$, where Φ is the distribution function of the standard normal distribution and h is a bandwidth which converges to zero as the sample size increases. Using this approximation, a smoothed log-likelihood function can be defined by replacing $\mathbf{W_i}$ in the definition of $\mathbf{W}$ in (17) with

$$\widetilde{\mathbf{W}}_{\mathbf{i}} = \begin{bmatrix} \Phi(\frac{w_i-c}{h}) \; b_i \times \Phi(\frac{w_i-c}{h}) \\ \Phi(\frac{w_i-c}{h}) \; b_i \times \Phi(\frac{w_i-c}{h}) \\ \vdots \qquad\qquad \vdots \\ \Phi(\frac{w_i-c}{h}) \; b_i \times \Phi(\frac{w_i-c}{h}) \end{bmatrix}_{n_i \times 2},$$

therefore the smoothed log-likelihood function of θ is given by

$$sl(\theta|\mathbf{Y}, \mathbf{X}, \mathbf{Z}) = -\frac{1}{2}\left\{ \log(2\pi) + n \log \sigma^2 + \right.$$

$$\left. \log|\mathbf{H}| + \frac{(\mathbf{Y} - X\beta - \widetilde{W}\eta)'\mathbf{H}^{-1}(\mathbf{Y} - X\beta - \widetilde{W}\eta)}{\sigma^2} \right\} \tag{19}$$

where $\widetilde{\mathbf{W}} = [\widetilde{\mathbf{W}}'_1, \widetilde{\mathbf{W}}'_2, \cdots, \widetilde{\mathbf{W}}'_\mathbf{n}]'$. The maximum smoothed likelihood estimates (MSLE) of θ can be obtained by maximizing the smoothed log-likelihood function (19). Based on this estimate, a treatment-sensitive subset of patients can be defined as $\{i : I(w_i > \hat{c})\}$, where $\hat{c}$ is an estimate of c, if η_2 is found significantly different from 0 based on its estimate and associated variance estimate.

4 Discussions and Future Work

Most of the methods reviewed in this article assume a specific statistical model for the clinical outcomes of the study. For example, the Cox proportional hazards models were assumed when the clinical outcomes are survival times and longitudinal outcomes are required to be normally distributed because of assumptions underlying the linear mixed models. The proportional hazards assumption behind the Cox model and the normality assumption required for linear mixed models may not be satisfied by the data. Some more robust methods with more realistic assumptions may be preferred. For example, since quality of life scores are restricted to an interval, a linear mixed model with beta (Hunger et al. 2012) or simplex (Qiu et al. 2008) distributions may be more appropriate. For patients with early stage of cancer, some of them may be cured by the treatment they received and, therefore, cure models may be more useful for the observed survival times (Othus et al. 2012). Extensions of the methods reviewed in this article to these models may be of interest. When the cutpoint of a single biomarker is known and pre-specified and survival times are the clinical outcomes of a study, a nonparametric measure of interaction was proposed recently by Jiang et al. (2016). Development of statistical methods which use this measure of interaction to identify treatment-sensitive subsets of patients may also be of interest but can be difficult when there are multiple biomarkers.

In many clinical studies, both survival times and longitudinal measurements are collected but they are usually analyzed separately. Joint analysis of longitudinal outcomes and survival times may identify treatment-sensitive subsets of patients for both of these outcomes. But technically this may be more difficult because additional random effects are required to connect the Cox proportional hazards with linear mixed models, which will require novel computation methods to make inferences on the parameters in both of these models.

When the clinical outcomes are longitudinal, only the case where a single covariate is available to define the subsets of patients has been considered. Similar procedures as that presented in Sect. 2.3 would be generalized from the case where the clinical outcomes are survival times to the case where longitudinal outcomes are outcomes of interest to combine multiple covariates or biomarkers when they are available.

There is so far no systematic comparison between the treatment-sensitive subsets of patients identified from different approaches. As noted by Janes et al. (2015), accuracy measures such as sensitivity, specificity, and positive and negative predictions employed for the comparison of statistical procedures for the identification of prognostic groups are difficult to define for the comparisons of statistical procedures for the identification of treatment-sensitive subsets. A consensus is required among medical researchers and statisticians on the measures which could be used for the comparisons.

References

Andrews, N., & Cho, H. (2017). Validating effectiveness of subgroup identification for longitudinal data. *Statistics in Medicine, 37*, 98–106.

Bezjak, A., Tu, D., Seymour, L., Clark, G., Trajkovic, A., Zukin, M., Ayoub, J., Lago, S., de Albuquerque Ribeiro, R., Gerogianni, A., Cyjon, A., Noble, J., Laberge, F., Chan, R. T. T., Fenton, D., Pawel, J., Reck, M., & Shepherd, F. (2006). Symptom improvement in lung cancer patients treated with erlotinib: quality of life analysis of the National Cancer Institute of Canada Clinical Trials Group study BR.21. *Journal of Clinical Oncology, 24*, 3831–3837.

Blazeby, J. M., Brookes, S. T., & Alderson, D. (2001). The prognostic value of quality of life scores during treatment for oesophageal cancer. *Gut, 49*, 227–230.

Brown, B. M., & Wang, Y.-G. (2007). Induced smoothing for rank regression with censored survival times. *Statistics in Medicine, 26*, 828–836.

Broyden, C. G. (1970). The convergence of a class of double-rank minimization algorithms 1. general considerations. *IMA Journal of Applied Mathematics, 6*, 76–90.

Chen, B. E., Jiang, W., & Tu, D. (2014). A hierarchical Bayes model for biomarker subset effects in clinical trials. *Computational Statistics & Data Analysis, 71*, 324–334.

Cox, D. R. (1972). Regression models and life-tables. *Journal of the Royal Statistical Society: Series B (Methodological), 34*, 187–202.

Cox, D. R. (1975). Partial likelihood. *Biometrika, 62*, 269–276.

Fletcher, R. (1970). A new approach to variable metric algorithms. *The Computer Journal, 13*, 317–322.

Ge, X., Peng, Y., & Tu, D. (2020). A threshold linear mixed model for identification of treatment-sensitive subsets in a clinical trial based on longitudinal outcomes and a continuous covariate. *Statistical Methods in Medical Research, 10*, 2919–2931.

Goldfarb, D. (1970). A family of variable-metric methods derived by variational means. *Mathematics of Computation, 24*(109), 23–26.

Hartley, H. O., & Rao, J. N. K. (1967). Maximum-likelihood estimation for the mixed analysis of variance model. *Biometrika, 54*, 93–108.

He, Y., Lin, H., & Tu, D. (2018). A single-index threshold cox proportional hazard model for identifying a treatment-sensitive subset based on multiple biomarkers. *Statistics in Medicine, 37*, 3267–3279.

Henningsen, A., & Ott Toomet, O. (2011). MaxLik: A package for maximum likelihood estimation in R. *Computational Statistics, 26*, 443–458.

Hunger, M., Döring, A., & Holle, R. (2012). Longitudinal beta regression models for analyzing health-related quality of life scores over time. *BMC Med Res Methodol*, 144: https://doi.org/10.1186/1471-2288-12-144.

Janes, H., Pepe, M. S., McShane, L. M., Sargent, D. J., & Heagerty, H. J. (2015). The fundamental difficulty with evaluating the accuracy of biomarkers for guiding treatment. *Journal of National Cancer Institute, 107*, djv157.

Jiang, W., Freidlin, B., & Simon, R. (2007). Biomarker-adaptive threshold design: a procedure for evaluating treatment with possible biomarker-defined subset effect. *Journal of the National Cancer Institute, 99*, 1036–1043.

Jiang, S., Chen, B., & Tu, D. (2016). Inference on treatment-covariate interaction based on a nonparametric measure of treatment effects and censored survival data. *Statistics in Medicine, 35*, 2715–2725.

LeBlanc, M., & Crowley, J. (1993). Survival trees by goodness of split. *Journal of the American Statistical Association, 88*, 457–467.

Moineddin, R., Butt, D. A., Tomlinson, G., & Beyene, J. (2008). Identifying subpopulations for subgroup analysis in a longitudinal clinical trial. *Contemporary Clinical Trials, 29*, 817–822.

Othus, M., Barlogie, B., LeBlanc, M. L., & Crowley, J. J. (2012). Cure models as a useful statistical tool for analyzing survival. *Clin Cancer Res, 18*, 3731–3736.

Patterson, H. D., & Thompson, R. (1971). Recovery of inter-block information when block sizes are unequal. *Biometrika, 58*, 545–554.

Qiu, Z., Song, P., & Tan, M. (2008). Simplex mixed-effects models for longitudinal proportional data. *Scandinavian Journal of Statistics, 35*, 577–596.

Shanno, D. F. (1970). Conditioning of quasi-newton methods for function minimization. *Mathematics of Computation, 24*, 647–656.

Shultz, D. B., Pai, J., Chiu, W., Ng, K., Hellendag, M. G., Heestand, G., Chang, D. T., Tu, D., Moore, M. J., Parulekar, W. R., & Koong, A. (2016). A novel biomarker panel examining response to gemcitabine with or without erlotinib for pancreatic cancer therapy in NCIC Clinical Trials Group PA.3. *PloS One, 11*, e0147995.

Su, X., Zhou, T., Yan, X., Fan, J., & Yang, S. (2008). Interaction trees with censored survival data. *The International Journal of Biostatistics, 4*, 2.

Verbeke, G., & Molenberghs, G. (2009). *Linear mixed models for longitudinal data.* Springer Science & Business Media.

Wells, C., O'Callaghan, C., Karapetis, C. S., Jonker, D., Tu, D., Liu, G., Shapiro, J., Simes, J., Siu, L., Tebbutt, N., & Price, T. (2008). Outcomes of older patients ($\geq$ 70 years) treated with targeted therapy in metastatic chemorefractory colorectal cancer: Retrospective analysis of NCIC CTG CO.17 and CO.20. *Clinical Colorectal Cancer, 18*, e140–e149.

Index

A

α−folding transformation, 227–229, 231, 232
α−transformation, 226, 228–233
Alzheimer's Disease Neuroimaging Initiative
(ADNI), 150

B

Bag-of-words (BOW), 102–108, 111, 113, 115
Bayesian analysis, 277, 283–286, 290–292
Bernstein polynomials, 183, 192, 194, 206

C

Censored data, 23–51, 182, 206, 207
Clinical trials, 160, 313, 316, 320
Clusters, 5, 82, 91, 103–117, 161, 260, 276,
281–287, 289, 290
Comment ranking, 98–118
Complex survey design, 282, 292
Compositional data, 225–233
Cosine similarity, 103–107
Current status data, 181–222

D

Data integration, 5, 19
Design of experiments, 182, 295–307
Discrete and continuous longitudinal
responses, 161, 162, 177–178
Distance correlation, 24–27, 32, 33, 43
Dynamic ARCH model, 236, 242

E

Efficient estimation, 166, 186–189, 205
Errors in variables, 236, 242, 244

F

False discovery rate (FDR), 19, 55–67
Finite mixture model, 70, 71, 81
Functional linear model (FLM), 138–141

G

General entropy, 101, 102, 108–114, 116–118
Generalized estimating equations (GEE),
161–170, 172, 177, 286, 290, 291, 320
Generalized method of moments,
161
Generalized semiparametric varying-
coefficient additive model, 159–178

H

High-dimensional data, 23, 55–67, 122, 128
High-dimensional theory, 121–122

I

Interaction, 3–19, 35, 312, 314, 316–320, 322,
324, 327
Inverse Fourier transformation, 25, 30, 43,
45
Isometric log-ratio transformation, 226,
227

K

Kullback–Leibler (K-L) divergence, 102, 108, 112–114, 116

L

Latin hypercube design, 296–300
Least angle regression, 55–67
Left-truncated data, 181–222
Linear transformation model (LTM), 181–222
Local linear smoothing, 177
Longitudinal data, 159–178, 271, 320

M

Measurement error, 23–51, 139, 141–149, 152, 235–254
Minimum distance estimator, 71–80
Modal regression, 257–272
Mode, 261, 269
Multilevel model, 275–292, 312, 320–322

N

Nearly orthogonal design, 304
Network analysis, 18

P

Pairwise composite likelihood, 286, 291, 292
Partially observed functional data, 137–157
Penalized maximum likelihood estimator, 79–80
Predictive function, 313, 323, 324

Principal components, 138, 141, 144, 145
Profile estimation, 159–178

Q

Quadratic inference function, 161, 162, 167–168
Quasi-likelihood approach, 167

R

Regularization, 56, 142, 295, 315
Robustness, 5, 8, 9, 18, 63, 71, 84–90, 93, 122–130, 265

S

Screening, 23–51, 63, 271, 279
Semiparametric time-varying coefficient, 150–178
Sensitivity, 41, 42, 44, 55–67, 327
Skewed data, 257–272
Statistical inference, 5, 56, 90, 316

U

Ultrahigh-dimension, 23–51

V

Variable selection, 55–57, 271, 295, 297, 307

W

Wasserstein distance, 69–97
Within-subject correlation, 159–178
word2vec, 103, 105, 106, 109, 114

CPSIA information can be obtained
at www.ICGtesting.com
Printed in the USA
LVHW080707021122
732179LV00003B/14